Living the Low Carb Life

Living
the
Low Carb
Life

CONTROLLED
CARBOHYDRATE EATING FOR
LONG-TERM WEIGHT LOSS

JONNY BOWDEN, M.A., C.N.S.
FOREWORD BY BARRY SEARS, PH.D.

STERLING PUBLISHING
New York

Published by Sterling Publishing Co., Inc.
387 Park Avenue South, New York, NY 10016

©2004 by Jonny Bowden
Revised Edition 2005

Distributed in Canada by Sterling Publishing
c/o Canadian Manda Group, One Atlantic Avenue, Suite 105
Toronto, Ontario, Canada M6K 3E7
Distributed in Great Britain by Chrysalis Books
64 Brewery Road, London N79NT, England
Distributed in Australia by Capricorn Link (Australia) Pty. Ltd.
P.O. Box 704, Windsor, NSW 2756, Australia

Library of Congress Cataloging-in-Publication Data

Bowden, Jonny.
  Living the low carb life from Atkins to the Zone :
choosing the diet that's right for you / Jonny Bowden ;
foreword by Barry Sears.— Rev. ed.
     p. cm.
  Includes index.
  ISBN 1-4027-1860-8 (pbk. : alk. paper)
  1. Low-carbohydrate diet. I. Title.
  RM237.73.B69 2005
  613.2'83--dc22
                              2005002367

Book Design by HRoberts Design
Illustrations by Steven Arcella

Printed in York, Pennsylvania, by The Maple-Vail Book Manufacturing Group

10 9 8 7 6 5 4 3 2 1

Some of the diet plans discussed in this book are not appropriate for people with kidney, liver, or gall bladder problems, for pregnant or nursing women, for people on medication to control cholesterol, blood pressure, fluid retention, or blood sugar, or for those who have abnormal heart rhythms or have had a heart attack in the past six months. People with these conditions must not begin such diet plans without a physician's guidance and close supervision.

While the publisher and the author have used best efforts in writing this book, they make no representations or warranties as to its accuracy and completeness. They also do not make any implied warranties of merchantability or fitness for a particular purpose. Any advice given in this book is not guaranteed or warranted, and it may not be suitable for every factual situation. The information contained in this book is not intended to replace the services of trained health professionals or be a substitute for medical advice. You are advised to consult with your health care professionals with regard to your health, and before beginning any diet or fitness program. Neither the publisher nor the author shall be liable for any losses suffered by any reader of this book.

For Anja

who gave me wings

Contents

Foreword

There are three things in life that induce powerful visceral responses—religion, politics, and nutrition. Each is based on assumptions, and the adherents of each believe in their hearts that they are right. Of course, they don't want to be confused by the facts. In the world of nutrition, nothing has generated as much heartburn as low-carbohydrate diets. To the nutrition establishment, they are the moral equivalent of devil worship. To the medical establishment, they are the cause of massive increases in chronic disease and death. To the millions of people who use them, they seem to be the key to actually losing weight.

Obviously, there is a disconnect between fantasy and reality. Are low-carbohydrate diets safe? And exactly what is a low-carbohydrate diet? Is a low-carbohydrate diet the same as a high-fat or high-protein diet? Are there any supplements that can make you magically lose excess body fat? Into this quagmire of controversy steps Jonny Bowden.

I first met Jonny nearly eight years ago. I had just written my first book, *The Zone*, and I was speaking about it in New York City. At the time, Jonny was a very well recognized nutritionist working with clients ranging from those seeking weight loss to fitness enthusiasts to bodybuilders. Like most New Yorkers, he was skeptical of anything new, especially when it concerned diet, and his skepticism was particularly high because my book recommended low-carbohydrate diets not only for patients with diabetes and heart disease but also for world-class athletes. After all, Jonny had been training athletes for years using high-carbohydrate diets, and here was some pointy-head scientist telling him that all of his nutritional advice for athletes was wrong. Needless to say, he was ready to rake me over the coals…until he heard my lecture. For the first time, Jonny was introduced to the nuances of hormone control theory using food as a drug. Although there was a lot of endocrinology (the science of hormones) being thrown around in the lecture (after all, I am still a pointy-head scientist), Jonny devoured every bit of information. After the lecture he asked if we could talk, and for the next two hours I went into great detail (probably more than lesser nutritionists would have wanted to know) on the intricate dance of the hormones controlled by diet. Jonny then said to me, "If you are right about this, then everyone in nutrition is probably wrong." My reply was "yes."

My statement was not as self-serving as it appears. Some thirteen years earlier, I was one of the leading researchers of intravenous drug delivery systems for cancer drugs. I had a very cushy job at MIT, played basketball in my leisurely two- to three-hour lunch breaks, and of course spent a good deal of time in the faculty club. (And you thought being an academic was a tough life.) Then I had a bizarre thought that I could apply the principles of intravenous drug delivery systems to controlling the hormones generated by the food we eat. I left to form my own company and went from being considered a boy wonder at MIT to being thought a charlatan in a six-month period of time. It was a very humbling experience.

For more than a decade, I wandered in the wilderness of nutrition science, constantly ridiculed for my outlandish idea that eating too many carbohydrates could be dangerous. I knew when I embarked on this journey that I would be taking some heat, but I had not realized just how contentious the arguments could get. Clearly, conventional doctors and nutritionists were not ready to admit the possibility that carbohydrates were anything but a gift from the gods. After being battle tested for thirteen years, my answer to Jonny was not a flip response.

While Jonny was intrigued, he remained skeptical but open minded. Because he was also an academic with a background in psychology and statistics, I knew that any references I gave him on low-carbohydrate diets (there wasn't much) and the science behind them (there was a lot) would be thoroughly read and analyzed. As a result, Jonny has become not only exceptionally well educated in the nutritional science of low-carbohydrate diets, but also my friend. I consider Jonny to be one of the better science writers I have ever met. That's why this book is so important for the general public. He outlines the history of low-carbohydrate diets, explaining in clear and concise language the underlying hormonal principles, and addresses the common misunderstandings surrounding these diets, all in an entertaining and lively style.

As Jonny correctly points out, there is no single diet that is right for everyone, since we are all genetically different. However, the hormonal principles behind choosing an appropriate diet are unvarying. Once you understand the hormonal rules that govern low-carbohydrate diets, you are in a position to become the master of your future. This book is the starting point of that journey to good health.

Barry Sears, Ph.D.
Author of *The Zone*

Preface to the Revised Edition

In the year since *Living the Low Carb Life* was published, I've had many extraordinary experiences, but none so telling and important to the message as the following encounter. I was lecturing to a large audience in the Midwest on the topic of low-carb nutrition when a woman in the audience stood up. "I lost 70 pounds on the Atkins diet," she said. "I went to my doctor when I was almost 100 pounds overweight and he read me the riot act. He told me the danger I was putting myself in and how important it was for me to lose weight. He wanted to put me on some medication, but I wanted to try it on my own. I went on Atkins, and over the course of the next year I lost almost 70 pounds." Delighted, I asked her what happened next. "Well," she said, "I went back to my doctor. He could hardly believe how different I looked. He did a blood test. My triglycerides had dropped to under 100, my cholesterol ratio was way improved, and my blood sugar was normal."

"Then what happened?" I asked.

"Well, he was just thrilled. He told me that what I had accomplished was amazing and that I should be very proud of myself. And then he asked me how I had done it. I told him I had gone on Atkins."

"And?"

"He said to me, 'oh, you've got to get off that immediately. That diet is *dangerous.*'"

The woman asked me what you say to a doctor like that. I replied, only half kidding, that you respectfully ask him to stop practicing medicine.

How do we change this kind of thinking? The kind of thinking demonstrated by this lovely lady's physician is closer to religious conviction than it is to a scientifically held position, and we know how hard it is to change religious beliefs. People who will not budge from their position that low-carb eating is dangerous simply have not looked at the emerging science—and many refuse to. Fortunately, more and more health-care practitioners are beginning to open their minds and take a second look at the dietary strategy that, up until a few short years ago, was considered nutritional heresy.

In the last few years, some thirty-plus studies or papers have been published investigating various aspects of low-carb regimens. Some of these have looked at weight loss; some have looked at serum biomarkers (triglycerides, HDL, and so on). Some have looked at inflammatory markers (C Reactive Protein). Many have looked at cholesterol, and not just the total number (which is fairly meaningless) but at the different fractions, HDL and LDL and the ratios. Some have even looked at the emerging data on LDL particle size, which tells us even more. The results are pretty clear. Low-carb diets perform as well as low-fat ones on virtually every parameter. In many cases, they perform better in terms of weight loss. In virtually all cases, low-carb eating lowers triglycerides (which in my opinion is a far more important risk factor for heart disease than cholesterol). In a very large number of cases, it improves the overall cholesterol ratio, or at least the triglyceride to HDL ratio (an important measure for heart disease risk). It frequently improves glucose control in diabetics and brings down a diabetic risk factor called hemoglobin A1c.

Folks, low-carb living is not dangerous.

And it works.

Maybe not for everybody. Maybe not in every situation. (Remember, I'm the guy who has been preaching for the last fifteen years that everybody's different and that no one diet works for everyone). But a low-carb diet works for many, many people. A large percentage of the people who are consciously controlling their carbs report that they find the diet easy to stay with. The enormous number of new lower-carb products on the market has afforded us more choices and variety. (Of course, we need to use those products responsibly—they're not a free lunch—but that's another story).

Low-carb isn't a fad. In fact, when I hear people say that I'm always amused, because when you think about it, controlled- (or lower-) carb eating is what we humans have done for the vast majority of our time on the planet. For goodness sake, agriculture was only "invented" ten thousand years ago (the human genus has been around for 2.4 million years!) Our Paleolithic ancestors didn't eat low-fat woolly mammoths or low-fat caribou. The artificially low-fat, high-carb diet, from the point of view of anthropology and history, is the true "fad" diet, and it's been less than a rousing success.

I believe that the future of low-carb eating is that it will simply become part of good nutritional practice. Our dietitians and nutritionists will no longer be wary of saying outright that sugar is bad for you and, despite political pressures, we'll begin to reject the products of "Big Food" that result in a per capita consumption of around 150 pounds of sugar a year. Already there is a nascent movement to remove garbage foods from the snack machines in our schools. And rumor has it that upscale restaurants are beginning to serve smaller (i.e., normal) portions instead of the obscenely supersized "mine is bigger than yours" servings we've been getting for the past few decades. Protein is making a comeback, and people are finally no longer afraid of whole eggs. There is progress.

A recent—and terrific—scholarly article in *The American Journal of Clinical Nutrition* thoughtfully suggested that we ought to reconsider saturated fat before we make the same mistake that we made in the 1980s with regard to fat in general. Many saturated fats are extremely healthy. And while no one suggests eating a diet abnormally high in saturated fats, we should not be so quick to talk about "healthier" versions of low-carb diets that eliminate saturated fat, for saturated fat is far from the villain it has been portrayed to be by some diet authors. The best approach is to incorporate a reasonable amount of saturated fat and balance it with other great fats and oils, especially omega-3s from fish and flaxseed, and omega-9s from olive oil and macadamia nut oil. In fact, one of those thirty-plus studies I mentioned earlier did exactly that, replacing starch with saturated fat in a diet that was already nice and heavy on the omega-3s and 9s, and they got improvement in almost every measured health parameter. (For a complete, updated list of studies supporting the statements in this book, don't forget to click on What's New? on jonnybowden.com and go to For Your Doctor.)

The point is this: low-carb eating is not a fad— it is here to stay, and none too soon. Obesity is quickly catching up to smoking as the number one preventable cause of death in America. Diabetes is approaching epidemic proportions. Nearly two thirds of Americans are overweight and a third of them are obese.

Low-carb living can help.

I am honored to have received hundreds of letters from people around the country thanking me for writing *Living the Low Carb Life*. I am especially honored to have heard from doctors whose minds have been changed by it, and by one who told me it was the only nutrition text he needed to have. All that feels really good.

But nothing feels as good as knowing that people are using *Living the Low Carb Life* to empower themselves and to take control of their health.

Remember, when you improve your body you improve your health. And when you improve your health you are improving your life. In taking control of your health, you regain a great deal of personal power.

Enjoy the journey.

Acknowledgments

Two sets of thanks here.

First . . . to my personal "brain trust," who gave so generously of their time. If this book is good, it's largely because of their stunning knowledge base.

Stacey J Bell, Ph.D. • Susanne Bennett, D.C. • C. Leigh Broadhurst, Ph.D. • Mary Enig, Ph.D. • Joseph Evans, Ph.D. • Oz Garcia, M.S. • Colette Heimowitz, M.S. • James Haig, M.A. • John Hernandez, M.D. • Malcolm Kendrick, M.D. • Ann Louise Gittleman, M.S., C.N.S. • Susan Lark, M.D. • Emily Lapkin • David Leonardi, M.D. • Shari Lieberman, Ph.D., C.N.S. • Linda Lizotte, R.D. • Lyle McDonald • Joe Mercola, D.O. • Liz Neporent, M.S. • Harry Preuss, M.D. • Uffe Rasvnskov,.M.D., Ph.D. • Donald S Robertson, M.D., M.Sc. • Ron Rosedale, M.D. • Alan Schwartz, M.D. • Diana Schwarzbein, M.D. • Barry Sears, Ph.D. • Stephen Sinatra, M.D. • Allan Spreen, M.D. • Anton Steiner, M.D. • Jeff S. Volek, PhD, R.D

A special thanks:
- to Dr. Anton Steiner for sharing his wealth of knowledge about the neurochemistry of pharmaceuticals and his invaluable help with the section on weight loss medications.
- to my dear friend Dr. Dave Leonardi, who put up with my endless medical questions at all hours of the day and night and served as my personal *Merck Manual* of diabetes.
- to the brilliant Dr. C. Leigh Broadhurst, a walking encyclopedia of biochemistry and nutrition, who generously read and tweaked entire sections.
- to Dr. Mary Enig, for making sure I knew my fats!

And a really special "general principles" thanks to Jeffrey Bland, Ph.D., Alan Gaby, M.D., Jonathan Wright, M.D., and especially to my friend and teacher Robert Crayhon, M.S., all of whom have spent their professional lives making a difference by educating physicians, nutritionists, chiropractors, and other health practitioners, challenging their boundaries and expanding their horizons.

They certainly did mine.

And second . . . to my family—chosen and otherwise—the special people in my life without whom I might have still written books, but without whom I would not be who I am.

Adrian Zmed, Aleta St James, Anja Christy, Billy Stritch, Cadence Bowden, Carol Meltzer, Cassandra Creech, Christopher Duncan, Danny Troob, Elliott Bowden, Howard Stern, Jeanine Tesori, Jeffrey Bowden, Kelly Wixted, Kimberly Wright, Lauree Dash, Lee Knapp, Liz Neporent (both lists!), Lynn Pentz, Max Creech-Bowden, Molly Fox, Nancy Fiedler, Oliver and Jennifer, Oz Garcia (both lists!), Pace Bowden, Peter Breger, Randy Graff, Richard Lewis, Scott Ellis, Sky London, Susan Wood, Tigerlily Creech-Bowden, Tom Leykis, Vivienne Bowden, Werner Erhard, Woodstock Creech-Bowden

And a warm thanks to my first agent, Linda Konner, who put me on the map.

And to my current agent, Coleen O'Shea, who kept me there.

And to my editor, Susan Lauzau, who had the patience to allow me to rant and rave about every comma change, most of which she was right about anyway.

And especially to Michael Fragnito, who had the vision to imagine this book, the editorial skills to shape it, and an unfettered belief in me that allowed me to do the best work I've ever done.

And to the superstar of publicists, who does more on an off-day than most people do on their best, Heidi Krupp of Krupp Kommunications, and her entire staff, especially Chris Capra.

Also to the support team at Barnes & Noble, especially Lindsay Herman.

And to my mother, Vivienne Simon Bowden.

And a special thanks to A.L.G.

Living the Low Carb Life

How to Use This Book

*T*he high-carbohydrate, low-fat diet has been the longest uncontrolled nutritional experiment in history.

The results have not been good.

Perhaps you've noticed.

Perhaps you have been one of its victims. You're unable to lose weight, or if you have lost, it certainly hasn't been easy. You found yourself constantly fighting cravings, you were hungry a lot of the time, and you suffered with feelings of deprivation. You felt fatigued, like you were running on empty, and were still always battling the bulge, mostly unsuccessfully.

Maybe, like a lot of low-fat, high-carbohydrate dieters, you've noticed that your hair is dry, your nails brittle, your energy low, and your vitality sapped. And guess what? For all that, the weight *still* doesn't come off, or if it does, it comes back on with a vengeance and you're right back where you started, except this time you feel even more discouraged.

Or maybe you're lucky enough to have never been on this delightful seesaw that I'm describing. Maybe you're just curious about all the fuss that's being made over low-carb diets and you want to learn more about how they work. Maybe you're thinking that you could stand to knock off a few pounds and are interested in low-carb dieting but don't know where to start. Or maybe you're already convinced that low-carb diets are for you but are concerned about some of the health implications that well-meaning people have warned you about.

Well, you've come to the right place.

Living the Low-Carb Life will help you understand three things:

1. **what** low-carb diets actually do *to* and *for* your body and how they do it
2. **why** some programs work for some people (and don't for others)
3. **how** you can adapt what you discover in this book to your own lifestyle

While I'd love to think that everyone who reads this book will devour it from cover to cover (for its scintillating content and wealth of information), realistically I know that, with the possible exception of my girlfriend and my mother, few people will approach it that way. So I have designed *Living the Low-Carb Life* to be used like the *I Ching*—open it anywhere and it will give you information you want.

I imagine that some of you will be interested in understanding more about the different popular diet plans, how they work, how they differ from one another, and what they offer. You guys should go straight for chapter 3—Seventeen Low-Carb Diets and What They Can Do for You— find the plan or plans you are interested in, and read about them. You may find that reading further will spark some questions, which you're likely to get answered in chapter 6, Frequently Asked Questions. Maybe, as you dig deeper into the book, you'll find yourself wanting to know more about the hormonal mechanisms in the body that drive weight gain and weight loss; you will find those issues addressed in chapter 2, Why Low-Carb Diets Work.

Some of you may have already been on one of the plans discussed in chapter 3 but want more in-depth information about the questions, concerns, and controversies you have been hearing about, for example, cholesterol or ketosis or bone loss or kidney problems. You might head straight for chapter 5, The Five Biggest Myths About Low-Carb Diets. When you get those concerns addressed, you may want to go back to chapter 2, Why Low-Carb Diets Work, to read more about the science behind low-carb eating and how it actually does its good work in the body.

The permutations are endless.

I also expect that there will be some dyed-in-the-wool low-carbers who have already experienced a myriad of health benefits, including weight loss, and simply want some tips for staying motivated, not getting bored, finding new things to eat, or breaking plateaus. All that information will be found in chapter 6, Frequently Asked Questions, and chapter 7, Tricks of the Trade: The Top 50+ Tips for Making Low-Carb Work for You.

Because I have designed this book to be extremely user-friendly and because I want you to be able to skip around as you like, some of the information and issues will be discussed in more than one place. For example, the subject of ketosis, which is so central to the Atkins diet and has been such a focus of criticism from the establishment and misunderstanding in the media, is discussed in three places. You will get a brief overview of ketosis in chapter 2, but a much more in-depth discussion, which answers the criticisms leveled at ketogenic diets, appears in chapter 5. You will also find an abbreviated discussion of ketosis in chapter 7, since ketosis is definitely one of the topics about which I get the most questions when it comes to low-carb dieting.

Here's a brief guide to what you will find in *Living the Low-Carb Life*.

Chapter 1: The History and Origins of Low-Carb Diets

Guess what? Low-carb dieting did *not* begin with Atkins! Low-carb diets actually date back to 1864, when William Banting wrote his famous *Letter on Corpulence* (in essence the very first commercial low-carb diet). But Banting's diet wasn't known as a "low-carb" plan; in fact, there was no such label until the USDA decreed in its 1992 food pyramid that the perfect healthy diet for Americans includes six to eleven servings of grains and starches per day. From that time on, any program that disagreed with this extremely elevated high-carb orthodoxy of the dietary establishment was by definition disparaged as "low-carb."

This chapter covers the breadth and evolution of low-carb diets over the decades, including the discovery in 1940 by Dr. Alfred Pennington that some individuals simply cannot metabolize carbohydrates as efficiently as other people do; Dr. Herman Taller's *Calories Don't Count* (the high-protein reaction to the fashionable mania for counting calories); Dr. Irwin Stillman's *The Doctor's Quick Weight Loss Diet*; and, of course, the introduction in 1966 of the CEO of all low-carb plans, the Atkins diet. Told against the background of "mainstream" nutrition, the chapter also considers the philosophy of the über-dean of high-carb proselytizers, Nathan Pritikin, and his heir apparent, Dean Ornish.

I hope you'll also begin to see why stances on nutrition can be so political, and gain a better understanding of where the lines in the sand are currently drawn regarding theories of weight loss and healthy diet.

Chapter 2: Why Low-Carb Diets Work

Low-carb diets are based on the fact that food has a profound effect on hormones—including the fat storage and fat release hormones. The hormone that gets the lion's share of attention, with good reason, is insulin, but there are others that come into play. The foundation of the low-carbohydrate movement has been the theory that controlling these hormones with your food choices is *at least* as important for weight loss as calories are (the establishment continues to insist that "it's the calories, stupid"). This chapter discusses:

- how insulin operates and why regulating it is central to the theory behind all low-carb diets
- controlling blood sugar
- insulin resistance
- the role of insulin in heart disease and why a low-carbohydrate diet can reduce your risks
- hypertension (high blood pressure) and how it can be reduced with low-carbohydrate eating
- obesity and how low-carbohydrate diets can help
- type 2 diabetes and low-carbohydrate diets

Chapter 3: Seventeen Low-Carb Diets and What They Can Do for You

In this chapter, seventeen of the best-known and most popular diet plans are exhaustively analyzed and compared. Not all of them are truly low-carb programs (for instance, the Zone diet), but if they have been portrayed that way in the press, you'll find them in this section. At the end of this chapter, you will know the exact differences among the various programs, and you'll have a much better idea of which ones speak to you and which ones leave you cold. The format for each discussion allows you to see what the plan is in a nutshell and gives an in-depth look at how the plan works and the theory behind it. You'll also learn whom it might be good for (and who should look elsewhere). Finally, I give you my evaluation of each plan (Jonny's Lowdown) and a rating of zero to five stars.

The seventeen plans and their architects are:

1. The Atkins Diet—Robert Atkins, M.D.
2. The Carbohydrate Addict's Diet—Rachael Heller, M.D., and Richard Heller, M.D.
3. The 7-Day Low-Carb Rescue and Recovery Plan—Rachael Heller, M.D., and Richard Heller, M.D.
4. Curves—Gary Heavin and Carol Colman
5. The Fat Flush Plan—Ann Louise Gittleman, M.S., C.N.S.
6. The GO-Diet: The Goldberg-O'Mara Diet Plan—Jack Goldberg, Ph.D., and Karen O'Mara, D.O.
7. The Hamptons Diet—Fred Pescatore, M.D.
8. The Lindora Program: Lean for Life—Cynthia Stamper Graff
9. Neanderthin—Ray Audette
10. The Paleo Diet—Loren Cordain, Ph.D.
11. Protein Power—Michael Eades, M.D. and Mary Dan Eades, M.D.
12. The Scarsdale Diet—Herman Tarnower, M.D.
13. The Schwarzbein Principle—Diana Schwarzbein, M.D.
14. Somersizing—Suzanne Somers
15. The South Beach Diet—Arthur Agatston, M.D.
16. Sugar Busters!—H. Leighton Steward et al.
17. The Zone—Barry Sears, Ph.D.

Chapter 4: Supplements and Diet Drugs

In this chapter, we'll review the major drug treatments for obesity and overweight—phentermine, Meridia, and Xenical—and consider the arguments for and against them, as well as review the supporting science. We'll examine the vast number of vitamins and supplements that are marketed for weight loss, such as 5-HTP, chromium, and L-carnitine. Which ones actually work and which are bogus? And if they *do* work, *how* do they work? What exactly do they do in the body? Here you'll find the science behind the advertising and discover whether there are any specific vitamins and minerals recommended for people following a low-carb lifestyle. You'll get the real scoop on controversial herbs like ephedra as well as information about the new "ephedra-free" fat-burning formulas. And you'll find out the *number one supplement for weight loss.*

Chapter 5: The Five Biggest Myths About Low-Carb Diets

There are a lot of common beliefs about the dangers of high-protein or high-fat diets. Does a high-protein diet cause osteoporosis? How about damage to the kidneys? Is ketosis a dangerous condition that should be avoided at all costs? Doesn't eating all that fat lead to heart disease? What about cholesterol?

In this chapter, I'll share what the science *really* shows.

Chapter 6: Frequently Asked Questions

Got cravings? Constipated? Bored with chicken and vegetables? This chapter reviews some of the methods that low-carb dieters use to combat common problems and make their program work for them. We'll talk about the use of glutamine to fight sugar cravings, mineral supplements such as potassium to fight muscle cramps, how much is enough when it comes to water, and if any of the "fat-burning" supplements on the market actually work. For easy reference, FAQs are organized by topic, including ketosis, food and water, plateaus, exercise, and more.

Chapter 7: Tricks of the Trade: The Top 50+ Tips for Making Low-Carb Work for You

The tips are organized into several categories, including food and drink, motivation, and general topics. You'll find more than fifty of the best insider tricks for making the low-carb lifestyle—and a weight loss program in general—easier to stick with and more enjoyable, too.

Chapter 8: Controlled-Carbohydrate Eating: Putting Together Your Program

Now that you know the nuts and bolts and have decided that low-carb living is for you, how do you put it all together? Many of the authors of the top low-carb diet books disagree vehemently on some issues—coffee, artificial sweeteners, the number of grams of allowable carbohydrate, the need for ketosis, and the timing of meals, just to mention a few—and agree on others. But there are many basic principles that can be extracted from the literature as a whole. These principles can be used to craft an individual lifestyle program that incorporates the basic tenets of low-carb eating for vibrant good health and ongoing weight loss and maintenance. This chapter tells you how to individualize and customize your own plan to create a personalized low-carb lifestyle using the principles discussed in *Living the Low-Carb Life*, as well as how to put the low-carb lifestyle into practice in the real world.

Resources and Support for a Low-Carb Lifestyle

In this section, you will find the most exhaustive and complete listing of resources and information pertaining to low-carbohydrate living ever assembled. Virtually every website worth visiting has been written up, and you'll find an amazing guide to the personal sites of people who have successfully transformed their lives and their bodies with a low-carb lifestyle. (Make sure you check out some of the before-and-after pics!) You'll find sources for research; ways to calculate your body mass index; food databases in which you can look up calories, carbs, fat, protein, and fiber; articles about cholesterol and cooking oils; information on exercise; an extensive reading list; suggested newsletters; and a comprehensive section related to food, recipes, and cookbooks both online and in print. You'll also discover dozens of Internet support groups that exist for the low-carb dieter, with comments on what to expect when you get there.

CHAPTER 1

The History
and Origins of
Low-Carb Diets

The first bona fide low-carb diet book came out in 1864, and it happened only because William Banting thought he was going deaf.

Banting was a prosperous London undertaker of sixty-six who was so overweight that he couldn't tie his own shoelaces. At five feet five inches in his stocking feet, he weighed in at 202 pounds and was so fat that he had to walk downstairs backward. On top of that, his eyesight was failing and he was having problems with his hearing. In 1862, Banting took himself to an ear, nose, and throat surgeon named Dr. William Harvey, who examined him and promptly decided that Banting's problem wasn't deafness; it was obesity. His fat was pressing on his inner ear.

Here's what Banting was eating: "bread and milk for breakfast, *or* a pint of tea, with plenty of milk and sugar, and buttered toast; meat, beer, and much bread and pastry for dinner; more bread and milk at tea time; and a fruit tart *or* bread and milk for dinner."

Harvey promptly put Banting on a diet, and by December 1862, Banting had lost 18 pounds. By August 1863, he was down to 156 pounds. In a little less than a year, he had dropped almost 50 pounds and 12½ inches from his waistline. Banting also reported feeling better than he had at any time in the previous twenty-six years. His sight and hearing were normal for his age, and his other bodily ailments had become "mere matters of history."

Here's what he ate *now*.

Breakfast (9 AM): five to six ounces of either beef, mutton, kidneys, broiled fish, bacon, or cold meat of any kind except pork or veal. One small biscuit or one ounce of dry toast. Large cup of tea or coffee without milk or sugar.

Dinner (2 PM): five or six ounces of fish, poultry, game, or meat, and any vegetable except potato, parsnip, beets, turnips, or carrots. One ounce of dry toast. Fruit. Two or three glasses of good claret, sherry, or Madeira (no champagne, port, or beer)

Tea (6 PM): two or three ounces of fruit. Toast and tea with no milk or sugar

Supper (9 PM): three or four ounces of meat or fish as for dinner. A glass or two of claret or sherry.

Night cap (if required): a tumbler of gin, whisky, or brandy with water but no sugar, or a glass or two of claret or sherry.

The man did like to drink.

Here's what he did *not* eat: milk, sugar, beer, potatoes, or pastry. And what he ate *way* less of: bread (3 ounces total, about 1 slice).

The calorie as a measurement was unknown at that time, but we know now that Banting was eating about 2,800 calories a day—not exactly a low-calorie diet. Banting may not have known much about the science and chemistry of food and weight, but he knew enough to observe that the *amount* of food he was eating didn't seem to be the determining factor in his weight loss. In Banting's words, "I can now confidently say that *quantity* of diet may be safely left to the natural appetite; and that it is the *quality* only which is essential to abate and cure corpulence."

In other words: it's *what* you eat, not how much, an idea that even then flew in the face of conventional wisdom.

Banting became a man on a mission. Excited and inspired by his results on this high-calorie, low-carbohydrate diet—which was made up almost entirely of protein, fat, alcohol, and what was then called "roughage"—he published, at his own expense, the first commercial low-carb diet book, *Letter on Corpulence*.[1]

Banting identified sugar as the main cause of his own obesity, and his physician, Dr. Harvey, promptly put both flour and sugar on the forbidden list.

It worked.

The book eventually went into four editions, with the first three selling 63,000 copies in England alone, and it was translated into French and German and sold heavily in those countries, as well as in the United States. The fourth edition included letters of testimony from at least 1,800 readers who had written to Banting to support his assertions and praise the diet.

Once I did some reading, I realized that low-carb diets aren't brand new—they've been advocated by some forward-thinking scientists for more than a century.

—Gary S.

Banting, by the way, kept the weight off and lived comfortably until the age of eighty-one.

With Banting's book, the nascent debate—is it *what* you eat or *how much* you eat that makes you fat?—was born, and it continues, alive and kicking, to this day. But the controversy didn't gather its full steam until Wilbur Atwater figured out how to measure calories.

It's the Calories, Stupid! The Dominating Hypothesis in Weight Loss Is Born

Sometime between 1890 and 1900, an agricultural chemist named Wilbur Atwater got the bright idea that if you stuck some food in a mini-oven called a calorimeter and burned the food to ash, you could *measure* the amount of heat it produced. He called the unit of measurement a calorie (technically, the amount of heat it takes to raise the temperature of 1 gram of water from 14.5 to 15.5 degrees centigrade). He went to town. He constructed vast tables of the caloric content of various foods. (It's important to remember that calories are not actually found *in* food; they're a measure of how much heat or energy can be *produced by* food.) The idea that the human body behaves exactly like the chamber used in Atwater's experiments—that we all "burn" calories exactly the same way and our bodies behave like calorimeters—has been the dominating hypothesis in weight loss to this day.

And man, is it wrong. (More coming—stay tuned.)

Later, some enterprising scientists extended the calorie theory even further. They began to measure how much heat was produced (read: how many calories were "burned") in the course of daily activities, from resting to vigorous exercise, from sleeping to digesting food to running marathons.

It was now possible to form an equation: calories in vs. calories out. The guiding concept of weight management was officially born.

That theory is called the energy balance theory, and it goes something like this: if you take in more calories than you burn up, you'll gain weight. If you burn up more calories than you take in, you'll lose weight. It doesn't matter where those calories come from. It's as simple as balancing a checkbook: spend more than you make, and you're calorically in the red (and dipping into your fat stores to make up the difference); make more than you spend, and you're in the black (and buying bigger jeans).

It was the first law of thermodynamics in action. What goes in must either come out in some other form (like heat) or stay in (in the form of fat or muscle). What it *can't* do is simply disappear.

Yet Banting, unscientific though he was, had made an interesting observation, which was that *what* he ate made more of a difference to his fat cells than *how much* he ate. This notion was heresy to the calorie theorists who believed, to paraphrase Gertrude Stein, a calorie is a calorie is a calorie. It wasn't until much later that the idea surfaced that calories from certain kinds of food (or combinations of food) might have a greater tendency to be stored in the body than others, or that people might vary widely in their metabolic ability to "burn" calories as opposed to "saving" them, or that the type of food eaten might actually trigger bodily responses that say "stay" or "go."

Meanwhile, calorie counting had taken off with a vengeance. In 1917 (the same year, coincidentally, in which the ultraconservative American Dietetic Association was founded), an L.A. physician named Dr. Lulu Hunt Peters published what had to be the first calorie counting book ever, *Diet and Health, with a Key to the Calories*. She sold 2 million books, making it the first best-selling diet book in America. And here's the thing: by making calorie counting equivalent to weight control, she also injected her own view of morality into the equation. People who couldn't control their calories (and therefore their weight) just lacked self-discipline. We can thank Dr. Peters for popularizing the concept that being overweight is a sign of moral weakness. And the idea that people are fat simply because they lack self-control is still very much alive and well today—witness, for example, the recent work of Dr. Phil McGraw.[2]

Calories in/calories out remains the dominant view of most mainstream weight loss experts to this day, and it is even embraced to a degree by some of the gurus of the low-carb movement, albeit not nearly to the extent as the mainstreamers, who have made it a virtual religion. All of the low-carb theorists have to be seen against the backdrop of this calorie-counting orthodoxy. But throughout the twentieth century and into the twenty-first, observations have indeed been made—and experiments performed—that have cast huge doubts on whether the calories in/calories out theory was the whole story or even the most important part of the story (no one claims it is not *part* of the story—the argument is about how *big* a part).

Eat and Grow Thin: Low-Carbing Reappears on the Scene

In 1914, Vance Thompson, a nonscientist and the husband of a famous actress of the day, published a book called *Eat and Grow Thin*,[3] which touted the virtues of a low-carb diet. It suggested that corpulence was caused by eating the wrong *kinds* of food, not merely the wrong amounts, and singled out "starches, sugars, and oils" as particular culprits—pretty much what you'd expect from a guy whose most famous saying was "To the scientist there is nothing so tragic on earth as the sight of a fat man eating a potato." His list of forbidden foods included the fattiest meats (like bacon); bread, biscuits, crackers, macaroni, and anything else made from the flour of wheat, corn, rye, barley, or oats, which included all breakfast foods and cereals; rice; potatoes, corn, dried beans, and lentils; milk, cream, butter, and cheese; oils and grease of any kind; pies, cakes, puddings, pastries, custards, ice cream, sodas, candies, bonbons, and sweets; and wines, beers, ales, and spirits.

One can only imagine how many times he was asked the question we hear so often today: *so what's left to eat?*

As it turns out, a lot. According to Thompson, the only things that had really been taken away were sugar, starch, oil, and alcohol. The rest of his book consisted of menus that included:

- all kinds of meat (except pig in any form)
- all kinds of game
- all kinds of seafood—fish, lobsters, oysters, etc.
- all kinds of fruit (except bananas and grapes)
- all kinds of salad
- virtually all vegetables

The low-carb gurus of today would have loved this, except they would have added some good fat to the mix.

The book also contained this little caveat: "Never, under any circumstances—even when you have reduced to the desired weight and have, to some degree, discontinued the diet—*eat potatoes, rice, white bread, macaroni, or sweets.*"

Calories were never once mentioned in Thompson's book, which went through 113 printings by 1931 and was still in circulation when a little problem arose at the DuPont company.

The Problem at the DuPont Company: The Work of Alfred Pennington, M.D.

DuPont executives were getting fat.

Really fat. No kidding.

Shortly after World War I, the medical department of E.I. DuPont, a large American chemical firm, became concerned about the growing obesity problem among the staff. The company hired Dr. Alfred Pennington and entrusted him with the job of finding out why the traditional low-calorie diets of the time were bombing when it came to losing weight. Pennington applied his considerable brain power to an analysis of the scientific literature and came to the conclusion that our old friend—the formerly fat undertaker William Banting—was right all along: obesity was due not to overeating, but instead to the body's inability to use carbohydrates for anything other than making fat.

Pennington put the DuPont executives on a high-fat, high-protein, low-carbohydrate, *unrestricted-calorie* diet. He limited their carb intake to 60 grams a day, allowed them at least 24 ounces of meat and fat (more if they wanted it), and restricted them to *one portion a day* of any one of the following: potatoes, rice, grapefruit, grapes, melon, bananas, pears, raspberries, or blueberries.

Pennington published a number of articles in prestigious journals such as *The New England Journal of Medicine,*[4, 5] but he summed up his results with the fat executives best in an interview he gave to *Holiday Magazine.* I've added the italics for emphasis.

> Of the twenty men and women taking part in the test, all lost weight on a diet in which the total calorie intake was unrestricted. The basic diet totaled about 3,000 calories per day, *but meat and*

fat in any desired amount were allowed those who wanted to eat still more. The dieters reported that they felt well, enjoyed their meals and *were never hungry between meals.* Many said they felt more energetic than usual; none complained of fatigue. Those who had high blood pressure to begin with [no longer did]. The[se] twenty obese individuals lost an average of twenty-two pounds each, in an average time of three and a half months. The *range of weight loss was from nine pounds to fifty-four pounds,* and the range of time was from about one and a half months to six months.[6]

Chalk up another one for the low-carb approach to weight loss.

Then, in 1928, something really interesting happened at the dietetic ward of Bellevue Hospital in New York City. But to understand why it happened, you have to understand the experiences of a rugged young explorer named Vilhjalmur Stefansson.

Stefansson and the Eskimos: All Meat, All Fat, All the Time

Kicked out of school at age twenty-three for inciting a protest within the student body, Vilhjalmur Stefansson picked up the pieces of his life and entered the world of his true love, anthropology. By 1906 he had managed to get a master's degree at Harvard, where he became an assistant professor of anthropology and got really interested in the diets of other people. Not much for city life, Stefansson dumped Harvard and decided that it would be more fun to join the Anglo-American Polar Expedition and travel to the Arctic. A couple of years after his first foray, he persuaded the American Museum of Natural History in New York to give him the money to do it again, and he departed on his second expedition in 1908; this time, he stayed four years. He discovered a previously isolated group of natives called the

I've always found it easier to stay on a low-carb diet than on any other kind of diet. I just never feel as hungry so I don't really feel like I'm dieting.
—Doug M.

Copper Inuit (so named because they used copper tools), and he lived with them for his entire stay. His third and final expedition began in 1913 and lasted for five years.

Later, he wrote: "In 1906 I went to the Arctic with the food tastes and beliefs of the average American. By 1918, after eleven years as an Eskimo among Eskimos, I had learned things which caused me to shed most of those beliefs."[7]

One of the beliefs Stefansson took to the Arctic was the prevailing notion that the less meat you ate, the better off you'd be. The view then—as now—was that if you ate a lot of meat, you would develop, among other things, hardening of the arteries, high blood pressure, and, very likely, a breakdown of the kidneys.

But this is what he found: the Eskimos he lived with ate a diet that consisted almost exclusively of meat or fish and fat. And they were as healthy and robust as a bunch of wild horses. High blood pressure, coronary infarctions, and strokes were virtually unknown. The women rarely suffered with breast-feeding problems, complications in pregnancy, or difficult births. And prior to their contact with mainstream civilization, Eskimos seldom suffered from cancer. (Today, about a century after their contact with "civilization" and the modern diet, they routinely suffer from all of the above.)

Ever the anthropologist, Stefansson lived with an Eskimo family for much of his time in the Arctic, and adopted all their eating habits. Though he had hated fish all his life, he ate it night and day. He ate it raw, baked, and boiled. He ate the heads and the tails. He even came to like the Eskimo delicacy of rotten fish, which he likened to his first taste of Camembert. It was the beginning of an aggregate of five years on a diet that consisted almost exclusively of protein, fat, and water.

According to the prevailing dietary wisdom of the times, he should've been dead.

He wasn't. And, by the way, he never gained weight. He also never saw a fat Eskimo. He wrote:

> Eskimos, when still on their home meats, are never corpulent—at least, I have seen none who were. Eskimos in their native garments do give the impression of fat, round faces on fat, round bodies, but the roundness of face is a racial peculiarity and the rest of the effect is produced by loose and puffy garments. See them stripped, and one does not find the abdominal protuberances and folds which are so in evidence on Coney Island beaches and so persuasive an argument against nudism.[8]

The guy did have a sense of humor.

By the way, lest anyone think that Eskimos were somehow genetically or racially immune to getting fat, Stefansson was quick to point out how quickly they fattened up when they ate mainstream American or European diets. In other words, they stay nice and slim on a high-fat diet, but as soon as they start eating starch and sugar, guess what happens?

Stefansson was genuinely curious to see if this strange diet had produced any ill effects that he perhaps hadn't noticed. And there were plenty of doctors who were just as curious as he. A committee was convened and Stefansson was put through as rigorous an examination as a potential astronaut would get today. The findings were published in *The Journal of the American Medical Association* on July 3, 1926, in an article titled "The Effects of an Exclusive Long-Continued Meat Diet." The result? The committee had failed to find even *one trace of evidence* of all the supposed harmful effects of the diet.

This brings us to the dietetic ward of Bellevue Hospital in 1928. Stefansson and Dr. Karsten Anderson, a colleague who had been on one of the expeditions with Stefansson, agreed to act as human guinea pigs in a two-person experiment. Stefansson had not only survived but thrived on a diet that was supposed to have killed him, but this experience had never really been verified under scientific conditions. So Stefansson and Anderson agreed to live in the dietetic ward of Bellevue Hospital under the strictest of medical supervision, eating an exclusive diet of meat, for one solid year. The aim of the project was not to "prove" something, but merely to get at the facts and answer the prevailing questions of the time: Would the men get scurvy? Would they suffer from other deficiency diseases? What would be the effect on the circulatory system? On calcium levels? On the kidneys? On their weight?

Lest anyone think this was a quaint little "experiment" supervised by a couple of country quacks, let's look at the committee assembled to supervise this dietetic experiment: from Harvard University, Dr. Lawrence Henderson, Dr. Ernest Hooton, and Dr. Percy Howe; from Cornell University Medical College, Dr. Walter Niles; from the American Museum of Natural History, Dr. Clark Wissler; from John Hopkins University, Dr. William McCallum and Dr. Raymond Pearl; from the Russell Sage Institute of Pathology, Dr. Eugene DuBois and Dr. Graham Lusk; from the University of Chicago, Dr. Edwin O. Jordan; from the Institute of American Meat Packers, Dr. C. Robert Moulton; and a physician in private practice, Dr. Clarence W. Lieb.

Not exactly "The Gang That Couldn't Shoot Straight."

This is how the experiment went: For the first three weeks, Stefansson and Anderson were fed the standard diet of the time: fruits, cereals, bacon and eggs, and vegetables. (Notice that there were no fast foods, no snacks, and no vending machine fare available then, so by today's standards, the "ordinary" diet was already light-years better than what we eat now.) During those first three weeks, the two guys were given preliminary checkups and were basically free to come and go as they pleased. After the first three weeks, they went on the all-meat diet and were more or less under house arrest. Neither of them was permitted at any time, day or night, to be out of sight of a supervising doctor or a nurse.

One interesting sidebar: Anderson was able to eat anything he liked as often as he wanted, provided that it came under the experimental definition of meat: steaks, chops, brains fried in bacon fat, boiled short ribs, chicken, fish, liver, and bacon. But because Stefansson had reported in one of his books, *My Life with the Eskimo*, that he had become very ill when he had to go two or three weeks on just *lean* meat ("caribou so skinny that there was no appreciable fat"), DuBois, who headed the experiment, suggested that for a while they try a *lean-meat only* diet on Stefansson to contrast the results with those of Anderson, who was eating whatever mix of fat and meat he felt like. They continued to give Anderson as much fat as he liked, but Stefansson was limited to chopped fatless meat.

Stefansson wrote:

> The symptoms brought on at Bellevue by an incomplete meat diet (lean without fat) were exactly the same as in the Arctic, except that they came on faster—diarrhea and a feeling of general baffling discomfort. Up north the Eskimos and I had been cured immediately when we got some fat. DuBois now cured me the same way, by giving me fat sirloin steaks, brains fried in bacon fat, and things of that sort. In two or three days I was all right, but I had lost considerable weight. If yours is a meat diet then you simply must have fat with your lean; otherwise you would sicken and die.[9]

For the rest of the year, both men were kept on a diet of meat and fat in whatever proportion they liked, and the experiment went off without a hitch. Every few weeks, with DuBois supervising, they would run around the reservoir in Central Park, then run up to DuBois' house, going up the stairs two or three at a time, after which they would plop down on cots and have their breathing, pulse rate, and other measurements taken. These tests showed that their stamina increased the longer they stayed on the meat diet.

In 1930, DuBois and associates published the results of the study in the *American Journal of Biological Chemistry*. The title of the paper was "Prolonged Meat Diets with Study of Kidney Functions and Ketosis." Here's a summary of what they wrote: Stefansson, who was about ten pounds overweight at the beginning, lost his excess weight in the first few weeks on the all-meat diet. His total caloric intake ranged from 2,000 to 3,100 calories per day. His metabolic rate rose—from 60.96 to 66.38 calories per hour during the period of the weight loss, indicating an increase of almost 9 percent. His blood cholesterol at the end of the year was 51 milligrams lower than it had been at the start. He wound up choosing a ratio of somewhere around 3:1 (in grams) of lean meat to fat. He continued the diet a full year, with no apparent ill effects.

> *Everyone warned me that if I went on a high-protein diet my cholesterol and triglycerides would go through the roof. Meanwhile, the exact opposite happened.*
> —Pamela R.

Stefansson wrote about his experiences in a fascinating and very long three-part piece called "Adventures in Diet" in *Harpers Monthly Magazine* between November 1935 and January 1936. His conclusions were surprisingly moderate: "So you *could* live on meat if you wanted to; but there is no driving reason why you *should*. Apparently you can eat healthy on meat without vegetables, on vegetables without meat, or on a mixed diet."

What he did not say, but undoubtedly would have had he been alive today, was this: you *cannot* eat healthily if most of your food comes from 7-Eleven.

The low-carbers of today would've loved him.

A postscript: it seems that in the twenty-or-so-year interim between his days in the Bellevue dietetic ward and his life in the 1950s as a scholarly (and relatively sedentary) academic, Stefansson suffered a mild cerebral thrombosis, put on a few pounds, and became quite a grump. According to Mrs. Stefansson, her husband had mostly recovered from the thrombosis but couldn't dump the extra weight. Her words: "By will power and near starvation, he had now and then lost a few [pounds] but [they] always came back when his will power broke down." Mrs. Stef also noted that he had become a real pain in the butt. As she delicately put it, "Stef had grown a bit unhappy, at times grouchy."[10]

Stef asked Mrs. Stef if she wouldn't mind if he went on the "Stone-Age Eskimo sort of all-meat diet" he had thrived on during the most active part of his Arctic career. Mrs. Stef was not exactly a stay-at-home wife. She lectured, she wrote books about the Arctic, she was the director of a course called the Arctic Seminar, and she sang in madrigal groups. She had better things to do with her time than to prepare two different menus. But she bit her tongue and said, "Of course, dear. That will be fine."

So back it was to *all meat, all fat, all the time* in the Stefansson household.

Mrs. Stef wrote:

> When you eat as a primitive Eskimo does, you live on lean and fat meats. A typical Stefansson dinner is a rare or medium sirloin steak and coffee. The coffee is freshly ground. If there is enough fat on the steak we take the coffee black, otherwise heavy cream is added. Sometimes we have a bottle of wine. We have no bread, no starchy vegetables, no desserts. Rather often we eat half a grapefruit. We eat eggs for breakfast, two for Stef, one for me, with lots of butter.
>
> Startling improvements in health came to Stef after several weeks on the new diet. He began to lose his overweight almost at once, and lost steadily, eating as much as he pleased and feeling satisfied the while. He lost seventeen pounds; then his weight remained stationary, although the amount he ate was the same. From being slightly irritable and depressed, he became once more his old ebullient, optimistic self.
>
> An unlooked-for and remarkable change was the disappearance of his arthritis, which had troubled him for years and which he thought of as a natural result of aging. One of his knees was so stiff he walked up and down stairs a step at a time, and he always sat on the aisle in a theatre so he could extend his stiff leg comfortably. Several times a night he would be awakened by pain in his hip and shoulder when he lay too long on one side; then he had to turn over and lie on the other side. Without noticing the change at first, Stef was one day startled to

find himself walking up and down stairs, using both legs equally. He stopped in the middle of our stairs; then walked down again and up again. He could not remember which knee had been stiff!

Conclusion: The Stone-Age all-meat diet is wholesome. It is an eat-all-you-want reducing diet that permits you to forget you are dieting—no hunger pains remind you. Best of all, it improves the temperament. It somehow makes one feel optimistic, mildly euphoric.[11]

A post-postscript: Stefansson remained married to the former Evelyn Schwartz Baird (Mrs. Stef) for twenty-one years; continued his research, writing, and public speaking at Dartmouth College; and died, by all accounts happy, on August 26, 1962, at the age of eighty-three.

Meanwhile, back at the ranch . . .

In 1944, cases of obesity were being treated at New York City Hospital by a cardiologist named Blake Donaldson. After a year of unsuccessful results with traditional low-calorie diets, he decided to investigate alternative methods. He took himself to the American Museum of Natural History, and using teeth as an indicator of both body condition in general and diet specifically, he hit the mother lode when he looked at skeletons dug from Inuit burial grounds. Looking further into Inuit diets, he consulted with Vilhjalmur Stefansson and became convinced that a meat-only diet was the answer for his obese patients. Donaldson allowed his patients to eat as much as they liked, but the *minimum* was one 8-ounce porterhouse steak *three times a day*, with a cooked weight of 6 ounces lean meat and 2 ounces fat, the same 3:1 ratio of lean to fat that had worked so well in the Stefansson-Anderson experiment (and the same one that Pennington had used with his DuPont execs).

Foreshadowing many of the low-carb diets of the 1990s, Donaldson kept his patients on a strict version of the diet until they reached their target weight, at which point they could add back certain "prohibited" foods, unless they began to put on weight again. Donaldson treated some 15,000 patients and claimed a 70 percent success rate using this diet. He also claimed that the 30 percent who were unsuccessful failed to lose weight not because of any fault in the diet but because they couldn't stay on it. He wrote a book in 1960 called *Strong Medicine*,[12] so named because Donaldson knew that his diet was not for the faint of heart—it took a lot of willpower and dedication to stick with it, and he knew that not everybody would be up for the challenge.

Then came a seminal moment in the history of low-carb theory, one that served as an acknowledged inspiration to the main guru of the low-carb movement of the late twentieth century, Robert Atkins. It happened in the 1950s and 1960s, and it happened in London.

Inspiration for Atkins

Professor Alan Kekwick was director of the Institute of Clinical Research and Experimental Medicine at London's Middlesex Hospital, and Dr. Gaston L.S. Pawan was senior research biochemist of the hospital's medical unit. These two researchers joined forces in the middle of the twentieth century to perform some visionary experiments.[13-15] They wanted to test the theory that different proportions of carbs, fat, and protein might have different effects on weight loss *even if the calories were kept the same*.

In one study, they put obese subjects on a 1,000-calorie diet but varied the percentages of protein, carbs, and fat. Some subjects were on a diet of 90 percent protein, some 90 percent fat, and some 90 percent carbs. The subjects on the 90 percent protein diet lost 0.6 pounds per day, the ones on the 90 percent fat diet lost 0.9 pounds per day, and the ones on 90 percent carbs actually gained a bit.

In another study, subjects didn't lose anything on a so-called "balanced" diet of 2,000 calories, but when these same subjects were put on a diet of primarily fat with very low carbohydrate, they were able to lose even when the calories went as high as 2,600 per day. The February 1957 issue of the American journal *Antibiotic Medicine and Clinical Therapy* reported, "If . . . calorie intake was kept constant . . . at 1,000 per day, the most rapid weight loss was noted with *high-fat diets*. . . . But when the calorie intake was raised to 2,600 daily in these patients, *weight loss would still occur provided that this intake was given mainly in the form of fat and protein*." (Emphasis mine.)

Still, the criticism from the medical establishment was enormous—this work contradicted the mantra that a calorie is a calorie is a calorie. One of the criticisms leveled at the two researchers was that the weight their patients lost was "just water weight." So Kekwick and Pawan did water-balance studies that showed water loss to be only a small part of the total weight lost. Interestingly, as recently as 2002, a very well-designed study done at the University of Cincinnati and Children's Hospital Medical Center[16] compared weight loss on a very low-carbohydrate diet to weight loss on a calorie-restricted low-fat diet, and found again that the greater weight loss experienced by the low-carb dieters was *not* due to water loss. The exact words: "We think it is very unlikely that differences in weight between the two groups . . . are a result of [water loss] in the very low-carb dieters." Yet to this day, the myth persists that the majority of weight lost on low-carbohydrate diets is mainly from water.

Eat Fat and Grow Slim and the Theory of Metabolic Disorder

The dietary establishment remained firmly convinced, as it does to this day, that the only thing that mattered when it came to weight reduction was calories, but there were pockets of dissent popping up throughout the 1950s, '60s, and '70s. One of the leaders of this dissent was Dr. Richard MacKarness, who ran Britain's first obesity and food allergy clinic and who in 1958 wrote *Eat Fat and Grow Slim* (which was revised and expanded in 1975).[17] He argued that it was *carbohydrates,* not calories, that were the culprit in weight gain. The following lines, from the foreword to the book, give the reader some idea of what's coming. They were written by Sir Heneage Ogilvie—a consultant surgeon at Guy's Hospital in London, the editor of *The Practitioner*, and a former vice-president of the Royal College of Surgeons, England.

> There are three kinds of foods—fats, proteins, and carbohydrates. All of these provide calories. *But the carbohydrates provide calories and nothing else.* They have none of the essential elements to build up or to repair the tissues of the body. *A man given carbohydrates alone, however liberally, would starve to death on calories.* The body must have proteins and animal fats. *It has no need for carbohydrates,* and, given the two essential foodstuffs, it can get all the calories it needs from them.

You heard it here first, folks. And you'll be hearing it again throughout this book: *the body has no physiological need for carbohydrates*. You cannot live without protein. You cannot live without fat. But you can survive perfectly well without carbohydrates. No one is saying you *ought* to, or that you *have* to—just that you *can*. This is simple, basic human biochemistry. There is no "minimum daily requirement" for carbohydrates—

which raises the question worth keeping in the back of your mind as you read through the rest of the book: why would the dietary establishment—including the American Dietetic Association—continue to insist that the only healthy diet consists of one in which *the majority* of the calories come from the *one macronutrient for which we have no physiological need*?

But I digress.

Sentiments similar to those of Ogilvie were echoed in the MacKarness book's introduction, written by Dr. Franklin Bicknell:

> The cure of obesity . . . can be, of course, achieved by simple starvation, but as Dr. MacKarness explains, this is both an illogical and an injurious treatment, while [a treatment] based on eating as much of everything one likes except starches and sugars and foods rich in these, is both logical and actively good for one's health, quite apart from the effect on one's weight. *The sugars and starches of our diet form the least valuable part and contribute nothing which cannot better be gained from fat and protein foods like meat and fish, eggs and cheese, supplemented by green vegetables and some fruit.* Such a diet provides an abundance . . . of vitamins, trace elements, and essential amino acids—an abundance of all those subtle, yet essential, nutrients which are often lacking in diets based largely on the fat-forming carbohydrates.

A little context: ever since 1829, when William Wadd, Surgeon-Extraordinary to the Prince Regent, proclaimed that the cause of obesity was "an over-indulgence at the table" (i.e., eating too darn much!), the conventional wisdom was that fat people are fat because they eat too much food. Period. This view, that only the quantity and not the quality of food that people eat makes a difference, had a stranglehold on mainstream medicine—a stranglehold that continued through the twentieth century with the cooperation of the sycophantic American Dietetic Association and is only now, in the twenty-first century, beginning to loosen.

To give you a sense of the spirit of the era, the medical correspondent of *The London Times*, on March 11, 1957, wrote at the time of MacKarness' book: "It is no use saying as so many women do: 'But I eat practically nothing.' The only answer to this is: "No matter how little *you imagine* you eat, *if you wish to lose weight you must eat less.*" (Emphasis mine.)

MacKarness comes out swinging, right in his author's introduction, leaving no doubt what "side" of the quality vs. quantity argument he's on: "Starch and sugar are the causes of obesity. Particularly modern refined and processed starches and sugars, the ever ready, highly publicized carbohydrate foods of twentieth-century urban man." He puts forth the interesting argument—foreshadowing much of what we hear today in the discussions of metabolic type—that there are two kinds of people, whom he characterizes as Mr. Constant-Weight and Mr. Fatten-Easily.

According to MacKarness, if you give both types the same exercise and feed them the same food, one will stay the same weight while the other will gain. When Mr. (or Ms.) Constant-Weight—people we hate who seem to be able to eat anything and not gain an ounce—take in too much carbohydrate, the extra food simply causes a revving-up in their metabolism that burns the extra calories consumed, and they stay the same weight. Nothing is left over for laying down fat. "But," MacKarness writes, "when Mr. Fatten-Easily eats too much bread, cake, and potatoes, the picture is entirely different: his metabolic rate does not increase. Why does he fail to burn up the excess? The answer is the real reason for his obesity: Because he has a defective capacity for dealing with carbohydrates."

MacKarness was suggesting a metabolic disorder, and he was on to something. He was really the first diet-book author to postulate some sort of metabolic defect in the way some people process food (especially carbohydrates) that causes them to send much of what they eat to their fat stores. Dr. Alfred Pennington (of the DuPont execs study) had come to the same conclusion. Summing up a 1953 paper called "Obesity: Over-nutrition or Disease of Metabolism?" published in the *American Journal of Digestive Diseases*, Pennington wrote, "Analysis of the results . . . appear[s] to necessitate an explanation of obesity on the basis of some intrinsic metabolic defect."

Writing for the general public, MacKarness had a simpler way of putting it. He came up with a great analogy: the steam engine.

The orthodox view is that a fat man's engine is stoked by a robot fireman, who swings his shovel at the same pace whether fat, protein, or carbohydrate is in the tender. This is true for Mr. Constant-Weight, but as he does not get fat anyway, it is only of academic interest to us. It is certainly not true for Mr. Fatten-Easily, with whom we are concerned. Mr. Constant-Weight has a robot stoker in his engine. The more he eats—of whatever food—the harder his stoker works until any excess is consumed, so he never gets fat. Recent research has shown that Mr. Fatten-Easily's stoker is profoundly influenced by the kind of fuel he has to shovel. On fat fuel he shovels fast. On protein slightly less fast *but on carbohydrate he becomes tired, scarcely moving his shovel at all.* His fire then burns low and his engine gets fat from its inability to use the carbohydrate which is still being loaded into the tender. *Mr. Fatten-Easily's stoker suffers from an inability to deal with carbohydrate.*

At the back of his book, MacKarness lists foods that can be eaten without reservation, which are meat, poultry, game, fish and other seafood, dairy products, fats and oils, most vegetables, and some fruits; foods that can be eaten in moderation with some caution, including nuts and higher-carb vegetables and fruits; and foods that could be eaten once a day, such as beans, beets, corn, potatoes, and bananas. While some low-carb theorists of today might quibble with the inclusion of dairy, what's more interesting is the MacKarness list of "Never eat" foods. Are you ready? Don't shoot the messenger.

- breakfast cereals
- bread and rolls
- biscuits and crackers
- macaroni products, noodles, spaghetti, and other pastas
- rice
- jellies, jams, and preserves
- ice cream, cakes, pies, and candy
- sauces and gravies thickened with flour or cornstarch
- beer
- sweet wines and liqueurs
- sodas (and all "sweetened fizzy drinks")
- sugar

The MacKarness diet suggests that carbs be kept as low as possible—no more than 60 grams a day for most people (and in some cases 50 grams or fewer a day). This figure is in the ballpark of the recommendations of many low-carb diet books of today (*Life Without Bread*[18] recommends a maximum of 72 grams a day, and the ongoing weight loss and maintenance programs of the Atkins diet and Protein Power are in the MacKarness range, as is the beginning program for overweight sedentary people adhering to the Schwarzbein Principle. It is also practically identical to the generic program for beginners that I recommend in chapter 8.)

We should not leave MacKarness without mentioning that he was one of the first to note the emotional and psychological component of overeating. Here's what he said, in words that will undoubtedly ring true for thousands of people today.

> So far, then, two big factors in the production of obesity have emerged.
> A *defect in dealing with carbohydrates* which makes a person fatten easily on an ordinary mixed diet;
> Overeating, especially of sugars and starches as a result of *loneliness, fear or emotional dissatisfaction.*
> When the two factors are present, weight is gained very rapidly.
> *So anyone who finds himself tempted to overeat for emotional reasons and who shows a tendency to get fat, should be careful to choose low-carbohydrate foods.*[19]

Overeaters Anonymous

MacKarness was not the only one to notice the emotional component of overeating. Interestingly, on the other side of the ocean, in 1959—less than a year after the publication of MacKarness' book and twenty-four years after the founding of Alcoholics Anonymous—two women in Los Angeles began the fellowship now known as Overeaters Anonymous. A spiritual program to address compulsive overeating, it was based on the same twelve-step principles as its predecessor, but with one significant difference. While alcoholics and drug addicts could abstain from their drug of choice, compulsive overeaters could not. They had to eat to survive.

This presented an entirely different set of issues, since for overeaters, complete "abstinence" from their "drug" (food) was not possible. Many of the original participants in OA attended because they were terribly overweight, but most understood that there was a compulsive emotional component to their overeating that could not be addressed by simple diets or by the prescription drug of the day, dextroamphetamine, sold under the brand name Dexedrine. What's especially interesting for our purposes is a particular sub-group of OA that developed in Los Angeles in the early sixties. This group had noticed that, even though many people lost weight in Overeaters Anonymous, many were nibbling their way back to obesity and that certain foods seemed to feed the compulsion to eat more than others.

Can you guess what the culprits were?

Yup.

By 1963 there was a very vocal minority of OA members who were convinced that carbohydrates sabotaged any weight loss plan because they produced cravings and addictive eating behavior. The OA contingent called them "binge foods." One of the founders of this faction—which later came to be known as the Grey Sheet Group—wrote "I wonder if we have an *allergy of the body* too. Are we going to help the Doctors understand obesity just as the alcoholic had to educate the medical profession?"[20]

From that time on—although it is little known—there has always been a faction of OA that believes strongly that "abstaining" from carbohydrates (with a very low-carbohydrate diet) is a necessary component of emotional sobriety when it comes to food, just as it is a necessary strategy for weight loss in carbohydrate-sensitive individuals. Could this be another case of the patient profoundly understanding the disease far in advance of the medical professionals?

Calories, Carbs, or Just Plain Fat? The Roaring '60s

In the 1960s, two books came out in favor of the low-carb approach, both of which got a lot of attention. One of them deserved it; the other did not. The one that did was a thoughtful, if somewhat misguided, treatise called *Calories Don't Count* by a New York doctor named Herman Taller. Taller had been a fat man all his life, at one time almost 100 pounds over his ideal weight. He described himself as one of those who "only had to look at a platter of spaghetti to gain [weight]." He struggled with every version of the low-calorie diet available with virtually no results. A physician friend of his was sure that Taller had to be lying about how much he was eating, so Taller hatched a plan. Reading his experience will no doubt produce quite a number of nodding, sympathetic heads.

> I proposed an interesting vacation test [to the physician who was certain I was cheating]. We would go away together for ten days, stay in each other's company continually, eat and drink the same things, and check the results. He accepted, and we went off to a resort. I followed what was then the accepted method of weight control: a low-calorie diet. I concentrated on salads,

which I now know was a mistake, ate fat sparingly, another mistake, and, since this was a vacation, drank a cocktail each night before dinner. My physician friend, who was slim, did the same. At the end of the vacation, he had lost a pound or two and I had gained nine pounds. "I don't understand it" he said as we drove back to New York. Neither did I.[21]

Taller didn't reject the calorie theory at all. On the contrary, he wrote, "No one, least of all myself, would dispute the concept that led to the calorie fad. Any person will lose weight when he burns up more energy than he eats. This is a simple chemical law. Why, then, didn't a low-calorie diet work? Why did people lose weight on high-calorie, high-fat diets?" Taller postulated that all calories are not the same and that carbohydrates present a different problem to the body *at least for some people*. He rightly pointed out that low-fat diets were by nature high in carbohydrates, thus stimulating insulin and creating more fat, particularly in people who were sensitive to carbohydrates. (It is noteworthy that, almost four decades later, Eleftheria Maratos-Flier, director of obesity research at Harvard's prestigious Joslin Diabetes Center, said, "For a large percentage of the population, perhaps 30 to 40 percent, low-fat diets are counterproductive. They have the paradoxical effect of making people gain weight.") Taller completely agreed that the underlying reason people get fat is an imbalance between calories taken in and calories burned. But he suggested that for some people there is a disturbance in the metabolism, with three results, none of them good: (1) the body *forms* fat at a rate that is faster than normal; (2) the body *stores* fat at a rate that is faster than normal; and (3) the body *disposes* of stored fat at a rate that is *slower* than normal. Taller summed up: "The crux of the matter is not how many calories [we] take in, but what [our bodies do] with those calories."[22]

Taller did not recommend a diet devoid of carbohydrates—in fact, a typical day's menu contained up to three slices of "gluten bread," something no low-carb advocate today, including myself, would recommend (there are far more healthy starchy carbs to choose from, including sprouted-grain or gluten-free breads). The rest of the day's food came from meat, poultry, seafood, and plenty of vegetables as well as some oils. There was no counting of calories.

Now here's where it gets interesting.

In the '50s and '60s, when Taller was writing, a scientist named Ancel Keys had begun studying heart disease and diet—research that culminated in what has come to be known as the diet-heart hypothesis. Keys concluded that cholesterol is a cause of heart disease, saturated fat causes a rise in cholesterol, and therefore saturated fat causes heart disease. Keys' seven-country study[23] became the basis for dietary policy for more than three decades, indirectly birthed the fat phobia of the '80s, and directly spawned an entire bureaucracy devoted to lowering cholesterol (i.e., the National Cholesterol Education Program) and to producing some of the most profitable pharmaceutical drugs in history (see chapter 2). Note for now that there are serious problems with this theory, and it is finally being reexamined.[24-26]

Taller, a product of the time, accepted the demonization of cholesterol and believed that if you could reduce it in the diet, you could significantly lower heart disease rates. He was very concerned about the saturated fat in the low-carb diets of the past, so he came up with what he thought was a perfect solution: his version of the diet would incorporate tons of polyunsaturated fats. Problem was, he lumped all unsaturated fats together. He was correct in pointing out how healthy marine fats are (the famous omega-3s from fish and flaxseed), but he was dead wrong in advocating excessive amounts of man-made refined vegetable oils like safflower, sunflower, and corn oils, which we now know are associated with a host of diseases, inflammatory conditions, and cancers.[27-30]

Taller's book went through eighteen printings and ultimately had more than a million copies in circulation, but his career came to an unfortunate end when he was convicted of six counts of mail fraud for using the book to promote a particular brand of safflower capsules, which the court called "a worthless scheme foisted on a gullible public."[31] Too bad. By all reports, he was a good guy and very sincere in his efforts to bring healthy low-carb living to the masses.

The other low-carb book published in the '60s—also against a backdrop of the fledgling no-fat madness started by the flawed Keys research—was one that didn't deserve much attention, though that little detail didn't stop it from selling 5½ million copies. *The Doctor's Quick Weight Loss Diet*,[32] otherwise known as the Stillman diet, put forth a high-protein solution that attempted, at the same time, to satisfy the low-fat contingent. On the Stillman diet, you ate nothing—and I mean *nothing*—but protein with every drop of fat trimmed from it. You could eat all you wanted from the following selection: lean meats with all possible fat trimmed; chicken and turkey without skin; all non-fatty fish; eggs made in nonstick pans without butter, margarine, oil, or other fat; cottage cheese and other soft cheeses made only from skim milk; and at least eight glasses of water a day. We know from the Stefansson experiment that this diet, if followed for any length of time, would make you very sick precisely because of the *absence* of fat.

The Stillman diet was a dumb idea and should not be followed for any reason. Although the Stillman all-protein plan was in fact a low-carb diet, it's important to remember that not all low-carb diets are *high-protein* diets. Even the Atkins diet, which will be discussed at greater length in chapter 3, is not necessarily high-protein. In fact, the average protein content of all three major phases of the Atkins diet is only 31 percent (the average *fat* content is 56 percent); and during the Atkins maintenance phase, the average protein content is only 5 percent higher than Weight Watchers (25 percent vs. 20 percent)![33] Some of the diets discussed in this book don't even approach high-protein—for example Barry Sears' Zone diet (see chapter 3) has often been called a high-protein diet by magazine writers who have either not read his books or not understood them, and by members of the American Dietetic Association, who have frequently done neither. The point is that *low-carb does not necessarily equal high-protein*, and the Stillman diet is Exhibit A in making the case that all low-carb diets are not the same.

Atkins, Yudkin, and the Question of Sugar

By 1970, the Keys research had been published and was being picked up by the media; the low- or no-cholesterol brigade was gearing up for an assault on the consciousness of the American public. In 1972, Robert Atkins published the first edition of the *New Diet Revolution*, the Cadillac of low-carb diet plans, which became the de facto poster child for the low-carb movement two decades later.

Atkins was the first popular diet-book author to seriously focus on insulin as a determinant in weight gain. He preached the virtues of something he called "the metabolic advantage": benign dietary ketosis (a process that, because it is so central to the discussion of low-carb diets and so misunderstood, will receive much further attention in chapter 5). Because his high-fat, high-protein, low-carb diet went so dramatically against the conventional "wisdom" of the times, Atkins was attacked mercilessly in the press and vilified by the medical mainstream, who turned him into a pariah in the medical community. His voice was drowned out by the low-fat, no-cholesterol, calorie-counting establishment, and although he remained active, he didn't catch on big time until the early 1990s, when an updated edition of the *New Diet Revolution* was published.

The public, with their rapidly expanding waistlines, was growing weary of the low-fat dogma and beginning to realize that their low-fat diets were accomplishing very little in the way of weight loss; people were finally ready to look elsewhere for a solution.

In the same year in which Atkins published the first edition of his book, which firmly took the position that carbohydrates and not fat were the problem in obesity, a brilliant English doctor named John Yudkin was making waves by politely and reasonably suggesting to the medical establishment that perhaps their emperor, while indeed cholesterol-free and low-fat, was nonetheless naked as a jaybird. A professor of nutrition at Queen Elizabeth College, London University, and the Surgeon-Captain of the British Royal Navy, Yudkin was a highly respected scientist, nutritionist, and possessor of both an M.D. and a Ph.D., with dozens of published papers in such august peer-reviewed journals as *The Lancet, Cardiovascular Review, British Medical Journal, The Archives of Internal Medicine, The American Journal of Clinical Nutrition*, and *Nature* to his credit.

Yudkin was typically portrayed by his detractors as a wild-eyed fanatic who blamed sugar as the cause of heart disease, but in fact he was nothing of the sort. In his 1972 book, *Sweet and Dangerous*, he was the embodiment of reason when he called for a reexamination of the data—which he considered highly flawed—that led to the hypothesis that fat causes heart disease. (These data, as you will recall, came originally from a study of six[34] and then seven countries[35] published by Ancel Keys, studies that conveniently omitted a substantial amount of data that did not fit his hypothesis.)[36]

Yudkin pointed out that statistics for heart disease and fat consumption existed for many more countries than those referred to by Keys, and that these other figures didn't fit into the "more fat, more heart disease" relationship that was evident when only the six selected countries were considered. He pointed out that there was a better and truer relationship between *sugar consumption* and heart disease, and he said that "there is a sizable minority—of which I am one—that believes that coronary disease is *not* largely due to fat in the diet." (Three decades later Dr. George Mann, an associate director of the Framingham Study, arrived at the same conclusion and assembled a distinguished group of scientists and doctors to study the evidence that fat and cholesterol cause heart disease, a concept he later called "the greatest health scam of the century."[37] Around the same time, the brilliant Danish scholar Uffe Ravnskov, M.D., Ph.D., reanalyzed the original Keys data and came to the identical conclusion. His exemplary scholarship is supported by hundreds of referenced citations and studies from prestigious, peer-reviewed medical journals and can be found in book form[38] and at the website www.ravnskov.nu/cholesterol.htm.)

While Yudkin did not write a low-carb diet book per se, he was one of the most influential voices of the time to put forth the position that sugar was responsible for far more health problems than fat was. His book called attention to countries in which the correlation between heart disease and sugar intake was far more striking than the correlation between heart disease and *fat*. And he pointed to a number of studies—most dramatically of the Maasai in Kenya and Tanzania—where people consumed copious amounts of milk and fat and yet had virtually no heart disease. Interestingly, these people also consumed almost no sugar.[39]

Yudkin patiently explained that sugar consumption is *one* of a *number* of indices of wealth. Heart disease is associated with many of these indices, including fat consumption, overweight, cigarette smoking, a sedentary lifestyle, and television viewing. It is *definitely* associated with a high intake of sugar. He never said that sugar *causes* the diseases of modern civilization, just that a case could easily be made that it deserved attention and study, certainly as much, if not more so, than fat consumption. (Yudkin himself did several interesting studies on sugar consumption and coronary heart disease. In one he found that the median sugar intake of a group of coronary patients was 147 grams, twice as much as it was in two different groups of control subjects who didn't have coronary disease; these groups consumed only 67 and 74 grams, respectively).[40]

As Yudkin put it, "It may turn out that [many factors including sugar] ultimately have the same effect on metabolism and so produce coronary disease by the same mechanism." What is that mechanism? Fingers are beginning to point suspiciously to an *overload of insulin* as a common culprit at the root of at least some of these metabolic and negative health effects like heart disease; controlling insulin was the main purpose of the original Atkins diet and has become the raison d'être of the low-carb approach to living. (In the next chapter, we will explore some of the connections between high levels of insulin and heart disease, hypertension, obesity, and diabetes.)

Cholesterol Madness

Yudkin's warnings against sugar and Atkins' early low-carb approach to weight loss were mere whispers lost in the roar of antifat mania. By the mid-1980s, fat had been utterly and completely demonized, and fat phobia was in full bloom, with hundreds of no-cholesterol foods being foisted on a gullible public (despite the findings that dietary cholesterol had little or no effect on serum cholesterol, a fact acknowledged even by Ancel Keys himself, who, in 1991, said that dietary cholesterol only mattered if you happened to be a rabbit!).[41] In November 1985, the National Heart, Lung, and Blood Institute launched the National Cholesterol Education Program with the stated goal of "reducing illness and death from coronary heart disease in the United States by *reducing the percent of Americans with high blood cholesterol.*"[42] (Emphasis mine.)

Though high cholesterol *doesn't* cause heart disease and, in fact, has turned out to be a relatively poor predictor of it, the juggernaut was already in full swing, and the cry of "hold the butter" was heard all over America. Fat-free foods were everywhere. Snackwells replaced Oreos as the best-selling cookie in America. In 1976, Nathan Pritikin opened his Pritikin Longevity Center in Santa Barbara, California, and for the next decade preached the super-low-fat dogma to all who would listen, which included most of the country. Jane Fonda ushered in a new generation of aerobicized exercise fanatics whose motto was "no pain, no gain" and who looked upon fat of any kind as a Tootsie Roll in the punch bowl. (Later, Apex, a supplement company based in California, got a strong foothold in health clubs as nutrition "experts" largely by being the handmaiden of the American Dietetic Association, and Apex's people taught gullible trainers and their clients the dogma of high-carbohydrate diets for weight loss while they railed against the "dangers" of high protein and ketosis.)[43] It became a point of pride to exorcise any hint of fat from the diet; egg-white omelets became de rigueur on every urban menu, and waiters across America became accustomed to orders without butter, oil, or fat of any kind.

Pritikin died in 1985, but his mantle was quickly taken up by Dr. Dean Ornish. Ornish's reputation—and much of the public's faith in the low-fat diet approach—was fueled by his famous five-year intervention study (the Lifestyle Heart Trial), which demonstrated that intensive lifestyle changes may lead to regression of coronary heart disease.[44] Ornish took forty-eight middle-aged white men with moderate to severe coronary heart disease and assigned them to two groups. One group received "usual care," and the other group received a special, intensive five-part lifestyle intervention consisting of (1) aerobic exercise, (2) stress management training, (3) smoking cessation, (4) group psychological support, and (5) a strict vegetarian, high-fiber diet with 10 percent of the calories coming from fat.

When Ornish's study showed some reversal of atherosclerosis and fewer cardiac events in the twenty men who completed the five-year study, the public perception—reinforced by Ornish himself—was that the results were largely due to the low-fat diet. This is an incredible leap that is in no way supported by his research. The fact is that *there's no way to know* whether the results were due to the low-fat diet portion of the experiment (highly unlikely in the view of many), the high fiber, the whole foods, the lack of sugar, or some combination of the interventions. It is entirely possible that Ornish would have gotten the same or better results with a program of exercise, stress management, smoking cessation, and group therapy plus a whole foods diet of high protein, good fats, high fiber, and low sugar. (Interestingly, critics of low-carb diets frequently proclaim with great righteousness that the only reason a low-carb diet works is because it is a low-calorie diet in disguise. They never level that criticism at Ornish, whose diet, in a recent analysis, turned out to be *lower* in calories (1,273 calories) than the Atkins ongoing weight-loss phase (1,627 calories), the Atkins maintenance phase (1,990 calories), the Carbohydrate Addict's Diet (1,476 calories), Sugar Busters! (1,521 calories), the Zone (approximately 1,500 calories), and even Weight Watchers (1,462 calories).[45]

The Tide Turns: A Reexamination of the Low-Carb Solution

By the 1990s, it was pretty obvious that low-fat dieting wasn't getting results. The country was fatter than ever, diabetes was becoming epidemic, and people were getting more and more frustrated and confused. The time was right for another look at the low-carb wisdom that had been around in one form or another since Banting's day in the 1800s. To the chagrin of the medical establishment and the American Dietetic Association, Atkins resurfaced with a vengeance with his newly updated *New Diet Revolution* in 1992, followed by perhaps the most influential nutrition book of the 1990s, Barry Sears' *The Zone*, in 1995, a year that also saw the publication of the brilliant *Protein Power* by Drs. Michael and Mary Dan Eades.

After massive resistance by the establishment, serious research was finally comparing low-carb diets to traditional diets, and the results were impressive. While it would be incorrect to say that low-carb diets always produced greater weight loss than the traditional kind, they *often* did; they frequently produced it faster (a huge motivating force for many people); and they almost always produced better health outcomes such as blood lipid profiles, precisely the measures that the anti-low-carb forces had predicted would be disastrous on these regimens (see chapter 2). In what will

probably turn out to be a signal event in the death of the high-carb dicta-
torship, Dr. Walter Willett—chairman of the department of nutrition at
Harvard University's School of Public Health and one of the most
respected mainstream researchers in the country—recently came out pub-
licly against the 1992 USDA Food Pyramid, which for a decade had promoted six to eleven servings a day of grains, breads, and pastas.[46–48]

Internecine battles among advocates of different diets were hardly
something new. What was different this time was that the arguments were
finally taken public. On February 24, 2000, the U.S. Department of Agriculture hosted a major symposium, "The Great Nutrition Debate," which
featured, among others, Dr. Robert Atkins (the Atkins diet), Dr. Barry
Sears (the Zone diet), low-fat advocates Dr. Dean Ornish and Dr. John
McDougall, and various representatives of the dietary establishment.[49]
Then, on July 7, 2002, *The New York Times* published a cover story in its
Sunday magazine section titled "What If It's All Been a Big Fat Lie?" in
which Gary Taubes, a brilliant science journalist and three-time winner of
the National Association of Science Writers' Science in Society Award,
brought to the table massive evidence that the low-fat diet had been the
dumbest experiment in dietary history. The article created a predictable
uproar, with defenders of the faith rallying to discredit Taubes—not an
easy task, I might add—and the low-carbers beaming ear to ear with I-
told-you-so grins. An interesting side note: on the Dietitian Central website (a dietitian Internet community), the following post was found on July
14, a week after the Taubes article appeared: "Please, dietitians, download
from the *NY Times Magazine* section from last Sunday, July 7, the article
'What If It's All Been a Big Fat Lie?' by Gary Taubes. *It is full of information
that could rock our world.* As dietitians, we need to be prepared and
informed re: changes that may be completely different from what we have
learned and have been educating people about."

Low-carbing had come back, but this time with a clarity and a scientific validation that had simply not been present in previous decades. It's
time now for a reassessment of the twin sacred cows of dietary commandments—*high carbohydrates* and *low fat*—and for a clearer look at just what
could be gained in terms of health and weight loss by following a diet
more like the one that sustained the human genus for 2.4 million years
and sustained modern man for at least 50,000 years.

It's time to revisit the low-carb wisdom of the past, evaluate the
wisdom of the present, and see what they have to teach us about living
healthily in the twenty-first century.

CHAPTER 2

Why Low-Carb Diets Work

In other fields, when bridges do not stand, when aircraft do not fly, when machines do not work, when treatments do not cure, despite all the conscientious efforts on the part of many persons to make them do so, one begins to question the basic assumptions, principles, theories, and hypotheses that guide one's efforts.

—Arthur R. Jensen, Ph.D.
Professor of psychology at the University of California at Berkeley, in Harvard Educational Review, *winter 1969*

On November 1, 1999, Woody Merrell—the Muhammad Ali of doctors, loved, respected, and admired across the entire political spectrum of medicine and nutrition—wrote an article in *Time* magazine about weight loss. This is how it started:

"In my 25 years of medical training and practice in Manhattan, I've seen a wide range of diets come and go. *Virtually none of them work.*"

A few paragraphs later, Merrell wrote, "For most of my professional career, I adhered to the generally recognized dictum of weight management. *I advised my patients to count their calories and follow a low-fat diet.*"

He then talks about his experience with a few patients who weren't getting anywhere no matter what they tried. Skeptically, he put them on a low-carb diet.

Finally he wrote, "I have become a convert. Carbohydrates . . . are often prime saboteurs of our weight. [O]f all the diets I've seen over the past few decades, the moderate-fat, lower-carbohydrate ones are the most successful. *They stress not how much food you eat but what kinds. Calorie counting is not as important as carbo counting.*" (All emphases mine.)

The article is titled "How I Became a Low-Carb Believer."[1]

What convinced Merrell—and what is convincing more and more of his colleagues—is the fact that lower-carbohydrate diets *really work* for many, many people. The evidence of the senses is hard to argue with. People lose weight, feel better, and, equally important, have major improvements in their health. Chronic complaints and ailments have been known to disappear. Some of these people had tried every possible diet, had adhered to every conventional cholesterol-lowering, fat-reducing program, and wound up in exactly the same place as when they started—and sometimes were even worse. Yet on lower-carb diets, they do great.

How can something that is so counterintuitive work? (And it *is* counterintuitive for most of us—after all, even Gary Taubes, in his seminal article "What If It's All Been a Big Fat Lie?",[2] said he couldn't quite get over the feeling that the bacon and eggs on his plate were going to somehow jump up and kill him.) We need to remember that low-carb eating is counterintuitive precisely *because* we have all been taught a number of "truths" that we have internalized as nutritional gospel but which may in fact be nutritional hogwash.

We "know" low-carb diets can't work because they are often high in fat or cholesterol (which we "know" causes heart disease), are often high in protein (which we "know" causes heart disease, bone loss, and possibly cancer), and may be higher in calories (which we "know" causes weight gain). Yet people eating the low-carb way are losing weight and lowering their risk for heart disease, hypertension, diabetes, and obesity. There is even some indication that they may be lowering their risk for some cancers.[3, 4] How do we

> **My doctor kept telling me not to try a low-carb diet because he thought it was so dangerous. Then his wife lost 50 pounds on Protein Power and now he's really done a 180.**
>
> **—Adele P.**

explain this? It is as though all three of Christopher Columbus' ships returned home with great bounty from the New World, but the people back in Spain shook their heads in disbelief, saying, "How can this be? It must be a trick. The ships had to have fallen off the earth because we *know* the earth is flat!"

I've got news for you: low-fat is the flat-earth theory of human nutrition.

See, all theories of weight loss fit into one of two major categories of thought—*all of them*. There is no exception to this rule. If you understand the two categories, you're immediately better informed than half the population on the subject of dieting and weight loss.

Let's call category one the Thermodynamic View. It comes from the first law of thermodynamics, which basically says that what goes in must come out. Applied to weight loss, it means simply this: you eat a certain number of calories, and you burn up a certain number of calories. If you eat *more* than what you need, you *gain* weight. If you eat *less* than what you need, you *lose* weight. I call this the checkbook theory. If I deposit more money than I write checks for, I have some extra cash (i.e., I gain weight). If I spend more than I take in, I have to dip into that cash (i.e., I lose weight). If what I deposit exactly equals what I spend, I have a zero balance (i.e., my weight stays the same).

Let's call category two the Telephone Theory of weight loss, based on the game of Telephone you may have played as a child. You line ten people up, then whisper something in the ear of the first person. That person whispers it to the second person, and so on down the line, until the words are repeated to the last person, who then says them out loud. What usually happens is that you start out with something like "A rose is a rose is a rose" and you wind up with "Gardenias don't grow on the planet Mars." Applied to weight loss, the theory goes something like this: the stuff that goes on *in between* the calories coming in and the calories going out is *much* more important than the actual number of calories involved. There are so many enzymes, cofactors, energy cycles, hormones, neurotransmitters, eicosanoids, genes, and other variables in the human body that determine the fate of the food coming in that it is impossible to predict what's going to happen to someone's weight just by knowing the number of calories that go in. It would be like predicting the outcome of Telephone simply by knowing the phrase that was originally said. Sure, if everything goes perfectly, "A rose is a rose is a rose" comes out as "A rose is a rose is a rose." More often, though, it comes out as "Madonna's latest movie stinks."

The Thermodynamic View, known as the energy balance theory, has been the dominant theory of weight loss for years. The entire low-fat movement has been built on it: take in fewer calories and burn more, and you will lose weight. You have probably been hearing this advice for years. While this view is not entirely without merit, it's so far from the whole picture as to almost constitute dietary malpractice.

The thinking behind low-carbing belongs to the second category of theories about weight loss, the Telephone Theory. This view asks a critical question: what goes on inside the body once those calories are taken in? Why do some people store everything as fat and others don't? What *determines* whether what you eat goes on your hips or is burned up as energy and disappears as heat into the atmosphere?

The answer is one word: hormones.

Hormones control just about every metabolic event that goes on in your body, and you control hormones via your lifestyle. Food—along with several key lifestyle factors such as stress—is the drug that stimulates hormones, and those hormones direct the body to store or burn fat, just as they direct the body to perform a gazillion other metabolic operations. (Dr. Barry Sears has said that "food may be the most powerful drug you will ever encounter because it causes dramatic changes in your hormones that are hundreds of times more powerful than any pharmaceutical.") Hormones are the air traffic controllers determining the fate of whatever flies in. *If your food is stimulating the wrong hormones or creating a hormonally unbalanced state, you will find it extremely difficult, if not impossible, to lose weight and keep it off.*

In this chapter you will learn why it is so vitally important to balance your hormones if you want to lose weight. It is probably as important or *more* important than counting calories, and it is *certainly* more important than reducing dietary fat. But managing our hormones has even bigger consequences. Insulin—the hormone most targeted by the low-carb diet plans discussed in this book—is at the hub of a significant number of diseases of civilization. When you control insulin, you hugely increase the odds that you will be able to control your weight. But, as you will see, you *also* reduce the risks for heart disease, hypertension, diabetes, polycystic ovary syndrome, inflammatory diseases, and even, possibly, cancer.

So let's get to know the players in our hormonal dance. If I've done my job, at the end of this chapter you'll have a much better understanding of what has now come to be popularly known as "endocrinology 101": how the body *makes* fat, *stores* fat, and, finally, *says goodbye* to fat. You'll also understand why the same eating plan that helps you lose weight *also* has the positive "side effect" of preventing you from becoming a medical statistic.

THE STAR OF THE SHOW: EXPERTS WEIGH IN ON INSULIN

"Insulin is the key to the vast majority of chronic illness."
—Joe Mercola, D.O.

"There is an epidemic of insulin resistance in the world at large."
—Gerald Reaven, M.D.

"When you have excess levels of insulin, it's like a loose cannon on the deck of a hormonal ship."
—Barry Sears, Ph.D.

"Insulin sensitivity is going to determine, for the most part, how long you are going to live and how healthy you are going to be. It determines the rate of aging more so than anything else we know right now."
—Ron Rosedale, M.D.

The Good, the Bad, and the Ugly: Insulin and Its Discontents

Insulin, a hormone first discovered in 1921, is the star actor in our little hormonal play. It is an anabolic hormone, which means it is responsible for building things up—putting compounds (like glucose and amino acids) inside storage units (like cells). Its sister hormone, glucagon, is responsible for breaking things down—opening those storage units and releasing their contents as needed. Insulin is responsible for *saving*; glucagon is responsible for *spending*. Together their main job is to maintain blood sugar within the tightly regulated range it needs to be to keep your metabolic machinery running smoothly.

And to keep you from dying. Without insulin, blood sugar would skyrocket and the result would be metabolic acidosis, coma, and death, the fate of virtually every type 1 diabetic in the early part of the twentieth century prior to the discovery of insulin. On the other hand, without glucagon, blood sugar would plummet and the result would be brain dysfunction, coma, and death. So the body knows what it's doing. This little dance between the forces that keep blood sugar from soaring too high and those that prevent it from going too low is essential for survival. It's interesting to note that while insulin is the only hormone responsible for preventing blood sugar from rising too high, there are several other hormones besides glucagon—cortisol, adrenaline, noradrenaline, and human growth hormone—that prevent it from going too low. Insulin is such a powerful hormone that five other hormones counterbalance its effects.

How a High-Carbohydrate Diet Raises Both Cholesterol and Triglycerides

Let's follow the nutrients you eat on their journey through the body. When you eat food—any food—it mixes with acids and enzymes from the stomach, pancreas, and liver that break it down into smaller molecules. The nutrients are then absorbed through the intestinal walls, while the indigestible parts of the food pass through the digestive system as waste. Proteins break down into amino acids, carbohydrates into glucose, and fats into fatty acids. These pass through the intestinal walls into the portal vein, which is like their private passageway into the liver, the central processing plant of the body. After the liver works its magic, often repackaging these compounds into different forms, the new forms are released into the general circulation of the bloodstream, where they are transported to cells and tissues to be either used or saved for a rainy day.

As these smaller units pass through the portal vein en route to the liver, the pancreas immediately takes notice of the parade and responds by secreting our star player, insulin. It secretes *some* insulin in response to protein, but when it sees carbohydrates in the passageway, its eyes light up, and it brings out the big guns and goes to town. (Fat doesn't even rate a "hello" from the pancreas and has no impact on insulin.)

Under the influence of this incoming insulin, the liver does a number of things. First, it decides how much of the sugar coming in is excess. It makes that decision based largely on how much insulin the pancreas has decided to send along to accompany the payload. If there's a lot of insulin, the liver says, *"Woo hoo, we've got a truckload of sugar on our hands; let's get busy."* Some of the incoming sugar will pass right through (as glucose) to the bloodstream to be transported to muscle cells—which can use a hit of sugar now and then for energy—and to the brain, which needs sugar (or ketones, which we'll discuss in detail later) to think and do all the other good things that brains like to do. Part of the excess sugar will be converted to the

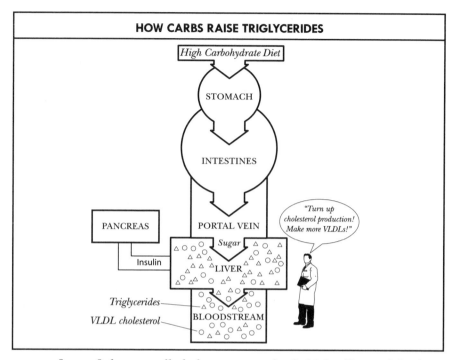

HOW CARBS RAISE TRIGLYCERIDES

storage form of glucose, called glycogen, much of which will stay right there in the liver. (Glycogen is also stored in the muscles, but muscle glycogen is like a private bank account that can be used only by the muscle in which it is stored.) The liver doesn't hold a lot of glycogen, so if there is *still* excess sugar, which there almost always is after a high-carbohydrate meal, it is packaged into triglycerides (fats found in the blood and in the tissues). The high level of insulin accompanying the high-carbohydrate meal stimulates the cholesterol-making machinery: the body starts churning out more cholesterol, which it then packages (together with triglycerides) into little containers called VLDLs (very low-density lipoproteins), most of which eventually become LDLs (low-density lipoproteins), or "bad" cholesterol. This is how a high-carbohydrate diet raises both triglycerides and cholesterol.

Which Is Worse, Sugar or Fat? No Contest!

Why, you may ask, does the liver feel this compelling need to get rid of the excess sugar, anyway? Why doesn't it just give it a pass and let it go into the bloodstream as is? Why create all this work for itself? Why bother to turn it into triglycerides in the first place?

That's a very good question, and the answer is central to understanding the health effects of a lower-carbohydrate diet: *sugar is far more damaging to the body than fat.* In a very real sense, what the liver is doing is *detoxifying* sugar into triglycerides.

As you just read, eating high-carb foods usually makes your cholesterol go up. Here's why: insulin turbocharges the activity of a particular enzyme—with the unwieldy name of HMG-coenzyme A reductase, or HMG-CoA reductase—that runs the cholesterol-making machinery in the body. (Glucagon inhibits the HMG-CoA reductase enzyme, so your body makes less cholesterol.) So high levels of insulin basically signal the liver to ramp up the production lines on cholesterol, and high levels of sugar signal it to ramp up the production of triglycerides. (Interestingly enough, if you ate a diet of almost 90 percent fat, your cholesterol numbers would probably drop, because there would not be enough insulin around to power the cholesterol-making machinery.) However, the American diet—high-fat *and* high-carbohydrate—virtually guarantees both high cholesterol *and* high triglycerides. Your Honor, the body had *motive, means,* and *opportunity.* Motive—to get rid of the excess sugar. Means—fat and sugar. Opportunity—tons of insulin to drive the works. Case closed: when there's plenty of excess sugar and insulin around, triglycerides skyrocket and so does cholesterol.

At this point, it may start to occur to you that since sugar is made into triglycerides, then maybe one of the reasons that blood levels of triglycerides are lowered on a low-carb diet is because there's less excess sugar coming in to require packaging into triglycerides in the first place. And you'd be absolutely, 100 percent right. (Cholesterol usually comes down as well, but as you'll see later, that doesn't matter nearly as much.) This lowering of triglycerides is one of the major health benefits of a low-carb diet—high triglycerides are far more of a danger sign for heart disease than high cholesterol ever was.

You may also be thinking that the higher levels of fat that are frequently (though not always) part of low-carb diet plans may not be so bad after all if they're not accompanied by the high insulin levels that go with high-carb diets. You'd be right on that count as well.

Insulin Prevents You From Losing Fat

An important thing to remember just from a weight loss point of view is that insulin isn't only responsible for getting sugar into the cells and out of the bloodstream. It's also responsible for getting *fat* into the fat cells *and keeping it there.* Insulin actually prevents fat burning. That's why a low-carb diet usually produces more weight loss than a high-carb, low-fat diet with the same calorie count. By lowering insulin, you open the doors of the fat cells and allow the body to release fat.

One of the ways insulin interferes with fat burning is by inhibiting carnitine, an amino acid–like compound in the body that is responsible for escorting fatty acids into the little central processing units of the muscle cells, where those fats can be burned for energy. By inhibiting carnitine, insulin inhibits fat burning. That's one reason you shouldn't eat a big meal before going to bed—the resulting high levels of insulin virtually ensure that your body will not be breaking down fat as you sleep but instead will be busy storing whatever is around in the bloodstream. (A side note: many years ago, an American health magazine decided to do a weight loss story on sumo wrestlers. The writers reasoned that the wrestlers knew everything there was to know about putting on weight, so if we could just learn what it was they did, we'd know what *not* to do if we wanted to slim down. One of the major rituals of the sumo wrestlers was eating a huge meal and then going right to bed.)

So on a high-carbohydrate diet, you've got all this sugar coming into your system—because all carbs eventually break down into sugar—and your liver can basically do one of three things with it:

1. Pass it right through and send it into the bloodstream.
2. Transform it into glycogen and store it (in the liver or the muscles).
3. Use it to make triglycerides.

Remember, as far as your body is concerned, the most important thing is to prevent blood sugar from getting too high. Your insulin may very well be able to keep your blood sugar in the normal range, but the high level of insulin needed to do the job—plus the high levels of triglycerides and VLDLs being created at the same time—are silently laying the foundation for future damage: you are slowly on your way to becoming overweight and/or insulin-resistant.

Insulin Resistance: The Worst Enemy of a Lean Body

Insulin resistance makes losing weight incredibly difficult and is a risk factor for heart disease and diabetes. It is not something you want, and you *can* do something about it. Here's how insulin resistance develops: the muscle cells don't want to accept any more sugar (this is especially true if you have been living a sedentary life). They say, "Sorry, pal, we're full, we don't need any more, we gave at the office, see ya." Muscle cells become *resistant* to the effects of insulin. But the fat cells are still listening to insulin's song. They hear it knocking on their doors and they say, "Come on in; the water's fine!" The fat cells fill up and you begin to put on weight.

Meanwhile, back in the bloodstream, those little packages called VLDLs that we talked about earlier are carrying triglycerides around trying to dump them. After the VLDL molecules drop off their triglyceride passengers to the tissues and the ever-expanding fat cells, most of them turn into LDL ("bad") cholesterol.

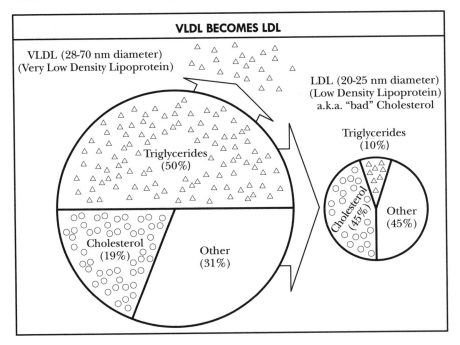

Now you're overweight, with high triglycerides, high LDL cholesterol, and *definitely* high levels of insulin, which the pancreas keeps valiantly pumping out in order to get that sugar out of the bloodstream. From here, two scenarios are possible, neither of them good.

In one scenario, your hardworking pancreas will somehow be able to keep up with the workload and keep your blood sugar from getting high enough for you to be classified as diabetic. But you will be paying the price for that with high levels of insulin and the increased risk factors for heart disease that go with them. In the other scenario, your poor pancreas will eventually become exhausted—even its most valiant efforts to shoot enough insulin into the system won't be adequate for the job. The sugar will run out of places to go, so it will stay in the blood and your blood sugar levels will rise. Now you'll have elevated insulin *and* elevated blood sugar, plus, of course, high triglycerides and abdominal obesity. If your blood sugar continues to rise even more, beyond the capacity of your insulin to reduce it, you'll eventually have full-blown type 2 diabetes.

Welcome to fast-food nation.

What's So Bad About a Little Sugar?

Obviously, the body knows how important it is to protect the tissues, the brain, and the bloodstream from excess sugar. So what exactly does sugar *do* that's so damaging to the body that the body is willing to risk the effects of large amounts of insulin and dangerously high levels of triglycerides just to prevent it?

Well, for one thing, excess sugar is sticky (think cotton candy and maple syrup). Proteins, on the other hand, are smooth and slippery (think oysters, which are pure protein). The slippery nature of proteins lets them slide around easily in the cells and do their jobs effectively. But when excess sugar keeps bumping into proteins, the sugar eventually gums up the works and gets stuck onto the protein molecules. Such proteins are now said to have become glycated. The glycated proteins are too big and sticky to get through small blood vessels and capillaries, including the small vessels in the kidneys, eyes, and feet, which is why so many diabetics are at risk for kidney disease, vision problems, and amputations of toes, feet, and even legs. The sugar-coated proteins become toxic, make the cell machinery run less efficiently, damage the body, and exhaust the immune system.[5] Scientists gave these sticky proteins the acronym AGES—which stands for **a**dvanced **g**lycolated **e**nd-products—partially because these proteins are so involved in aging the body.

For another thing, high blood sugar is also a risk factor for cancer—cancer cells consume more glucose than normal cells do.[6,7] Researchers at Harvard Medical School suggested in the early 1990s that high levels of a sugar called galactose, which is released by the digestion of lactose in milk, might damage the ovaries and even lead to ovarian cancer. While further study is necessary to definitively establish this link, Walter Willett, M.D.—chairman of the department of nutrition at the Harvard School of Public

Health and one of the most respected researchers in the world—says, "I believe that a positive link between galactose and ovarian cancer shows up too many times to ignore the possibility that it may be harmful."[8]

Sugar depresses the immune system. It makes the blood acidic, and certain white blood cells (lymphocytes) that are part of our immune system don't work as well in an acidic environment.[9–11] A blood sugar level of 120 reduces the phagocytic index—a measure of how well immune system cells gobble up bacteria—by 75 percent.[12] Since refined sugar comes with no nutrients of its own, it uses up certain mineral reserves of the body that are needed to metabolize it, which in turn throws off mineral balances and results in nutrient depletions.[13] (One of the minerals that refined sugar depletes is chromium, which is needed for insulin to do its job effectively!) Since minerals are needed for dozens of metabolic operations, these mineral deficiencies can wind up slowing down your metabolism and creating havoc with your energy level. Finally, sugar reduces HDL, the helpful, "good" cholesterol, adding yet another risk factor for heart disease to its résumé.[14]

Is it any wonder people drastically improve their health when they switch to a diet lower in sugar?

Why Should We Care About High Levels of Insulin?

Now you understand the problems caused by high levels of sugar in the blood. But what problems are associated with high levels of *insulin*? See, insulin doesn't just bring blood sugar down, call it a day, and go home. It affects many other systems as well. Bringing in a huge amount of insulin to fix the sugar problem is like importing twenty thousand workers to fix a broken power plant in a city. The city can't run efficiently without electricity—hospitals are in danger, computers shut down, there's no public transportation, and you can't cook. So the prime order of business is to fix the emergency. At first, city officials aren't thinking about the effect of that influx of workers on the *rest* of the city's business; they just want to get the immediate problem fixed. Yet all those workers are going to have a major impact: the roads will be overcrowded, pollution will increase, crime may go up, and there will be additional demands for housing and food. But the city is faced with a life-and-death situation, so it imports however many people are needed to fix the problem. The same thing happens when the body produces high levels of insulin to cope with high blood sugar: damn the torpedoes, full steam ahead—the body will worry about the consequences later.

Insulin and Heart Disease

One of insulin's many effects on the body is to make the walls of the arteries thicker. It does this by encouraging growth and proliferation of the muscle cells that line those artery walls. Insulin also makes the walls stiffer, reducing the "flow space" inside and increasing blood pressure. Smaller arteries are also more prone to plaque.

As we've seen, insulin also increases LDL cholesterol (the so-called "bad" cholesterol) in the blood. But despite what you may have heard, we don't really care about that until that LDL is deposited on the lining of the artery walls. In fact, we *still* don't need to worry about it unless that LDL becomes damaged. When it becomes damaged, then we have something to worry about. Damaged LDL attracts cells called macrophages, little Pac-Man–like creatures that come out to feast on the LDL like sharks on a bleeding carcass. When LDL is not damaged, the macrophages leave it alone, but as soon as damage occurs, the macrophages zoom in and feed, gorging themselves until they're full, at which point they're called foam cells. These foam cells group together and make a fatty streak, the first step in the formation of plaque.

How does the LDL get damaged in the first place? By two processes—oxidation, the interaction with oxygen that produces the same kind of "rusting" damage you see when you leave a cut apple out in the air, and glycation, bumping into sticky sugar. We just discussed how glycolated proteins cause all sorts of damage in the body. This same process of glycation damages LDL, and damaged LDL attracts macrophages like red flags attract bulls.

So insulin increases the amount of LDL in the system, and excess sugar damages the LDL, leading ultimately to plaque. If this were not enough to increase your risk for heart disease, you're also going to have lowered levels of magnesium, a mineral that is absolutely essential for the health of the heart. Why is your magnesium level lowered? Because insulin, in addition to storing sugar and fat in the cells, is also responsible for storing magnesium, so when your cells become resistant to insulin, you lose the ability to store some of that magnesium. Magnesium relaxes muscles, including those in the arterial walls. When you can't store magnesium, you lose it and your blood vessels constrict, causing a further increase in blood pressure. The loss of magnesium can also lead to heart arrhythmia and other cardiac problems.[15] And because magnesium is required for virtually all energy production that takes place in the cells, you may also find yourself with lower energy to boot.

How Does a Low-Carb Diet Lower Your Risk of Heart Disease?

There are numerous ways in which a low-carb diet can significantly lower your risk for heart disease. Lowering your insulin levels is certainly one of the most important. Raising your HDL cholesterol is another. A third— the importance of which it is difficult to overstate—is by lowering triglycerides. Researchers from the cardiovascular divisions of Brigham and Women's Hospital and Harvard Medical School, in a study led by J. Michael Gaziano, looked at various predictors for heart disease and found that the ratio of triglycerides to HDL ("good" cholesterol) was a better predictor for heart disease than anything else, *including* cholesterol levels. They divided the subjects into four groups according to their ratio of triglycerides to HDL and found that those with the highest ratio (i.e., high triglycerides to low HDL) had a *sixteen times greater risk of heart attack* than those with the lowest ratio (low triglycerides to high HDL).[16]

There's more. Most of us are familiar with "good" cholesterol (HDL) and "bad" cholesterol (LDL), but what is not as well known is that both types of cholesterol have subparts that behave very differently from one another. What *kind* of LDL you have turns out to be much more important than just the *amount* of LDL you have (an LDL-GGE test is now widely available to tell you about your LDL). For example, LDL cholesterol comes in two basic flavors: it can be a big, fluffy, cotton ball–like molecule (LDL-A type), or it can be more like a dense, tight, BB-gun pellet (LDL-B type). The big, fluffy LDL-As are pretty harmless. They are far less likely to become oxidized or damaged and cause problems. But the little LDL-Bs are a different story. Those are the ones that cause problems, and those are the ones you should be concerned about. The Gaziano study found that high triglycerides correlate strongly with high levels of the dangerous LDL-B particles. Low levels of triglycerides correlated with higher levels of the harmless LDL-As. In other words, the higher your triglycerides, the greater the chance that your LDL cholesterol is made up of the B-particles (the kind that is way more likely to lead to heart disease). The take-home point: reduce your triglycerides (and raise your HDL), and you reduce your risk of heart disease. (For for an updated list of journal articles showing that triglycerides and HDL improve on a low-carb diet, go to What's New? at JonnyBowden.com and click on For Your Doctor.

Insulin and Hypertension

As you saw in the previous paragraphs on heart disease, high levels of insulin can narrow the arterial walls which, in turn, will raise blood pressure, since a harder pumping action is required to get the blood through the narrower passageways. But there's an even more insidious way in which insulin raises blood pressure.

It talks to the kidneys.

Insulin's message to the kidneys is this: *hold on to salt*. Insulin makes the kidneys do this even if the kidneys would much prefer not to. Since sodium, like sugar, is controlled by the body within a very tight range, the kidneys figure, listen, if we have to hold on to all this salt, we'd better bring on more water to dilute it so that it stays in the safe range. And that's exactly what they do. Increased sodium retention results in increased water retention. More fluid means more blood volume, and more blood volume means higher blood pressure. Fully 50 percent of people with hypertension have insulin resistance.[17]

Insulin will also ultimately raise adrenaline, and adrenaline will raise both blood pressure and heart rate. We'll discuss the insulin-adrenaline axis a little more under obesity in the next section.

How Does a Low-Carb Diet Lower Your Risk of Hypertension?

Lowering insulin levels will intercept the message to the kidneys to hold on to salt. You will almost immediately lose water weight, and bloat and blood pressure will go down. Lowering insulin is actually such an effective strategy for lowering blood pressure that it sometimes works too well too fast. In rare cases, your blood pressure might dip too low, and you may experience lightheadedness or dizziness upon standing up. This is why some clinicians recommend increasing salty foods or adding a teaspoon of salt to your food on a daily basis if you find this happening to you.[18]

When the kidneys dump excess sodium, potassium sometimes gets caught in the crossfire and you wind up dumping potassium as well. This is even truer if you exercise and sweat a lot. You don't want to lose too much potassium, because that can cause muscle cramps, fatigue, and breathlessness. This is why I always recommend potassium supplements, especially during the first week of a low-carb diet, and particularly when you are on one of the very restricted carbohydrate plans such as the induction phase of Atkins or the first two weeks of Protein Power. Potassium supplements come in 99-milligram tablets, and you can get them at any drugstore or health food store. Take one or two at each meal. Foods rich in potassium, such as liver, broccoli, and avocados, are also a good idea, as is using over-the-counter salt substitutes like Morton's Lite Salt or NoSalt, which are both potassium salts.

Insulin and Obesity

The connection between a high-sugar diet, high levels of insulin, and becoming overweight or obese should be painfully obvious by now. The more sugar—i.e., carbohydrates—you take in, the more sugar you need to store and the more your insulin levels rise. The more your insulin levels rise, the less fat you burn and the more sugar you store in fat cells, along with those extra triglycerides that the liver made from excess sugar. The more you store, the fatter you get. The fatter you get, the more insulin-resistant you become.

When there are consistently high levels of insulin floating around, the body will put out more cortisol and adrenaline (the "breakdown" hormones) to counteract the "building up" effects of insulin and attempt to bring the body back into balance. Cortisol in part breaks down muscle, further reducing your metabolic rate. Too much adrenaline can eventually lead to even *more* insulin, as insulin will eventually be secreted to combat the effects of too much adrenaline! The interaction of insulin and cortisol/adrenaline is the particular aspect of low-carbohydrate dieting central to the metabolic healing work of Diana Schwarzbein, who feels that this kind of constant imbalance—often brought on by yo-yo dieting, high levels of stress, and a diet high in sugar—ultimately damages the metabolism. If getting off this particular seesaw sounds interesting to you, be sure to read about the Schwarzbein Principle in chapter 3.

Even if you don't remember the basic biochemistry discussed here, tattoo the following inside your eyelids: *insulin is the fat-storage hormone.* It is also the hunger hormone. When it finally does its job of lowering blood sugar, it causes blood sugar to go really low, setting you up for a cycle of craving (and eating) more high-carb foods. Result: higher blood sugar, more insulin, and more fat storage as the cycle continues.

How Does a Low-Carb Diet Help You Lose Weight?

When you eat a lower-carb diet, you stimulate less insulin but you *also* stimulate more glucagon, its sister hormone, which responds more to protein (remember that neither hormone is stimulated by fat). Glucagon liberates the fat from storage sites and gets it ready to burn for energy. Meanwhile, since you no longer have elevated levels of insulin, you are not suppressing carnitine, which, you may remember, is the compound in the body responsible for escorting fat into the central furnaces of the cells, where it can be burned for fuel.

Along with insulin and glucagon, a pair of enzymes plays a major role in the whole fat-storage/fat-release equation: lipoprotein lipase and hormone-sensitive lipase. Lipoprotein lipase is responsible for storing fats; it breaks down triglycerides in the bloodstream and shoves the fatty acid parts into fat cells. People who are trying to lose weight are not fond of this enzyme. It's very persistent; in fact, when people lose weight, the activity of lipoprotein lipase is ramped up, almost as if the body is fighting to hold on to fat. This is one of the reasons it's so difficult to keep weight off. (Lipoprotein lipase is also suppressed when you smoke and increases when you stop smoking, one of the reasons people usually put on a few pounds when they first give up cigarettes.)

Hormone-sensitive lipase, on the other hand, reaches into fat cells and releases fatty acids into the bloodstream when they are needed—for example, if you're doing a long aerobic exercise session and your legs need some fuel. Its ability to liberate fat is really intense. Consider this: there's a protein called perilipin that shields fat from the fat-burning effects of hormone-sensitive lipase. Mice that don't have any perilipin to protect their fat from hormone-sensitive lipase don't get fat no matter what they eat![19] The fat-burning effect of hormone-sensitive lipase is that intense.

Insulin and glucagon have profound effects on both lipoprotein lipase and hormone-sensitive lipase. Can you guess what effects they have? By now it should come as no surprise: insulin stimulates lipoprotein lipase (the fat-storing enzyme) and inhibits hormone-sensitive lipase (the fat-releasing enzyme). If you want your fat cells to let go of fat, you want all the hormone-sensitive lipase activity you can scrounge up—you certainly don't need high levels of insulin turning down the volume. Glucagon, on the other hand, has exactly the opposite effect on these enzymes. It *inhibits* the fat-storing enzyme and *stimulates* the fat-releasing one. This is just one more way that restoring a healthy balance between insulin and glucagon helps you to lose weight.

Fat Cells Know How to Protect Their Existence!

When you do lose weight, you stack the hormonal deck in your favor even more. We used to believe that fat cells were these inert little sacks of blubber that basically didn't do anything metabolically—they just took up space and held onto a gazillion calories' worth of energy that never got burned up fast enough. We now know that fat cells are anything *but* inactive. They are actually endocrine glands that releases a host of hormones—including estrogen—and other substances that can have a profound effect on our weight.

Many of the hormones that are released by the fat cells have one major purpose—to keep those fat cells in business! In this way, you might say that fat actually perpetuates its own existence by releasing hormones that make it harder for the body to get rid of it.

One of the hormones released by fat cells is resistin. The more fat cells you have, the more resistin that gets released into your body. Mice given extra dosages of resistin develop insulin resistance in two days[20,21] and, as we've just seen, insulin resistance is a major obstacle to fat loss. Another substance released by the fat cells is TNF-alpha 1, also known as tumor necrosis factor. This is a good guy: it's part of the immune system's arsenal, and as you can tell by the name, it's involved in destroying tumors. But TNF-alpha 1 is also found in fat tissue, and in the circulatory system it appears to act like a hormone. In low amounts, it *inhibits* the ability of insulin to lower blood sugar, essentially making insulin's job harder to accomplish and thereby forcing the pancreas to put out even more insulin to get the job done.[22] Once again, a hormonelike compound released by the fat cells raises insulin and makes fat loss difficult. As you can see, the fat cells *themselves* contribute to the difficulty in losing weight by releasing substances that offer "fat-protection insurance"—chemicals that, in essence, help your fat cells stay in business. By lowering your fat stores with a low-carbohydrate diet, you will also lower the amounts of these fat-protecting substances in the bloodstream.

A Low-Carb Diet Helps Reduce Insulin Resistance

When you are insulin-resistant, your cells stop making insulin receptors to import sugar and fat into the cells. This process is called down-regulation. Receptors are like job recruiters. When the market is flooded with unemployed workers, companies don't have to go hunting for job applicants because there are so many knocking at the door. When you're insulin-resistant, you've got a hell of a lot of insulin—applicants—knocking at the cell door. The cells figure there's enough insulin hanging around and beating on the doors, so they stop sending out "recruiters" to the surface of the cells. When you bring your insulin down with a low-carb diet, suddenly there's not so much insulin banging at the doors of the cells. Now you begin to lose weight. Eventually, the cells start to send up more receptors to bring in the fuel, a process called up-regulation. The cells are now gradually becoming more insulin-*sensitive*—a condition you most decidedly want. Insulin sensitivity always improves when you lose weight.

There are other ways in which a low-carb lifestyle will help you lose weight. One way has to do specifically with protein itself, which is usually more plentiful on lower-carb diets. Protein has less of an effect on insulin, has a greater effect on glucagon, and increases metabolic rate considerably more than carbohydrates do. Specific amino acids found in protein may also play a role in weight loss. Several papers by D.K. Layman demonstrated greater body-fat loss on a high-protein diet than on a high-carb diet,[23,24] and in one paper he argued that leucine—an amino acid— may be one of the reasons.[25] Other studies have also suggested the possible role of specific amino acids in weight loss. In one animal study, a diet deficient in the amino acid lysine resulted in the accumulation of larger amounts of fat both in the bodies of the animals and in their livers.[26] Increasing the proportion of protein to carbohydrates appears to be more *satiating* during weight loss—it makes you feel fuller.[27] And metabolic rate, technically called thermogenesis—the heat production in our bodies from burning calories—is turned up after eating protein. In one study, thermogenesis was 100 percent higher with high-protein meals—even two and a half hours after eating—in young, healthy women.[28]

You may have heard that it is easier to stay on a low-carb diet than it is to stay on a traditional high-carb, low-fat diet. Let me say one word about that: *appetite*. A low-carb diet contains built-in appetite controls—it's like having your own little diet pill built into the meals. Here's how it works. One of the major hormones involved in telling the brain that you are full is cholecystokinin (CCK), which is secreted in the intestines in response to a meal. (You may have also heard, correctly, that it takes about twenty minutes for this hormone to reach your brain and tell you you've had enough—another reason to listen to your grandmother and eat slowly if you want to lose weight!) But here's the thing: CCK, being part of our ancient digestive system, recognizes protein and fat very well because they've been the mainstay of our diet for as long as the human genus has been on the planet. But CCK does *not* respond to carbohydrates. It barely recognizes them! That's why it is so easy to overeat carbs—you really have no idea when you've had enough.

Insulin Resistance and Diabetes

Insulin resistance is a huge risk factor for the development of both heart disease and diabetes.[29] Eighty percent of the 16 to 17 million Americans who have diabetes are insulin-resistant.[30] Dr. David Leonardi, founder of the Leonardi Medical Institute for Vitality and Longevity in Denver, Colorado, insists that insulin resistance is reversible and that many type 2 diabetics can be cured. He says, "Diabetics die from *diabetes complications, all of which are a direct or indirect result of high blood sugar.* Normalizing the blood sugar prevents disease, normalizes life expectancy, and profoundly enhances quality of life. Cured or not, they're winners either way."

In case you hadn't noticed by now, low-carb diets are all about normalizing blood sugar. Insulin resistance *is* reversible. And it's hardly a rare phenomenon. The prevalence of insulin resistance has skyrocketed 61 percent in the last decade alone, according to Daniel Einhorn, M.D., cochair of the AACE Insulin Resistance Syndrome Task Force and medical director of the Scripps Whittier Institute for Diabetes.[31] In fact, the prevalence of insulin resistance has probably been underestimated from the beginning. Gerald Reaven of Stanford University did the original work on insulin resistance in the 1980s. Here's how he approximated the number of people who were insulin-resistant. He divided his test population—nondiabetic, healthy adults—into quartiles and tested their ability to metabolize sugar and carbohydrates. He found that while the top 25 percent of the population could handle sugar just fine, the bottom 25 percent could not—they had insulin resistance (or, in the parlance of researchers, impaired glucose metabolism). So for a long time, it was thought that the number of people with insulin resistance was one in four.

DIABETES AND COMPLICATIONS

- *80 percent of diabetics are insulin-resistant.*
- *2,200 people are newly diagnosed each day.*
- *Diabetes is the seventh leading cause of death in the United States.*
- *60–70 percent of diabetics have mild to severe forms of nerve damage.*
- *Diabetes is the leading cause of lower-extremity amputations in the United States.*
- *86,000 amputations a year are related to complications from diabetes.*
- *The five-year mortality rate after amputation is 39–68 percent.*
- *Diabetics are two to four times more likely to have heart disease.*
- *Heart disease is present in 75 percent of diabetes-related deaths.*
- *Diabetes is the leading cause of new cases of kidney disease.*
- *Diabetes is the leading cause of new cases of blindness in adults.*
- *Each year, 12,000–24,000 people lose their sight because of diabetes.*

Source: American Podiatric Medical Association, American Diabetes Association, CDC, American Association of Diabetes Educators, and National Diabetes Educational Program

But there's a problem.

What happened to the 50 percent of the people *between* those two extremes? It turns out they had neither the terrific glucose metabolism of the top 25 percent nor the full-blown insulin resistance of the bottom 25 percent; instead, they fell somewhere in between. One could easily argue that since only 25 percent of the population had flawless glucose metabolism, the rest of us—up to 75 percent of the population—have *some* degree of insulin resistance! Remember, too, that Reaven used young, healthy adults as subjects, and their numbers are definitely not representative of the population as a whole—the fact is, insulin sensitivity actually decreases as you get older. The take-home point: insulin resistance isn't just something that happens to other people. Recently, the American Association of Clinical Endocrinologists estimated that one in three Americans is insulin-resistant.[32]

There are approximately 17 million diabetics in the United States, of which 5.9 million are not yet diagnosed.[33] Approximately 80 percent of them are insulin-resistant. Even if you are insulin-resistant and somehow manage to dodge the diabetes bullet, you are still at serious risk for heart disease. Being overweight (having a body mass index of greater than 25 or a waistline of greater than 40 inches for men and 35 inches for women) is a risk factor for insulin resistance—a big one. So are hypertension (high blood pressure), elevated triglycerides, and low-HDL cholesterol.[34] It's estimated that 47 million Americans have some combination of these risk factors.[35,36] As you have seen in this chapter, *all* of them are related to insulin, and virtually *all of them improve substantially on a low-carbohydrate diet*.

How a Low-Carb Diet May Help Prevent—or Even Reverse—Diabetes

Dietary treatment for diabetes is currently one of the hottest topics of debate in the diabetes community.[37] Some factions are passionately holding on to the old recommendations of a high-carb diet, while other clinicians are making strenuous arguments for lower-carb, higher-fat, higher-protein diets.[38,39] The precise dietary treatment for full-blown type 2 diabetes is beyond the scope of this book, though it is a fascinating subject and in my opinion has great relevance for nondiabetics as well.* What can we say for sure? A number of studies have shown that people on low-carbohydrate diets experience increased glucose control, reduced insulin resistance, weight reduction, lowered triglycerides, and improved cholesterol. If you have been diagnosed with, or are at risk for, diabetes and your doctor is reluctant to put you on a low-carb diet, you can find updated references for relevant studies on my website, JonnyBowden.com.

---

*Diabetes expert Dr. Ron Rosedale of the Rosedale Center for Metabolic Medicine in Boulder, Colorado, states that everyone in this country is to some degree "pre-diabetic."

Excess Insulin and PCOS

One in ten women have polycystic ovary syndrome (PCOS), the most common reproductive abnormality in premenopausal women, which puts them at high risk for both cardiovascular disease and diabetes.[40] One of the major biochemical features of PCOS is insulin resistance and hyperinsulinemia (elevated insulin levels). Obese women with PCOS have significant impairment of their ability to use glucose and have a marked reduction in insulin sensitivity.[41]

When we talk about insulin resistance, we often forget that not all tissues and cells become resistant at the same time, and some do not become resistant at all. For example, overweight people may—at least in the beginning—have very nonresistant fat cells. Their muscle cells refuse to take any more sugar, but the fat cells still have open arms. These cells are said to be insulin-sensitive. The ovaries also tend to remain insulin-sensitive. If there's a genetic predisposition for these glands to overproduce androgen hormones—as there is with women who have PCOS—the excess insulin that's sent into the bloodstream to deal with the excess sugar bathes these nonresistant tissues in an ocean of insulin that is way too much for their needs. One of the responses to all that insulin hitting the ovaries is that they produce even more testosterone and androstene, which leads to hair loss, acne, obesity, infertility, and other symptoms of PCOS.

Interestingly, those affected with PCOS often have relatives with adult onset diabetes, obesity, elevated triglycerides, and high blood pressure.[42] Sound familiar? This is why a low-carb diet is the dietary treatment of choice for PCOS. It's a common enough problem that many of the community bulletin boards on the low-carb sites listed in the Resources section have specific areas for PCOS.

Excess Insulin and Inflammation

Essential fatty acids, notably members of the omega-6 and omega-3 family, are the parent molecules for an entirely different group of fascinating hormones called eicosanoids. Eicosanoids, formerly called prostaglandins, live in the body for only seconds and act on the cells that are in their immediate vicinity—they don't travel in the bloodstream. They are very, very powerful modulators of human health. Like many other systems in the body, they need to be in balance. Sometimes, as a shorthand, we'll talk about "good" eicosanoids (the prostaglandin 1 series, or PG1), which inhibit clotting, promote vasodilation, stimulate the immune response, and are anti-inflammatory, vs. the "bad" eicosanoids (the prostaglandin 2 series, or PG2), which have the opposite effects, promoting clotting, constriction, and inflammation. But this shorthand is not completely accurate, as you need a *balance* of the two. For example, if you clot too much and too easily, you can have a stroke, but if you didn't clot at all, you'd bleed to death from a hemorrhage!

Here, too, insulin leaves its mighty footprint. Insulin inhibits a critical enzyme called delta-6-desaturase, which is responsible for directing traffic into the production line for the "good," anti-inflammatory eicosanoids. Inflammation has been implicated in a host of conditions, from heart disease to Alzheimer's to arthritis to food allergies. In fact, the modulation of insulin for the purpose of controlling eicosanoid production and reducing the risk of heart disease was the major reason for the development of the Zone diet by Barry Sears. If you're interested in learning more about this diet, be sure to read about it in chapter 3.

Excess Insulin and Aging

"If there is a single marker for life span," asserts Dr. Ron Rosedale, "it's insulin sensitivity."[43] He's right. In 1992, researchers collected data on people who were both mentally and physically fit and were at least one hundred years old. The researchers looked carefully to find the factors these folks might have in common, the ones that could be predictors for a long and healthy life. They came up with three. The first was low triglycerides. The second was high-HDL cholesterol. Can you guess the third? A low level of fasting insulin![44] You've learned in this chapter how a lower-carbohydrate diet almost always improves all three of these variables. Since this kind of diet is what our ancestors ate for eons, it makes sense that we would live the longest and stay the healthiest by adhering to it.

By the way, the only dietary strategy shown to actually *increase* life span in laboratory animals has been calorie restriction. When we humans try calorie restriction on a standard high-carb, low-fat diet, we generally hate it—we're hungry all the time. With a diet higher in protein, higher in fat, and lower in carbohydrates—and high in fiber—we're more satiated and our appetite is much more under control. Insulin—the hunger hormone—is no longer out of control, blood sugar is manageable, and weight becomes stabilized. We can actually wind up eating fewer calories and feeling more satisfied in the bargain. That's a recipe for an antiaging, health-producing diet *without* creating cravings or hunger pangs.

Switching to a Fat-Burning Metabolism: The Meaning of Ketosis

When you go on a low-carbohydrate diet, you restrict the amount of sugar coming into your system. That's a good thing. But what happens when there's a severely reduced amount of sugar coming down the pike? What does the body use for fuel?

The body does have basic glucose (sugar) requirements. The brain, for example, needs about 150 to 200 grams of glucose daily. If you're eating only about 20 grams of carbs a day—probably the lowest amount you would consume on the first phase of the strictest diets—where does the other 130 to 180 grams of glucose come from? Equally important, where does the body get the *rest* of the fuel it needs for its many other metabolic activities, such as exercise and breathing?

Well, the body gets sugar from a process called gluconeogenesis, a word that literally means "the creation of new sugar." Gluconeogenesis is a metabolic process by which sugar is created from *noncarbohydrate* sources. For example, the body will make sugar by using the glycerol molecule in triglycerides (making sugar from fat). It will also make some sugar from protein (i.e., from certain amino acids). And here's the really good news for the overweight person: if carbohydrates in the diet are sufficiently limited, the majority of the fuel the body needs for its day to day operations will come from fat, specifically from a breakdown product of fat called *ketones.*

The body loves ketones. The heart works fine on them, and so does the brain. Here's how they work. Fats are oxidized, or broken down, by a process called beta-oxidation, in which the long chain of carbons that constitutes a fatty acid is split into pairs of two carbon molecules each, called acetyl fragments. These acetyl fragments join with a compound called CoA (coenzyme A) to form the appropriately named acetyl CoA. Incidentally, acetyl CoA is also the end product of the breakdown of carbohydrates, so both carbohydrates and fats eventually wind up as acetyl CoA.

When there are enough carbs in the pipeline, the acetyl CoA do-si-dos into something called the Krebs cycle, in which the acetyl CoA is burned for energy. But if there's not enough sugar, acetyl CoA doesn't get its all-access pass into the Krebs cycle. Instead, it accumulates at the door and eventually turns into three ketone bodies (first acetoacetic acid, then beta-hydroxybutyric acid and acetone, for the science-minded among you). Most of these ketone bodies are sent to the tissues—including the heart and brain—to be used for energy, and some are excreted in the urine and breath. This is what the low-carb diets that stress ketosis are talking about when they speak of changing from a sugar-burning metabolism to a fat-burning metabolism. Ketones are the by-product of fat breakdown.

Ketosis—which happens when there are enough of these ketones to be detectable in the urine—is a topic of such misunderstanding, controversy, and criticism that it will get a much fuller discussion in chapter 5. For now, let's just say that this process is a part of normal metabolism and is not— I repeat, *not*—dangerous.

Ketosis is not *necessary* for weight loss. You could be in ketosis and not lose weight, just as you could lose weight without being in ketosis. You won't burn your stored fat (and the ketone bodies made from it) if you have a surplus of fuel coming into the pipeline from the food you're eating. If you're eating 10,000 calories of fat and no carbs, you'll definitely be producing a ton of ketones but you won't lose a pound. However, if you are eating a moderate number of calories *and* you are in ketosis, it is a good sign that you are burning fat and not sugar as your primary energy source.

If you switch to a higher-fat, higher-protein, lower-carb (and higher-fiber!) diet, you won't have enough sugar coming in to burn as fuel, and your body will have to make its own, mostly from fat and certain amino acids, and/or happily use ketones, a metabolic by-product of fat break-down, as fuel. If calories are at reasonable levels at this point—which they probably will be because you'll be a lot less hungry and have a lot fewer cravings—you will lose weight. You will also improve your blood lipid pro-files (lower triglycerides, higher HDL) *and* your insulin sensitivity. Not only will you get slimmer, but your risk for heart disease, diabetes, and hypertension will plummet.

Not a bad deal, right?

How a Low-Carb Diet Keeps You Healthy and Slim

We've talked about what sugar does to the body and why eliminating it is such a good idea. Obviously, a low-carb diet removes a great deal, if not all, of the refined sugar you've probably been eating. The health benefits of this reduction are enormous. But a low-carb diet can also remove two other substances that are a huge problem, albeit for very different reasons. One is trans-fats. The other is wheat.

The subject of trans-fatty acids is one of the hottest topics in nutrition today and has been the center of a great deal of debate in the area of public policy regarding food and food labeling. It has been discussed extensively elsewhere, particularly in the writings of Dr. Mary Enig, a lipid biochemist widely considered to be the leading authority on trans-fats in the country, if not the world. For now, let's just say that in the opinion of many experts saturated fats have gotten a raw deal and have in fact been blamed for damage done, for the most part, by trans-fats. We know that trans-fats raise LDL cholesterol, probably way more than saturated fats do, and that these damaged trans-fats actually *increase* the risk for type 2 diabetes.[45] They also lower HDL cholesterol and raise the risk for heart disease. A prediction was made in the prestigious medical journal *Lancet* as far back as 1994 that trans-fats would turn out to be a major factor in insulin resistance[46]; that was the same year that the Center for Science in the Public Interest petitioned the FDA to require that Nutrition Facts labels disclose amounts of trans-fat. On July 10, 2002, the National Academy of Science's Institute of Medicine issued a report that concluded that "the only safe intake of trans-fats is *zero*." After much hemming, hawing, and stalling, the FDA has finally mandated that trans-fat content be listed on food nutrition labels, though the law won't go into effect until 2006.

> *After learning the dangers of trans-fats, I began avoiding fast-food lunches—it's better for me and my kids.*
> —Gina D.

The intelligent low-carb diet is almost *always* naturally low in trans-fats, which may be one of the many reasons it can impart such health benefits. Consider this: the top sources of trans-fats are baked goods, muffins, cakes, cookies, doughnuts, granolas, crackers, pies, fast food, french fries, anything deep-fried, partially hydrogenated vegetable oils, and most margarines. The intelligent low-carb diet naturally contains almost none of these foods, or if it does, they are present in extraordinarily low amounts. The health benefits of this alone are incalculable.

The other ingredient that is either missing in action or has an extremely low profile on the low-carb diet is wheat. Now, most people are probably under the impression that wheat and grains are "good" for you. Maybe; maybe not.

Certainly, foods made with whole grains—which are far harder to find than you might think and most certainly do *not* include most commercially available "wheat breads"—are better than foods made with the refined grains that constitute the vast majority of grains we eat. But grains, particularly wheat, have a high propensity for turning into sugar quickly, and wheat is also one of the foods most likely to be implicated in food sensitivities.[47] At one point it was believed that celiac disease—an intolerance of gluten, which is found in most grains—was fairly rare, affecting only 1 in 1,700 people. Estimates are now running closer to 1 in 85, with some estimates as high as 1 in 33.[48] And this doesn't include the hard-to-estimate number of people who have delayed food sensitivities, very often to grains in general or at the very least to wheat. A recent book by clinician James Braly, M.D., suggests that gluten insensitivity may affect tens of millions of Americans.[49]

Dr. Joseph Mercola, medical director of the Optimal Wellness Center in Illinois, contends that grains—along with starches and sweets—trigger a "hormonal cycle of grain and sugar addiction, weight gain, and diabetes."[50] And numerous studies link carbohydrates that have a high glycemic load—the tendency to turn into sugar quickly—with increased risk of coronary heart disease[51] and with risk of type 2 diabetes.[52] Most high-glycemic processed grains fall into this category, but these grains are virtually eliminated on low-carbohydrate diets.

Insulin: The Smoking Gun

Controlling insulin is the number one priority of all low-carb diets. The dietary approaches discussed in chapter 3 differ only in how they go about accomplishing it—what degree of carbohydrate restriction they believe is necessary to successfully control insulin, whether they emphasize protein or fat (or both) in the diet, what kinds of fat they recommend, other aspects of metabolism they stress, and whether or not they include a component on emotional eating and holistic self-care.

Once you understand what runaway insulin levels and unregulated sugar metabolism in general can do to your health, it's easy to understand why correcting those imbalances brings about not only weight loss but a myriad of wonderful health benefits.

In the next chapter, we'll explore exactly how a number of popular diet plans approach the issue of insulin control, and you'll be able to determine which one is best for you.

CHAPTER 3

Seventeen Low-Carb Diets and What They Can Do for You

E ach of the programs in this chapter was selected for one of three reasons: it is extremely popular, it is extremely good, or it has gotten a lot of attention by the media. One thing will become abundantly clear from reading these reviews: all low-carb diets are not the same! When I give a program a rave review, I've spelled out exactly why that is, and when I have reservations I've told you what they are—it's always up to you to decide if you agree with me or not. With very few exceptions, the programs have *something* to recommend them, and even in those cases where I've given a less than glowing overall review, I've tried to represent fairly the strengths of the program as well as detailed reasons for my reservations.

As you will see, the outlines and discussions of these diets are detailed enough that you should be able to get a very good idea of what the program entails and decide whether it is a good match for you, or at least determine whether or not you'd like to explore it further by reading the book on which it's based.

So that you can get a sense of the program at a glance, I've given you the "In A Nutshell" description; after that, there's a much more detailed explanation of the diet itself, followed by "Jonny's Lowdown." The programs are "rated" between one and five stars, but be sure to read the explanation in the lowdown to see how I chose the rating. Understand that the ratings are my own opinions, based on the information I've shared with you in the discussion, and reflect my personal biases. (I'm pretty sure that *my* biases are the correct ones, though I suppose that everyone else thinks *theirs* are correct as well!) That, as the saying goes, is what makes a horse race. Or a political election. Or even a diet plan.

Happy reading!

The Atkins Diet
The Carbohydrate Addict's Diet and The 7 Day Low-Carb Rescue and
    Recovery Plan
Curves
The Fat Flush Plan
The GO-Diet: The Goldberg-O'Mara Diet Plan
The Hamptons Diet
The Lindora Program: Lean for Life
Neanderthin
The Paleo Diet
Protein Power
The Scarsdale Diet
The Schwarzbein Principle
Somersizing
The South Beach Diet
Sugar Busters!
The Zone

THE ATKINS DIET

ROBERT ATKINS, M.D.

WHAT IT IS IN A NUTSHELL

An easy-to-follow, specific dietary plan in four distinct stages. Stage one is "induction": a very low-carb (20 grams or less) approach to jump-starting weight loss. You move through the four stages, adding more carbs in specific increments until you find the level of carbohydrate consumption at which you can continue to lose weight gradually and consistently. You stay at that level of carb consumption until you are within a few pounds of your goal, and then you transition into a lifetime maintenance plan.

About the Atkins Diet

The Atkins diet was introduced in 1972 with the first edition of *Dr. Atkins' Diet Revolution* and immediately became an object of scorn and disdain by the conventional medical establishment. Why? Because it went completely against the accepted dietary truths of the time. In many ways it still does, though cracks in the cement are beginning to show, and the dietary establishment is finally becoming less certain that its nutritional commandments are actually true. As you may remember from chapter 1, the conventional wisdom that Atkins opposed included the following:

- To lose weight, you must eat a low-fat, high-carbohydrate diet.
- High-fat diets cause heart disease.
- Low-fat, high-carbohydrate diets prevent heart disease.
- All calories are the same.

Dr. Robert Atkins, a cardiologist and something of a visionary, was the first to bring to popular attention the influence of the hormone insulin on weight loss and to introduce the notion that *controlling insulin effectively is the key to losing weight*. By now, if you've read chapters 1 and 2, you are familiar with the central role that insulin control plays in virtually every carbohydrate-restricted diet and the reasons it occupies center stage. But in 1972, virtually no one in America who wasn't either a diabetic or a doctor had heard of insulin, let alone understood its role in weight gain and obesity. And it was not until much later that the public began to get a glimmer of insulin's role in heart disease, hypertension, and aging.

Atkins explained that insulin causes the body to store fat, that some people are metabolically primed to put out more insulin than others in response to the same foods, that sugar and carbohydrates were the prime offenders when it came to raising insulin, and that elevated levels of this hormone invariably resulted in increased body fat. He argued that it is not *fat* in the diet per se that makes you fat, but rather *sugar*—even more precisely, fat *in combination* with high sugar—and the resulting insulin that leads to weight gain. Atkins took serious issue with the idea that fat causes heart disease and claimed that his diet would actually *improve* blood lipid profiles, measures that show up in blood tests as risk factors for heart disease. (Much research has borne this out—see chapter 5 and the For Your Doctor page on JonnyBowden.com.)

What is the actual diet that stirred such passionate controversy? Well, the Atkins diet is, and always has been, a four-stage affair, but most people think of it as synonymous with the first stage, induction. During induction, you eat all the fat and protein you want, but you limit carbohydrates to 20 grams per day—an extremely low level of carbohydrate consumption equal to about 2 cups of loosely packed salad and 1 cup of a vegetable like spinach, broccoli, Brussels sprouts, or zucchini. At stage one, there is absolutely *no* rice, potatoes, cereal, starch, pasta, bread, fruit, or dairy products other than cheese, cream, and butter.

To anyone who has read a diet book in the last ten years that wasn't written by low-fat guru Dean Ornish or his followers, this list of prohibited foods sounds pretty familiar. But you have to realize that in 1972, banning these foods for even two weeks was the nutritional equivalent of suggesting that every school and office in the country burn the American flag. These foods were the holy grail of the low-fat religion. Bagels were the breakfast of choice for health-conscious Americans. Oils, fats, butter, cheese, cream, steak, and the like were considered heart attacks on a plate, and here Atkins was making them the centerpiece of his eating plan.

The establishment thought him quite mad.

If this weren't enough, Atkins spoke in downright loving terms of something called ketosis, which he termed "the metabolic advantage" and compared to sunshine and sex. For Atkins, being in ketosis was the secret to unlocking your fat stores and burning fat for fuel. Ketosis was the desired goal of the induction phase. Being in ketosis was a virtual guarantee that you were accessing your stubborn fat stores and throwing them on the metabolic flame, using your fat for energy instead of your sugar. A big part of the program involved checking your urine for ketones, which are the by-product of this kind of fat breakdown.

The problem was that mainstream medicine considered ketosis to be not only undesirable but dangerous, a metabolic state to be avoided at all costs. For the most part, they still do—see chapter 5 for a full explanation of why the common belief that ketosis is dangerous is wholly without merit. The emphasis on ketosis, coupled with the recommendation to eat unlimited amounts of fat, was enough to make Atkins a complete pariah in the medical establishment, and it is only now, more than thirty years after the publication of the original book and shortly after his death, that we are beginning to see a slow turnaround in that evaluation.

Briefly, ketosis works this way: when there is not enough carbohydrate (sugar) coming into the body and when sugar stores (glycogen) have been essentially used up, the body is forced to go to its fat stores for fuel. Furthermore, because there isn't enough sugar to get fat into the usual slow-burning energy production cycles of the body (known as the Krebs cycle), the fat has to be broken down in another pathway, with the result that *ketones*—by-products of this incomplete fat burning—are made and used freely for energy by most of the tissues, including the brain and the heart. Forced to run on a fuel of fat, the body drops weight as the fat is burned off.

The advantages of this plan are twofold. First, the severe restriction of carbohydrates and sugar in the diet immediately brings down your level of insulin, the hormone that is released in response to carbohydrates (and to some extent protein). By dialing down insulin production, you are forced to burn your own fat, a situation Atkins referred to as biologic utopia. Since insulin is a "storage" hormone, less *insulin* means less *fat storage*. Dietary fat has no effect on insulin, so, Atkins reasoned, even if there *is* a lot of fat coming into the diet, there's not enough insulin to drive the "fat-storing" machinery.

Second, going into ketosis was a way of "tripping the metabolic switch" from a sugar-burning metabolism to a fat-burning one. Excess calories cause weight gain only when you're eating a lot of carbohydrates, said Atkins. Dump the carbohydrates, and the fat in your diet is not a problem. He also claimed, to the sputtering frustration of his detractors, that you could consume *more* calories on his program and *still* lose weight, precisely because the fat-storing hormone, insulin, remained at low levels.

Atkins argued that obesity exists when the metabolism is not functioning correctly but that metabolic disturbances have little to do with the fat we eat; rather, they are caused by eating too many carbohydrates. According to Atkins, if you've been overweight for a long time, it's a virtual certainty that your body has problems processing sugar.

Atkins also believed that the biggest reason people gain back weight lost on a diet is hunger, and that hunger is just about inevitable when you go on a reduced-calorie, high-carbohydrate, low-fat diet. On his program, hunger was virtually eliminated, as were cravings and blood-sugar instabilities. There are good physiological reasons that the appetite is suppressed on a low-carbohydrate diet rich in protein and fat—i.e., the release of the hormone CCK (which tells your brain you are full) and the possible suppression of a substance in the brain called neuropeptide Y, which stimulates appetite.

The rules of induction are straightforward and simple. You do not count calories. You do not count protein. You do not count fat. You *do* count grams of carbohydrate, and you can have up to 20 grams a day in the form of *either* 2 cups of loosely packed salad and 1 cup of uncooked vegetables chosen from a specific list *or* 3 cups of salad. Period. As mentioned earlier, you can't have starches, grains, sugar, fruit, or alcohol. You cannot eat nuts, seeds, or "mixed" foods (combinations of protein and carbohydrate) like beans, chickpeas, and legumes. It is also suggested that you avoid the artificial sweetener aspartame (Equal) and caffeine, the latter because it can lead to low blood sugar and stimulate cravings.

Weight loss in the induction phase is fairly quick and dramatic. Much, but not all, of the weight loss is water and bloat, largely because insulin's message to the kidneys to stockpile salt (and therefore water) is no longer being sent. But the induction phase is only meant as a jump start. Though Atkins felt it was perfectly safe to stay in the induction phase for a month or so, he encouraged dieters to progress to stage two, which he calls ongoing weight loss, or OWL.

The key to the success of OWL is finding what Atkins calls your *Critical Carbohydrate Level for Losing*, or CCLL. (Some version of this has been adapted by virtually every low-carbohydrate diet that uses the concept of "stages.") Here's how it works. After completing the initial induction phase, you slowly add back carbohydrates at a very specific rate of 5 grams *per week* (the amount of carbs in another cup of salad, half an avocado, or six to eight stalks of asparagus, for example). This would put you at 25 grams of carbs per week. If you continue losing, in the next week you go up to 30 grams. You continue this progression upward until your weight loss stalls, and then you cut back to the previous level. That level is what Atkins calls your CCLL.

The rules for OWL are simple: you still eat as much protein and fat as you want (stopping when you're satisfied, of course); you increase carbs by no more than 5 grams per week; you add one new food group at a time to see if it has any negative impact on cravings or symptoms (such as headaches, bloating, and so on); and you continue this way until you are close to your goal weight.

When you are within 5 to 10 pounds of your goal, you move to stage three, premaintenance. During premaintenance, you up your carbs by another 10 grams per week (typical 10-gram portions are ½ cup of almonds, filberts, or macadamia nuts; ¼ cup of yams or beans; and 1 cup of strawberries or watermelon). Again, you're looking for the level of carbohydrate consumption that will let you keep losing, albeit at a much slower rate. If you overshoot that level and stop losing completely or even start gaining, you drop back down a level. Simple.

Atkins stresses the importance of the premaintenance stage, but I imagine it's the one most people resist the most. Here's why: when you're within spitting distance of your goal, you are naturally tempted to keep doing what you're doing until you get there. Atkins wants you to actually *slow the weight loss down* during premaintenance to less than 1 pound a week for two to three months. Premaintenance is seen as a kind of driver's ed for lifetime maintenance. You're using this time to learn and master new habits of eating that will last the rest of your life. You need to do a great deal of experimenting and tweaking, as the difference between your Critical Carb Level for *Losing* and your Critical Carb Level for *Maintaining* is likely to be very small. Finally, when you do arrive at your goal, you increase the carbohydrate level—again in measured increments and very gradually and carefully—until you find the level that allows you to stay exactly at that weight. Now you're in stage four, maintenance; the number of grams of carbohydrate you're consuming is your Critical Carb Level for Maintaining, and that's what you continue eating to stay at your goal weight.

Atkins spent a lot of time discussing metabolic resistance to weight loss, which he defines as the inability to burn fat or lose weight. He identifies four major causes of metabolic resistance, which are discussed at length in chapter 20 of his *New Diet Revolution*. Obviously, excessive insulin and insulin resistance is one of the causes (see chapter 2 for a full discussion on insulin resistance). Prescription drugs or hormones are another, and an underactive or malfunctioning thyroid is another. The last is yeast.

Atkins' discussion of yeast is useful reading for everyone who has had trouble losing weight. I believe yeast is a far more common factor in weight loss problems than was previously thought. Atkins explains that yeast overgrowth is commonly found in conjunction with a sensitivity to mold, and that the combination may easily suppress metabolism. Dr. Alan Schwartz, medical director of the Holistic Resource Center in Agoura Hills, California, has said that yeast creates its own food source by literally demanding sugar to feed on (i.e., cravings), a theory that would dovetail nicely with Atkins'. Yeast, a living organism, also produces waste products and toxins, which can weaken the immune system and lead to food intolerances, another obstacle to weight loss. While the mechanisms are not completely understood, it's a good bet that Atkins was right about the yeast connection. Fortunately, the Atkins diet—at least the induction phase—virtually eliminates all of yeast's favorite foods, and the classic antiyeast diet looks a lot like Atkins' induction.

Atkins identifies what he calls three levels of metabolic resistance: high, average, and low. How easily your body responds to carbohydrate restriction defines your level of metabolic resistance. He suspected that most people with a high level of metabolic resistance would wind up with a maintenance level of somewhere around 25 to 40 grams of carbs a day. Those with a low level of resistance would be in the 60- to 90-gram range, and regular exercisers would be at 90-plus grams of carbohydrate per day.

Atkins has been one of the most misunderstood diet authors and has been the target of more attacks than any other low-carb proponent, probably because his was the first and the most commercially successful of the plans and also, to the constant chagrin of the establishment, because he simply wouldn't go away. While some of the larger criticisms of the Atkins diet are applicable to all low-carb diets and will therefore be dealt with in depth in chapter 5, some are specific to Atkins and are briefly addressed here.

One of the sources of misinformation about Atkins came because many people confused the *induction* phase with the whole program. Atkins was very clear that induction was for a limited time only. A common criticism of Atkins is that he doesn't allow you to eat vegetables and fruits. Actually, he said no such thing. Atkins was a nutritionist, and a very good one at that—he did not want you to miss the incredible nutritional benefits of the phytochemicals found in vegetables and fruits, which you add back to the program in the subsequent stages of his plan. He never said you couldn't eat vegetables and fruits. He *did* say you couldn't eat junk carbohydrates.

Another problem with the public's (and medical establishment's) perception of Atkins' program is that it was based solely on the first (1972) edition of his book. In that edition, where Atkins first put forth the radical proposition that cutting carbohydrates was the key to controlling insulin, he didn't pay as much attention to what you were *allowed* to eat, concentrating instead on the foods you were *not* allowed. Atkins in 1972 was like the doorman at an exclusive club who is given the order *"don't let in anyone wearing sneakers!"* and, as a result, is so focused on the ground that he doesn't realize he is letting in all kinds of other riffraff that just happen to be wearing shoes. Atkins revised the book twice (in 1992 and 2002), and with each edition he became more outspoken about the need to emphasize omega-3 fats, eliminate trans-fats, and include plenty of vegetables and fiber in the diet. But he could never shake the 1972 image as the diet doc who lets you eat pork rinds and lard.

Finally, it bears mentioning that the fully developed Atkins program is a three-pronged approach to health that involves not just carbohydrate management (he later called the diet a "controlled-carbohydrate approach to eating") but exercise and nutritional supplementation. In his New York clinic, only a small percentage of patients came in solely for weight loss. Atkins should be remembered for his marvelous work in the field of complementary and integrative medicine as well as for his pioneering work on diet.

The Atkins Diet as a Lifestyle: Who It Works for, Who Should Look Elsewhere

While his last book, *Atkins for Life*, is a pretty good template for healthy living that almost anyone could benefit from (and is not wildly different from the Zone or the last stage of the Fat Flush Plan), the Atkins diet proper is likely to be most successful with, and most appreciated by, those who really have a fair amount of weight to lose and have had a great deal of difficulty getting it off. People with 10 to 15 pounds to lose could certainly do the program, but the exacting and cautious approach to adding carbohydrates back 5 grams at a time is likely to be overkill for them.

In the next decade, I believe we will have a much better understanding of the nascent concept of metabolic typing, but even now it appears that there are some types who do very well on higher-protein, higher-fat diets and some who do not. Obviously the protein types are going to fare well on this diet and not find it nearly as difficult and restrictive as those with a different sort of metabolic blueprint.

JONNY'S LOWDOWN ★ ★ ★ ★ ★

Rereading the Atkins opus for the zillionth time in preparation for this book, I was once again struck by the disparity between what he actually said and what people think he said. The Atkins diet was never an "all-protein" diet; in fact, a recent statistical analysis put the induction phase at 35 percent protein and the maintenance phase at only 25 percent! *He stressed vegetables, talked about fiber, went to great lengths to emphasize individual responses and the need for customizing, and thought that both exercise and nutritional supplements were absolutely vital for optimal health. The later version of his book—as well as the breezier* Atkins for Life—*is heavily referenced with a superb bibliography of scientific studies.*

Atkins' only real mistake was in portraying ketosis as identical to fat loss, and making it seem as though calories didn't matter at all. He kind of boxed himself into a corner on this one. Ketosis doesn't cause fat loss; it is simply the by-product of fat burning. Yes, ketosis occurs when you are burning fat for fuel, but you will dip into stored fat only if you are not getting enough fuel from the diet. If your diet is 10,000 calories made up of 90 percent fat and 10 percent protein, you will most certainly be in deep ketosis, but you will gain weight like crazy.

I don't think everyone who needs to lose weight must go on Atkins, but it is certainly a viable option and likely to be quite helpful for people with carb addictions, resistant metabolisms, significant insulin problems, and a fair amount of weight to lose. It deserves every one of its five stars.

Books in the Series

Dr. Atkins' New Diet Revolution (revised in 2002)

Dr. Atkins' New Diet Cookbook

Dr. Atkins' New Carb Gram Counter

Atkins for Life: The Complete Controlled Carb Program for Permanent Weight Loss and Good Health

Dr. Atkins' Age-Defying Diet

The Vita-Nutrient Solution: Nature's Answer to Drugs

Dr. Atkins' Health Revolution: How Complementary Medicine Can Extend Your Life

Best Book to Start With

It's a toss-up between *Atkins for Life* and *Dr. Atkins' New Diet Revolution*, with *Revolution* getting the edge. There's less of a possibility of misunderstanding anything if you take the time to read *New Diet Revolution*. In addition, it will give you a terrific overview of the Atkins approach to many conditions besides being overweight, such as diabetes, heart disease, and hypertension, not only with diet but with supplements. *Atkins for Life* is breezier, friendlier, less argumentative, and much, much more concise. It summarizes the stages of the diet and tells you how to do them, but it doesn't go into nearly as much depth as the original book. Look at both and take your pick.

About the Author

Robert C. Atkins, M.D., was the founder and medical director of The Atkins Center, a world-renowned integrative medical practice located in Manhattan. A graduate of the University of Michigan and the Cornell University Medical School, Dr. Atkins specialized in cardiology and internal medicine and was a leader and innovator in the use of supplements and nutritional protocols for chronic diseases. He died at the age of seventy-three, at the height of his popularity, from an unfortunate fall in front of his clinic in 2003.

Website

The official Atkins site, atkins.com, is very well done and has a ton of information ranging from "How To Do Atkins" to "Food & Recipes" to "Advice & Inspiration." I particularly like the section "The Science Behind Atkins," which contains an impressive amount of research in support of the Atkins view on a number of controversies. The original research is referenced, and there is a nice little summary of each study written for the general public. In addition to the official website, there are all kinds of Atkins support boards and ad-hoc sites set up by his followers. See Resources for more information.

THE CARBOHYDRATE ADDICT'S DIET

RACHAEL HELLER, M.A, M.PH, PH.D., AND RICHARD HELLER, M.S., PH.D.

WHAT IT IS IN A NUTSHELL

Those with a sense of humor call this plan "Atkins with dessert." You eat two protein-and-vegetable meals a day and one "reward meal," during which you can eat anything you like. On most variations of the plan, there are no snacks.

About the Carbohydrate Addict's Diet

The Hellers are pretty much responsible for adding the term *carbohydrate addict* to the popular lexicon. They define carbohydrate addiction as follows: "A compelling hunger, craving or desire for carbohydrate-rich foods; an escalating or recurring need or drive for starches, snack foods, or sweets." Sound familiar? It does to a lot of people. Rachael Heller certainly recognized herself in that description. And she discovered the principles upon which the diet is based quite accidentally through a fortuitous experience in her own life.

At the time of her discovery, Rachael weighed 268 pounds. She had had a weight problem all her life, weighing more than 200 pounds by the age of twelve and more than 300 pounds by age seventeen. She spent the better part of twenty years on diets, on liquid fasts, in Overeaters Anonymous, you name it. She became a psychologist largely because she wanted to learn about the psychological causes of overeating. Her own eating was, to put it mildly, out of control.

One day, because a medical test that had to be done on an empty stomach was postponed from the morning to late afternoon, Rachael found herself not being able to eat until early evening. At dinner, she ate everything in sight, then got on the scale the next day and found, to her astonishment, that she had lost 2 pounds. Equally important—and somewhat surprising—was that on the day she *didn't* eat breakfast or lunch, she *also* wasn't particularly hungry. She tried the same routine the next day—no breakfast, no lunch, no hunger, big dinner—and boom, off came another pound.

She continued to experiment and add refinements to the diet (which thankfully included putting breakfast and lunch back into the mix), and ultimately lost 150 pounds, which she has kept off to this day. It was out of this experience that the carbohydrate addict's diet was born and the theory behind why it works was developed.

As with many low-carbohydrate diets, the theory centers around the activity of insulin, but with a slightly different twist. As we know from elsewhere in this book, there are many people who oversecrete insulin in response to food (particularly carbohydrates) and many who eventually become *insulin-resistant,* meaning that their cells no longer "pay attention" to the insulin in their bloodstream. This leaves them with elevated levels of blood sugar *and* of insulin (a situation that can easily precede diabetes and certainly precedes other health problems). We also know that elevated insulin *prevents* fat burning and *encourages* fat storage. The Hellers hypothesize one more chain in this link, which is critical to the understanding of the carbohydrate "addict." According to the Hellers, too much insulin in the bloodstream prevents the rise of the brain chemical serotonin. (Make sure you read Jonny's Lowdown for a discussion—in my opinion, this is a misreading of the science.) Serotonin is the neurotransmitter that is intimately connected with feelings of satisfaction (antidepressants like Prozac and Zoloft work by basically keeping serotonin hanging around in the brain). If serotonin levels fail to rise, which is what the Hellers hypothesize in this scenario, the carb addict will not feel satisfied and will attempt to satisfy the gnawing hunger by again consuming carbs, which of course will spark another release of insulin, and the cycle will start again. "The repetition of this cycle," say the Hellers, "forms the physical basis of what we call carbohydrate addiction."

Meanwhile, of course, the carb addict will get fatter and fatter.

According to the Hellers, a normal person can eat a carbohydrate-rich meal and be satisfied for four or five hours, whereas carb addicts, with their impaired carbohydrate-insulin-serotonin mechanisms, might feel hungry again in a couple of hours, or even less, and find themselves with a craving for more sweets.

Another premise central to the development of this diet was this: it isn't only the amount of carbs you eat that matters; it is how *frequently* you eat them. (Therein lies the reason that Rachael felt less hungry when she didn't eat until dinnertime on those first few days of experimenting.) The Hellers believe that any weight loss diet that prescribes three or more small meals each day that contain anything more than minor amounts of carbohydrates will ultimately fail with the carbohydrate addict. In the

Hellers' view, hyperinsulinemia (high levels of insulin) is the best explanation for recurring cravings and hunger and the body's tendency to store fat.

In summary, the following applies to the carbohydrate addict:

- For the amount of carbs consumed, too much insulin is produced.
- The constant excess of insulin eventually leads to insulin insensitivity.
- Serotonin (a feel-good brain chemical) does not rise enough to cause the addict to feel satisfied and to produce the signal to stop eating, so the addict continues to eat carb-rich food.
- Production of insulin rises with each subsequent carb intake.
- Greater and greater amounts of carbs may be consumed with no increase in satisfaction.

The Hellers use the addiction model throughout their book. In the patients they have worked with, they identified three levels of addiction, characterized by an escalating need for carbs and sweets as you move up the "ladder." In level one, you are simply interested in eating all the time, craving basically wholesome foods but lots of them; in level 2, there is an increased desire for carbs, especially breads and baked goods; and in level 3, there is a much greater reliance on snacks and sandwiches as staples of the diet, with a high contribution from cakes, candies, potato chips, popcorn, cookies, pies, and the like. This is also accompanied by more and more compulsiveness.

Addiction "triggers" can come from emotional events, day-to-day events, or food. Examples of emotional triggers include unexpressed anger, anxiety, depression, a sense of being out of control, excitement, and frustration. Examples of daily life triggers are stresses of any kind, PMS, illness, or a change in home life. Finally, food triggers are all the things dieters commonly report as deadly and that you would expect to be on a list like this: bread and other grain products, fruit, sweet desserts, snack foods, all kinds of pasta, french fries, and of course sugar.

Carbohydrate addicts have the greatest difficulty controlling their eating when they consume carbohydrates several times a day. According to the Hellers, when the *number* of carb meals (or snacks) is reduced, eating becomes far more controlled and there is a dramatic decrease in cravings. So here's the program they recommend:

- two low-carb meals per day (which they call "complementary" meals)
- one "reward" meal per day

Complementary meals are defined as high in fiber, low in fat, and low in carbs. They are basically made up of protein and vegetables (with no fat added). The protein can be either 3 to 4 ounces of meat, fish, or fowl *or* 2 ounces of cheese. You can have 2 cups of vegetables or salad, but you can't use the vegetables on the "higher-carbohydrate" list. The vegetables on that list have more than 4 grams of carbs per serving, and you *can* eat them, but only at the reward meal. (Some of the vegetables on the Hellers' list don't belong there, such as broccoli, which actually has only about 2 grams of effective carbohydrate* per serving, and avocado, which is not even a vegetable and in any case doesn't contain 4 grams of effective carbohydrate.) Other "high-carb per serving" vegetables not to be eaten during the complementary meals include potatoes and corn.

Reward meals, which happen once a day, usually at dinnertime, are made up of anything you like. Quantities are not limited. There are only three rules.

1. The meal must be equally balanced, in thirds, among protein, vegetables, and starch (or dessert).
2. The meal must be consumed within one hour of starting.
3. You can go back for seconds on this meal, but if you do, you have to eat equal amounts from all three categories.

There is a one-hour time limit for the reward meal because of the Hellers' understanding of what is called the biphasic release of insulin (more about this in Jonny's Lowdown). Insulin is released in two phases (hence the term *biphasic*). The first phase occurs within minutes of consuming carbs: the pancreas releases a fixed amount of insulin regardless of how much carbohydrate is being consumed at the time. The second phase of insulin release—according to the Hellers but to no one else in the field—takes place about seventy-five to ninety minutes after eating and is dependent on how much carbohydrate you actually ate at the meal. If the "initial jolt" of insulin release in phase one wasn't enough to handle the carb load, the second phase shoots out more. Thus, they maintain, you want to consume your entire reward meal within sixty minutes to prevent that "second surge" of insulin production.

---

*To get the "effective" (or "net") carb content of a food, you simply look at the label and subtract the number of grams of fiber from the total number of carbohydrates. What's left is the net amount of carbs, which is all you need to count. For a fuller discussion of effective/net carbs, see page 229.

Alcohol is not prohibited on this diet, but it needs to be consumed as part of the reward meal.

Artificial sweeteners are not permitted, and for a very good theoretical reason: it is hypothesized that insulin release might be subject to conditioned responses, much like salivation was conditioned in Pavlov's dogs, whose mouths watered when they heard a bell that had been rung every time dinner was served. The Hellers put forth the very interesting hypothesis that artificial sweeteners somehow trick the body into releasing insulin, probably because they taste sweet and because the body becomes used to secreting insulin when the taste buds and the brain notice the sweet stuff coming in. In addition, the sweetness keeps the addictive cycle going and keeps you wanting more.

No snacking is allowed between meals (except on a variation called Plan A, which allows one "complementary" snack per day). The Hellers explain that "one piece of fruit eaten other than during the reward meal can reverse the whole metabolic process that is emptying your fat cells. That apple or banana or whatever can be the difference between weight loss and weight gain."

There is a seventeen-item quiz you can take to determine whether this diet is for you. It's called the Carbohydrate Addict's Test, and it is also available in a shortened form (a ten-question "Quick Quiz") on the website. Your score identifies you as having "doubtful addiction," "mild carbohydrate addiction," "moderate carbohydrate addiction," or "severe carbohydrate addiction." The Hellers claim that they have refined the quiz so that it now identifies 87 percent of carb addicts and gives a "false positive" (i.e., mislabels a "normal person" as an addict) only 4 percent of the time. They also point out that their diet was not designed to address the eating patterns or problems of those with "doubtful addiction."

The Carbohydrate Addict's Diet as a Lifestyle: Who It Works for, Who Should Look Elsewhere

This program has a huge following and has helped many people. I suspect that those who score highest on the Carbohydrate Addict's Test are the best candidates for this diet. There are many people for whom the idea of giving up their favorite foods, even if it's not for the rest of their lives and even if it will result in demonstrably improved health and a great deal of weight loss, is simply too great a sacrifice to contemplate. This program has great appeal to people who feel that way and who find enormous comfort in the fact that they're never more than twenty-four hours away from any food they choose to eat. On the other hand, there are many people who are simply too carb-sensitive or sugar-addicted to be able to handle trigger foods in any amount, even if it is only once a day. If this is you, you should look for a more carb-restricted plan.

JONNY'S LOWDOWN ★ ★ ★ ☆ ☆

I have absolutely no doubt that there is such a thing as carbohydrate (and sugar) addiction, but I'm not at all sure that the mechanisms behind it are fully understood. The Hellers are very sincere, very kind people who have helped thousands of people, but the theory behind the program is, depending on where you stand, either really weak or completely false. While it seems pretty clear that there are both insulin and serotonin abnormalities in the obese, it's not at all clear that high levels of insulin depress levels of serotonin, as the Hellers hypothesize—in fact, the majority of the evidence points to the opposite response.

Current thinking is that it works like this: insulin not only removes sugar from the bloodstream, but also removes amino acids (protein). Tryptophan, the building block of serotonin, is a little runt of a molecule that is constantly competing with the other amino acids for "elevator space" into the brain, where it can be converted to serotonin. As Kathleen Des Maisons, Ph.D., author of The Sugar Addict's Total Recovery Program *and an expert on addictive nutrition, colorfully explains, it's as if a bunch of big bodybuilders and a little runty guy are standing around the gym, waiting for the bench press. All of a sudden a really great-looking chick walks into the gym and all the bodybuilders gravitate to her, leaving the bench press empty for the runty guy. Insulin functions in the body like the great-looking chick: it temporarily removes the competition, letting tryptophan get up into the brain.[2] Hence, it is thought that more insulin increases serotonin, not lowers it.*

The Hellers predict that the more insulin you have hanging around, the less serotonin in the brain, giving rise to all those terrible cravings. A recent article in the Journal of Clinical Epidemiology[3] *suggested exactly the opposite. It found that insulin sensitivity (which would mean lower levels of insulin) was positively related to suicide and accident rates—the authors postulated that accidents and suicide are frequently associated with lowered serotonin. In this model, less* insulin goes with less serotonin. The Hellers, remember, postulate the opposite: for them, insulin-resistant (higher levels of insulin) equals less serotonin. Calvin Ezrin, M.D., author of Your Fat Can Make You Thin, explains the mechanism rather well and shows why high levels of insulin lead to higher levels of serotonin, not lower ones.[4]

The two-shot, biphasic theory of insulin release seems to be completely misunderstood by the Hellers. According to Dr. David Leonardi, who lectures worldwide on diabetes and is the medical director of the Leonardi Medical Institute for Vitality and Longevity in Denver, Colorado, insulin is indeed released in two phases, but there is not a seventy-five- to ninety-minute gap between the two. "If you eat a bunch of carbohydrates in fifteen minutes, believe me, you're not going to have to wait sixty minutes to get that second phase of insulin release," he says, raising questions shared by many about the theory behind the one-hour time limit on the reward meal.[5–6]

Finally, I'm not comfortable with the short shrift exercise gets in this program. The Hellers are entirely right that exercise alone is not a great weight loss method, but it's vital to both maintaining weight and to raising metabolic rate.

But sometimes a program works well even if it is not for the reasons its designers believe. The Hellers have come up with something that works for a lot of people, even if they're not 100 percent correct about why.

Books in the Series

The Carbohydrate Addict's Diet

The Carbohydrate Addict's Healthy Heart Program: Break Your Carbo-Insulin Connection to Heart Disease explores the insulin connection to high blood pressure, atherosclerosis, risk-related blood fats, weight gain, insulin resistance, type 2 diabetes, and their link to heart disease.

Carbohydrate-Addicted Kids: Help Your Child or Teen Break Free of Junk Food and Sugar Cravings—for Life! shows how children can beat cravings for sweets and junk food and learn to take control of their weight, their feelings, and their behavior.

The Carbohydrate Addict's Lifespan Program: A Personalized Plan for Becoming Slim, Fit and Healthy in Your 40s, 50s, 60s and Beyond

The Carbohydrate Addict's Program for Success is a workbook for the program.

Healthy for Life: The Scientific Breakthrough Program for Looking, Feeling, and Staying Healthy Without Deprivation is a slow-change weight loss and health-promotion program with slightly less demanding guidelines and a wider variety of food choices than the other programs.

The Carbohydrate Addict's Cookbook details 250 low-carb recipes suitable for all carb-conscious diets.

In addition, the Hellers have a *Carbohydrate Addict's Gram Counter*, *Calorie Counter*, *Fat Counter*, and *Carb Counter.*

Best Book to Start With

Begin with either the original *Carbohydrate Addict's Diet* or the newer *Carbohydrate Addict's Lifespan Program.*

About the Authors

Dr. Rachael Heller has a Ph.D. in psychology and was assistant clinical professor at the Mount Sinai School of Medicine in New York. She was also assistant professor at the Graduate Center of the City University of New York's biomedical sciences program. Dr. Richard Heller has a Ph.D. in research biology and was professor at Mount Sinai School of Medicine and professor emeritus at the Graduate Center of the City of New York's biomedical sciences program. They have been codirectors of the Carbohydrate Addict's Center and Program since 1983.

Website

The official website, www.carbohydrateaddicts.com, is somewhat disappointing in that it appears to exist mainly to sell the Hellers' ever-expanding franchise of books. There is no "Contact Us" link or any other way to get in touch with the Hellers or their center. There is a description of each book, a FAQ section, stories of success, and the Quick Quiz mentioned above. That's about it. You can find a lot of forums and support for followers of this program at other locations (see Resources) but unfortunately not at this site.

THE 7 DAY LOW-CARB RESCUE AND RECOVERY PLAN

RACHAEL HELLER, M.A., M.PH., PH.D.,
AND RICHARD HELLER, M.S., PH.D.

WHAT IT IS IN A NUTSHELL

A six-step plan to get back on track if you've fallen off the low-carb wagon. Alternately, this could be seen as a nonthreatening, step-by-step approach to getting on the Carbohydrate Addict's Diet.

About the 7 Day Low-Carb Rescue and Recovery Plan

The dedication in the book that outlines this plan tells you a lot. It reads: "To all of us who have been told to 'just eat sensibly.'" According to the Hellers, who pioneered their theory in the Carbohydrate Addict's Diet, carbohydrate addicts are like nearsighted people in a farsighted world—the prescriptions that help others just don't apply. And the subtitle of the book reveals its intention: "For every low-carb dieter—on any program—who needs real help right now." That pretty much tells the tale. The 7 Day Low-Carb Rescue and Recovery Plan is about getting back on track.

The book is divided into three sections: the 7 day jump start plan, a section on tips, troubleshooting, and restaurant tactics, and a third section on recipes. The 7 day jump start plan has one purpose: to bring blood sugar and insulin level back into balance so that cravings drop and motivation soars. The Hellers believe you can accomplish this by making a small change each day that builds on the success of the previous day until, almost without trying, you are back in control and on track. Those changes are lovingly detailed in the 7 Day Plan.

The six steps are as follows:

1. Add protein to every meal.
2. Add vegetables and/or salad to lunch, dinner, and snacks.
3. Balance all meals (a la the Zone diet).
4. Eat only low-carb foods for all snacks.

5. Eat only low-carb foods for all snacks and at *one* meal.
6. Eat only low-carb foods for all snacks and at *two* meals.

Of course, if you follow these six steps you will wind up on—you guessed it—the Carbohydrate Addict's Diet!

The Hellers offer "Five Vital Clues Low-Carb Diet Doctors Miss," which is actually pretty thought-provoking, though in my opinion, most of the statements they make are hypothetical at this point. Let's take a look:

1. **Saturated fat can raise insulin**. According to the Hellers, a diet high in saturated fat (and/or trans-fats) is likely to increase your insulin levels (or increase insulin resistance), leading to more cravings and decreased weight loss. I think this statement is pretty controversial and I have not seen any science to support it. And while no one thinks that a diet that's healthy has a ton of saturated fat, I think the movement to have all saturated fat condemned as "unhealthy" and the idea that we should lower it as much as possible is not a wise one. Why not have a diet well balanced between saturated fats (many of which are actually downright good for you), omega-3s from fish and flax, and omega-9s from such foods as olive oil and macadamia nut oil?

2. **Sugar substitutes are carb act-alikes**. This is an interesting statement that is purely speculative, but, I must admit, bears further study. Isn't it possible that—like Pavlov's dogs, who salivated at the sound of a bell because they were conditioned to associate the bell with food—we have a conditioned response to sweet tastes? Maybe we are so conditioned to secrete insulin in response to something sweet that we might—just might—secrete insulin in response to foods that are sweet, even if they have no calories! And some new evidence suggests that the consumption of artificially sweetened foods (and beverages like diet sodas) could disrupt our innate ability to judge the caloric content of food and eat accordingly, leading us to eat more when we're consuming a lot of artificially sweetened stuff. Definitely food for thought. (The Hellers offer a quiz to determine if you are "addicted to diet drinks.") I think this idea actually has a great deal of merit.

3. **Glutamates are also carb act-alikes**. The Hellers point to a study that showed that applying MSG to the tongues of animals causes

them to release high levels of insulin within three minutes (MSG stands for monosodium glutamate, a flavor enhancer that's in a lot of food, including, but not limited to, Chinese food.) But MSG is far from the only glutamate. Food manufacturers add glutamates to a zillion things, including water-packed tuna. It's also frequently one of those innocuous-sounding "natural flavors" you see on labels. The Hellers make the point that glutamates are thought to be excitotoxins, and that if you've ever wondered why you can't stop eating something that tastes good, even when it's low in carbs, this might be the reason.

4. **How often you eat carbs matters.** Not surprisingly for authors who pioneered the concept of a "reward meal," the Hellers are of the belief that it is not just the total number of carbohydrates you eat in a day that makes a difference, but also the frequency with which you eat those higher-carb foods. They believe that when you decrease the number of times in a day that you eat high-carb foods (even if the total intake of high-carb food for the day is the same), you can keep your insulin levels lower and your body in "spending mode" for longer periods of time.

5. **You should eat toward your carbs**. The Hellers believe that the order in which you eat your food matters. If a meal contains a high-carb food—for example, the Reward Meal in their Carbohydrate Addict's Diet plan, or any other meal where you've decided to have a high-carb food—they feel you should eat it last. Their advice is to start the meal with the foods that are lowest in carbohydrates and finish with the foods that are highest. This advice makes sense on the face of it, i.e., you should stay away from the bread that comes before the main course, but it also seems to allow a meal of fish and vegetables to end with chocolate cake. This fifth "clue" is based on the Hellers' belief, which I discussed in my review of the Carbohydrate Addict's Diet—that the second surge of insulin happens about sixty minutes after you begin eating, so if you finish your food within an hour of beginning your meal, you will do less damage. Their thinking is that if you start with protein and low-carb foods like vegetables, you'll be satisfied before you get too enamored of the dessert.

The Hellers also discuss four very good "Carb Myths" (my favorite: "You should have seen what I *didn't* eat"), "troubleshooting," and "restaurant tactics" and include recipes.

The 7 Day Low-Carb Rescue and Recovery Plan as a Lifestyle: Who It Works for, Who Should Look Elsewhere

I'm not 100 percent sure this book was meant to be a lifestyle—after all, the Carbohydrate Addict's Lifespan Program is the Hellers' "rest of your life" plan—but it's excellent for those who want to try a lower-carb way of life without giving up their favorite foods. It's also terrific for devotees of the Carbohydrate Addict's Diet who have "strayed" and want to get back on track. For those who need more structure and whose bodies do well only on specific, measured amounts of net carbs, this plan might be too loosey-goosey.

JONNY'S LOWDOWN ★ ★ ★ ★ ☆

I like this book better than the original. I still have a lot of problems with some of the Hellers' biochemistry, but this book offers some theories—like the one about artificial sweeteners triggering hunger—that I think are both interesting and worth investigating.

I didn't agree with the Hellers about saturated fat in their other books, and I still don't. But I like the step-by-step approach to getting back on track, which can be used even by someone who wants to investigate a lower-carb lifestyle in a less rigorous way. And the tips section is quite good. I was going to give this plan three and a half stars, but I think the low-carb myths and the hypothesis about artificial sweeteners moves this plan into four-star range.

CURVES

GARY HEAVIN AND CAROL COLMAN

WHAT IT IS IN A NUTSHELL

An eating and exercise program targeted to "real women": thirty minutes of exercise three times a week combined with one of two eating plans: low-carb or low-calorie. Both plans have three phases: weight loss, transition, and maintenance.

About Curves

The Curves program was developed for women, and has a very definite sensibility. It targets "real" women, eschews the diet mindset that causes women to bemoan their inability to be a size two, and has the admirable goal of being easy to stick with while at the same time correcting metabolic problems created by a lifetime of dieting. How well does it succeed? As they say, "let's go to the videotape."

Heavin explains that dieting eventually lowers metabolic rate and causes the opposite of the desired effect—by lowering your metabolism you actually activate survival mechanisms, like your body's ability to run on fewer calories, that cause you to hold onto fat. He calls these mechanisms "starvation hormones" (more on that in Jonny's Lowdown). The Curves program promises to correct damaged metabolism, turning your body from a "food-burning machine" into a "champion fat-burning machine," and fixing your "slow metabolism" in the process. Sounds deliciously appealing. And certainly a worthwhile goal.

How does the Curves diet accomplish this metabolic sleight-of-hand? Heavin asserts that the secret of the program's success is that "we address the complicated biological issues that have been conveniently overlooked by conventional diets." This might be news to the other authors discussed in this book, many of whom have presented sophisticated and accurate discussions of the hormonal and biological issues involved in weight loss, but that's another story.

Curves is right on in its desire to "fix" (or, as Diana Schwarzbein would say, "heal") a damaged metabolism. Heavin states, however, that there are some people who have "destroyed" their metabolism through years of low-fat, low-calorie or yo-yo dieting and for these unfortunates, "Metabolic Magic" (his term, not mine) can't happen until they repair their metabolism and restore it to normal. For these people, he offers the "Metabolic Tune-Up," a rather convoluted regimen in which you "eat normally" (2,500 to 3,000 calories!), weigh yourself every day, and try to stay between your "low weight" and your "high weight." You should expect to gain 3 to 5 pounds during this phase. If you gain more, you're to go back to phase one for no more than three days to "burn off the fat." You repeat this cycle until it takes longer and longer to gain those extra 3 to 5 pounds and, consequently, you have fewer and fewer returns to phase one. At this point you can resume your weight-loss diet.

And what is the weight-loss diet? Actually, there are two plans—a low-carb version and a low-calorie version. (The book offers tests to help you determine which plan is right for you.) In the low-carb version, you can eat unlimited amounts of protein but you cut back on starchy and sugary carbohydrates. (The book states that "as long as you are eating the right foods, your caloric intake doesn't matter," which is complete nonsense and exactly the kind of silliness that gives thoughtful lower-carb plans a bad name). The low-calorie version allows you about 1,200 calories a day, but is higher in protein than most conventional low-fat diets. And the book is correct in touting the metabolism-raising properties of protein and disdaining high-glycemic carbs like bagels for just about everyone.

In the low-carb version of the program, there are three phases. Phase one is the strictest part of the program. If you have fewer than 20 pounds to lose, you follow it for a week. If you need to lose more than 20 pounds, you stick with it for two weeks. In phase one, you are limited to 20 grams of carbs a day (exactly like Atkins induction, which the author does not credit). You may eat unlimited amounts of protein (including lean meats, cheeses, eggs, seafood, and poultry), and in addition you are allowed unlimited amounts of Free Foods (which are basically all the greens recommended on Atkins induction). You are also allowed one protein shake a day, which is also counted as a Free Food (for reasons that are not explained), which can contain 20 grams of protein and 20 grams of carbs. During this time, you will probably be in ketosis, which, the author correctly points out, is not at all unhealthy if you don't have a preexisting kidney problem and you drink enough water. This phase, as expected, produces the most weight loss in the shortest time.

In phase two you add more food. You continue to eat an unlimited amount of protein, but you increase your carb intake to between 40 and 60 grams a day, (exactly like Atkins and Protein Power). Unlike those two plans, however, you continue to eat unlimited quantities of Free Foods and that one protein shake a day which, for baffling reasons, doesn't "count." During phase two you should lose 1 to 2 pounds per week. You stay on this phase until you reach your desired weight or until you want a break from dieting.

In phase three you have attained your goal weight and can basically be rid of the "diet." The author—astonishingly—recommends that you go back to a "normal" intake of 2,500 to 3,000 calories a day (!) and suggests that you can stop counting both calories and carbohydrates (more on this in Jonny's Lowdown). The "built-in" safeguard against gaining more weight is much like my 4-pound rule (see page 294 in chapter 8). If you gain more than a few pounds, you go back to phase one until you take it off, then go back to eating "normally."

On the calorie-sensitive version you eat 1,200 calories a day during phase one, and no more than 60 grams of carbohydrates. It's recommended that you get 40 percent of your calories from protein. As with the low-carb plan, you're allowed unlimited Free Foods and the inexplicable free protein shake daily. And in phase two you up the bar to 1,600 calories a day with the same freebies. You're also allowed to ramp up the carb intake to 60 grams (not counting, of course, the Free Foods and the carbs in the protein shake). Much like with the low-carb plan, phase three sets you free, telling you to eat "normally" and only return to phase one if your weight goes up more than 5 pounds or so.

The exercise program is on much more solid ground than the nutritional advice. The Curves workout incorporates strength training, cardiovascular training, and stretching in a simple thirty-minute routine that you do three times a week. Though there are Curves gyms all over the country where exercise leaders take you through the workout, the book provides a pretty darn good at-home version. The only equipment you need is an exercise tube, which is like a rubber rope with two handles, one on each side.

The workout is quite good: after a three-minute abdominal warm-up, you alternate a strength exercise with a cardio interval. There are eight such combinations, and each component is done for forty seconds. For example, you do as many reps of the chest press as you can do in forty seconds; then you do an "aerobic recovery" of forty seconds (this is anything that keeps your heart rate up—jogging in place, for example). You then move on to the second strength exercise (leg extension) and the second aerobic recovery interval. Continue until you've done all eight strength exercises (each followed by its "aerobic recovery") and then do the whole circuit of eight once again. You follow this with a cooldown and a few flexibility exercises and you're done. Thirty minutes out the door. As the British say, "Not too shabby!"

The rest of the book is devoted to meal plans, shopping lists, recipes, and some basic discussion of various health conditions.

Curves as a Lifestyle:
Who It Works for, Who Should Look Elsewhere

The program makes no bones about targeting busy women who want to get healthier and more fit, lose some weight, but not necessarily look like a model (honorable goals for sure!). The studies are pretty clear that thirty minutes of exercise three times a week—no matter how good the workout (and the Curves workout is good)—is probably not enough to make a real dent in your weight, but, in combination with a good eating program, it's certainly a huge step in the right direction. The fact that it is so doable is a tremendous plus, and if you really watch your food, you may get great results. If you're metabolically resistant, the low-carb plan may not be strict enough for you. On the other hand, the flexibility of the program is bound to appeal to many.

JONNY'S LOWDOWN ★ ★ ☆ ☆ ☆

I approached this book wanting to like it. I'd heard great things about Curves, and liked the "real women have curves" ethic of encouraging women to get fit, become happy with their bodies, and lose the aspiration to look like rail-thin models. I also liked what I had heard about the thirty-minute intense circuit-training workouts. And at first glance, the choice between two programs—one a low-carb program and one a "calorie-sensitive" program—sounded interesting.

So I really wanted to like this book. Unfortunately, it was hard to do. This is a textbook example of what happens when a businessperson writes a book on nutrition and fitness. It's so filled with god-awful voodoo nutrition and snake oil salesmanship that by page 23 I was downright angry. Want an example? The author talks about turning on "starvation hormones." I've been working with the top nutritionists and endocrinologists in the field for fifteen years and I've never heard the term "starvation hormones." Wanna know why? 'Cause they don't exist. The author claims that you can return to eating "normally" once you achieve your weight goal, "normally" being defined as 2,500 to 3,000 calories a day. Hello? This statement pretty much belongs in the same category of thinking as the "flat earth" theory. It's utterly ridiculous and very disingenuous. Virtually every study (including the highly respected National Weight Control Registry) has shown that caloric levels for weight maintenance for women are around 1,400 to 1,800 calories. In my experience, most women— members of the women's Olympic volleyball team and Laila Ali being possible exceptions—would get fat eating 3,000 calories a day.

The author also makes a statement right in the beginning that called his "expertise" into question. Here's what he says about other programs, from Atkins to Zone to Weight Watchers. Ready?: "These diets require you to make a lifelong commitment. I don't think this is realistic or fair—a diet should be temporary. It should not become a way of life." Yet if there's a single thing that every diet author agrees on—from those advocating the lowest low-carb to those promoting the lowest low-fat plan—it's that to stay successful you have to make lifestyle changes, and that these lifestyle changes have to be forever. Of course eating differently has to become a way of life. That's what the maintenance phases of all the plans are about. And the irony is that a page or so later, the author says, "The Curves program is designed with the knowledge that you are going to cheat." How can you cheat if there's no program to follow?

The book is not all bad, however. The exercise program is great, and very doable. There's some decent info about protein and cutting junk carbs, though nothing original. I can't get past some of the scientifically silly ideas like eating all the calories you want, or not "counting" certain foods, or advice to go back to "eating normally—2,500 to 3,000 calories a day." But many women have been helped a lot by the Curves philosophy of balance and the way its centers welcome and embrace women of all sizes and get them started on a very decent fitness program. And the idea of metabolic healing—though much better articulated by Dianne Schwarzbein, and with much greater scientific credibility—is a good one.

Books in the Series
Curves: Permanent Results Without Permanent Dieting
Curves on the Go is the companion book, and offers a journal to keep track of nutrition and exercise habits, as well as advice for eating out.

About the Authors

Gary Heavin is a self-taught nutritional counselor and fitness instructor who opened his first gym for women in 1974. He started the Curves franchise in Texas in 1992, and since then it has grown to become one of the largest fitness franchises in the world. Carol Colman has coauthored a number of books on health and medicine.

Website

The official website, www.curvesinternational.com, provides downloadable lists of free foods, the metabolic tune-up, and other basics from the program. It also helps you locate a Curves center near you and provides information if you're interested in purchasing a franchise.

THE FAT FLUSH PLAN

ANN LOUISE GITTLEMAN, M.S., C.N.S.

WHAT IT IS IN A NUTSHELL

A three-phase eating plan designed for both fat loss and detoxification. The idea is both to lose fat and to make your body more efficient at processing it effectively, largely by targeting a sluggish liver, the main organ for detoxification and fat metabolism in the body. The first phase is fairly (though not completely) carbohydrate-restrictive—you can still have two portions of fruit a day and a ton of vegetables—with each subsequent phase adding back more carbohydrates until you reach maintenance.

About the Fat Flush Plan

The Fat Flush Plan started life as a two-week eating program that was originally chapter 16 in Ann Louise Gittleman's pioneering book, *Beyond Pritikin*. Developed and expanded over the years, it eventually became the fully realized diet and lifestyle plan that is the cornerstone of this book.

Fat Flush brings a different spin to low-carb dieting by concentrating on what Gittleman calls the "five hidden weight gain factors": an overworked liver, lack of fat-burning fats, too much insulin, stress, and something that Dr. Elson Haas has called "false fat."

The Liver

In addition to being the main organ for detoxification in the body, the liver is also responsible for fat metabolism. Bile, for example, is made in the liver (and stored in the gallbladder) and is responsible for helping the liver break down fats. But bile can't work efficiently if it doesn't have the proper nutrients that make up the bile salts or if it is congested or thickened with toxins, pollutants, hormones, drugs, and other nasty stuff. Hence, inefficient bile production can slow weight loss.

Another example of how impaired liver function can slow weight loss is "fatty liver," a condition that many overweight people develop. It's not life-threatening, but it's also not something you want to put on your holiday wish list. A very early symptom of possible liver disease frequently seen in alcoholics, it basically means that fat is backed up in the liver like cars on a multilane freeway trying to get through a single toll booth.

Modern life puts a lot of stress on the poor overworked liver. The number of commonly used substances (including medications and even some herbs) that can harm the liver is enormous, and includes Tylenol, some cholesterol-lowering medications, some estrogens used in hormone replacement therapy and birth control pills, alcohol, and a host of other stuff.

Getting the liver in tip-top shape is one goal of the Fat Flush Plan, and that's something that virtually no other diet program addresses. Fat Flush does it by including well-known bile thinners like eggs (high in an amazing liver-supportive substance known as phosphatidylcholine, which also has the ability to break up fats in the bargain) and hot water with lemon juice.

Fat-Burning Fats

Gittleman was a pioneer in debunking the popular '80s notion that a no-fat diet was a good thing (*Eat Fat, Weigh Less*), and she was especially credible because she had been chief nutritionist at the Pritikin Center, which was (and still is) command central for the low-fat contingent. She specifically recommends supplementation with GLA (gamma linolenic acid, a fatty acid found in evening primrose oil, borage oil, and black currant oil) because it stimulates a special kind of fat in the body called *brown adipose tissue,* or BAT. BAT is metabolically active fat that surrounds vital organs and can actually help *burn off* calories.

Excess Insulin

Virtually every low-carb diet plan exists precisely because of the theory that too much insulin is the culprit behind weight gain for a huge number of people. The Fat Flush Plan addresses this with the now-familiar pre-scription of healthy fats, lean proteins, and low-glycemic carbohydrates.

Stress

The connection between stress and fat gain is mediated by excess production of the stress hormone cortisol, is firmly established by research, and is now making its way into the popular consciousness (which you know is happening once it hits the women's magazines), largely due to the pioneering work of Dr. Pamela Peeke. The connection is too lengthy to go into detail here—those interested should check out Dr. Peeke's excellent book, *Fight Fat After Forty*, or read the very good explanation of the stress-fat connection in the Fat Flush Plan. Here's the condensed version: *stress makes you fat*. The Fat Flush Plan addresses stress by offering suggestions on improving sleep, getting moderate exercise, and removing dietary cortisol boosters such as caffeine and sugar.

"False Fat"

People love this term. When I wrote about it for iVillage.com, my article got more hits than almost anything else I had ever written and was featured on the America Online home page. People are fascinated by the notion that they could actually be carrying around something that *feels* like fat, *looks* like fat, but maybe, just *maybe*, isn't *actually* fat at all! The term is the invention of the wonderful integrative physician and author Dr. Elson Haas, who wrote a book about it (*The False Fat Diet*), and Gittleman honorably credits him with the concept, which is central to her discussion of the five hidden weight gain factors.

Here's the deal: food sensitivities can trigger hormonal reactions in the body that lead to both water retention and cravings. Water retention happens because incompletely digested molecules or peptides from the food you're sensitive to enter the bloodstream and are perceived as invaders by the immune system, which then mounts a full-fledged Pac-Man–like attack, releasing histamine and flooding the area with extra fluid. (This extra fluid can be up to 10 to 15 pounds in some people—it's not really fat, but it sure feels like it, and it can easily make the difference between you being able to wear your "skinny clothes" and having to wear your "fat jeans.")

During this immune system response, the body also overproduces the hormones cortisol and aldosterone, which in turn increase sodium retention, attracting even more water to the cells and tissues. This whole immune cascade will cause you to release endorphins (natural "feel-good" opiates), which can, over time, easily give rise to a feeling that you're addicted to the very foods you're sensitive to. (Think of sugar, wheat, flour, and the like. Ever notice how no one ever says they're addicted to Brussels sprouts?) Finally, your levels of serotonin—the feel-good neurotransmitter—drop when the immune system goes into full alert, because the same white blood cells that carry serotonin are now too busy fighting off the invaders to bother with serotonin. Lower levels of serotonin almost always lead to increased cravings for high-carbohydrate foods, which in turn spikes your blood sugar, leading to a vicious circle of higher levels of insulin and more fat storage. Get it?

The Fat Flush Plan relies heavily on daily intakes of "cran-water," a mixture of unsweetened cranberry juice (not the "cocktail" stuff commonly found in supermarkets) and water. The juice contains arbutin, an active ingredient in cranberries that is a natural diuretic (as is the lemon in the hot water and lemon juice mix). The Fat Flush Plan also deals with the "false fat" issue by restricting the "usual suspect" foods that are likely to trigger food sensitivities: wheat, dairy, and sugar.

Phase one of the plan is about 1,100 to 1,200 calories (this is one of the few low-carb plans in which the author actually mentions the caloric intake) and is designed to jump-start weight loss. It's also meant to be a good cleansing program that supports the liver. You stay on it for two weeks; if you've got more than 25 pounds to lose, you can stick with it for a month, though it might get pretty boring.

In phase one, you avoid:

- hot spices (because of possible water retention)
- oils and fats (other than daily flaxseed oil and GLA supplementation)
- all grains
- all starchy vegetables (potatoes, corn, peas, carrots, beans, etc.)
- all dairy
- alcohol and coffee (you are allowed one cup of organic coffee in the morning)

Other than that, the diet is flexible. No counting carb grams, figuring out protein minimums, or counting calories. You eat:

- up to 8 ounces a day of almost any kind of protein
- *in addition*, up to two eggs a day
- one serving of whey protein powder (not in the book, but later added to the phase one food list on the website)
- unlimited amounts of almost any vegetable but the starchy ones (which get put back in during the next phase)
- up to two portions of fruit per day

You can sweeten with stevia (xylitol wasn't widely available when Fat Flush first came out, but I'm willing to bet that xylitol would be acceptable). Each day, you have a fiber supplement, a GLA supplement, flaxseed oil, and the cran-water mixture.

Phase two is for ongoing weight loss and ups the calories to between 1,200 and 1,500. You stay on phase two until you're at or near your goal weight. The main difference between phase one and phase two is that during phase two, you slowly add back some carbohydrates from the "friendly carb" list—one serving per day for the first week and two servings per day for the second week and beyond. The cran-water drink gets replaced with pure water, and most everything else stays the same.

Phase three is 1,500 (or more) calories per day and is designed for ongoing maintenance. There are more liberal choices in the oil and fruit categories, and you can now add dairy products as well as choose from a bigger list of "friendly carbs," working up to four servings a day. Most everything else remains the same—there are some minor changes in supplementation that are discussed.

The book also has sections on exercise (greatly expanded in the *Fat Flush Fitness Plan*), journaling, stress reduction, recipes, resources, and great FAQ.

The Fat Flush Plan as a Lifestyle: Who It Works for, Who Should Look Elsewhere

This is such an all-around sensible plan that it's hard to see how anyone wouldn't benefit from it. Within certain parameters (like the carb restriction and the prohibition on sugar), it's very flexible, and it's one of the few lower-carb plans where you can eat fruit right from the beginning. Gittleman seems to have a particular gift for writing for women, who appear to constitute the majority of her audience. Men do well on this plan, too, but need to make some adjustments. According to Gittleman, they should do phase one as is, but can usually jump to phase three so they can take in more carbohydrates right away. They also generally should increase the portion sizes of their protein and can double up on the whey protein powder.

People who need a lot of structure might find this plan too free-wheeling for their tastes, and the maintenance plan allows more carbs than some people might feel comfortable with. In addition, if you suspect you have a carbohydrate addiction, the amount of carbs allowed on the maintenance phase could conceivably trigger binges.

JONNY'S LOWDOWN ★ ★ ★ ★ ★

This is one of the half-dozen best low-carb approaches to health around. I have minor quibbles, emphasis on minor: there is a lot of talk about cellulite and how the plan can reduce it, which I think is highly speculative, as is the section on food combining. I'd like to have seen alpha lipoic acid mentioned as an important supplement for liver health. In my opinion, there is disproportionate emphasis on flaxseed oil and not enough on fish oil, which provides equally important omega-3s that are harder for the body to make on its own. But with that said, the basic template—limited starch, some fruit, unlimited vegetables, lean protein, and high-quality fats—is a great program and would benefit anyone. The phenomenal success and public acceptance of this program is well-deserved.

Books in the Series

The Fat Flush Plan: The Breakthrough Weight-Loss System That Melts Fat from Hips, Waist, and Thighs in Just Two Weeks and Reshapes Your Body While Detoxifying Your System

The Fat Flush Journal and Shopping Guide Journaling is a big part of this program. If you don't want to make your own journal, this one has it all laid out for you and comes with shopping lists.

The Fat Flush Cookbook is exactly what it says it is!

The Complete Fat Flush Program is a bundled package of *The Fat Flush Plan, Journal,* and *Cookbook.*

The Fat Flush Fitness Plan (with Joanie Greggains) is a very expanded version of the fitness program that was sketched out in *The Fat Flush Plan,* with lots of new information and a recap of how to use the fitness plan in conjunction with the original book. The fitness routines were designed by Greggains, a well-known fitness expert, author, and radio show host who has used the Fat Flush Plan with clients for years.

Best Book to Start With

The Fat Flush Plan

About the Author

Ann Louise Gittleman is the much-loved "First Lady of Nutrition" and has a dozen books to her credit, including *Beyond Pritikin*; *Eat Fat, Lose Weight*; *Your Body Knows Best*; and the *New York Times* best-seller *Before the Change*. Her advice to women on weight management is prominently featured on iVillage.com, and she has been featured in dozens of national magazines and appeared on as many television and radio shows, including a series of appearances on *The View* and a recent appearance on *Dr. Phil*. Gittleman holds a master's degree in nutrition education from Columbia University and the highly regarded credential of certified nutrition specialist from the American College of Nutrition. She was the nutrition director at the Pritikin Center.

Website

The official website, fatflush.com, features a great overview of the plan, an archive of articles, a store, and a "Fat Flush Forum," where you can post to moderated bulletin boards and get answers to your questions.

THE GO-DIET:
THE GOLDBERG-O'MARA DIET PLAN

JACK GOLDBERG, PH.D., AND KAREN O'MARA, D.O.

WHAT IT IS IN A NUTSHELL

Very low in carbs, high in fiber, and very high in monounsaturated fats. There is no counting of calories ever. Only carbohydrates, satu-rated fat, and fiber are measured. Daily total intake of carbs is 50 grams net carbohydrates, with no more than 12 to 15 grams eaten at any given meal (see more about net carbs in "About the GO-Diet," below). Other than this limitation on carb grams, you can eat as much as you like. There is a daily portion of yogurt, buttermilk, or kefir.

About the GO-Diet

The G in GO is Jack Goldberg, Ph.D., a clinical biochemist and researcher, and the O is Karen O'Mara, a board-certified specialist in internal medi-cine. They developed this program originally to deal with their own weight problems (as did a number of the authors discussed in this book). They mince no words in describing their target market: "Remember," they say early on, "the weight loss part of this diet is meant for fatties." It's a weight loss diet for people who have a BMI (body mass index) of greater than 25. (You can easily calculate your BMI on any of a dozen calculators available on the Internet—it takes about five seconds. See Resources for a reliable Web address, or type the words *body mass index* into a search engine.) The World Health Organization considers BMIs of up to 25 desirable, 25 to 29.9 as overweight, and 30 or greater as clinically obese.

The GO-Diet plan is short, sweet, and to the point. The authors spend a few pages reviewing the traditional methods of weight loss and discuss, very briefly, why these have not been successful. They air a dirty little secret that no one likes to hear: exercise, as beneficial as it is for health and as demonstrably important as it is for the *maintenance* of weight loss, is *not* a terribly effective way to *lose* weight if you don't accompany it with dietary overhaul. Restricting calories will produce weight loss, but the weight is usually regained. Even restricting carbohydrates—which this plan advocates—can be a problem because, according to Goldberg and O'Mara, it could lead to excess protein consumption, which is potentially harmful for people with liver and kidney problems (true, but what percentage of the population is that?), or it could lead to excess fat intake, which they claim can be harmful to people who are "fat sensitive" (up to 30 percent of the population, according to the authors). That they do not describe what they mean by "fat sensitive" or give any supporting data for that claim is one of my few criticisms of the book.

Goldberg and O'Mara lay the blame for our increasing fatness on two substances: sugar and saturated fat. One problem is our attraction to prepackaged, processed foods and their overabundant carbohydrate (in particular sugar) content. Sugar consumption, they say "both artificially added granulated sugar and corn syrup and 'naturally' enhanced sugars in our foods, is one of the major problems affecting weight gain." Right on. And it's nice that they mention the fact that even those who eat only fruits as sweets are not exempt from the sugar problem. Fruits today are definitely not the same fruits our ancestors ate. Our fruits have been bred and engineered for far more sweetness than the bitter little things that our Paleolithic ancestors gathered. And agribusiness, modern transportation, and processing have made these sweet fruits available year-round, not just during their traditional seasons. Add to this the high consumption of saturated fats *in the presence of high carbohydrates* (which is typical of the American diet), and you've set the stage for an array of health problems.

So what is the actual GO-Diet?

Number one: *it's very low-carbohydrate*. Drs. G and O use the now-standard way of identifying carbs as "net," or "effective." (To get the net or effective carb content of a food, you simply look at the label and subtract the number of grams of fiber from the total number of carbohydrates. What's left is the net amount of carbs, which is all you need to count.) The GO-Diet allows a total daily intake of 50 grams of net carbohydrate, with no more than 12 to 15 grams taken in at a meal. You *will* need to count the carbohydrates in all the foods that you eat. There are plenty of carb counters available (many of the diet authors in this book sell them), and some are already keyed for net, or effective, carbs (e.g., Protein Power and Atkins).

Number two: *it's very high in monounsaturated fat*. Fifty percent of your fat on this diet comes from monounsaturated fats, which include most nuts, seeds, olive oil, olives, and avocados. Lots of meats, like lean chicken and beef, already have close to 50 percent of their fat as monounsaturated.

Number three: *it has at least 25 grams of fiber a day* (more on how to incorporate that into your diet later).

Here's how the diet works.

Phase one, the first three days, is considered a transition. For most people, this will be a transition from the fat-free, high-carb lifestyle to one in which, as Drs. G and O say, "you can lose some serious weight." The purpose of the first three days is to concentrate on one goal and one goal only: *to get the carbohydrates out of your eating pattern.* Your goal is to force your body to switch from being mainly a sugar-burning engine to one that primarily uses fat for fuel. You can eat as much food as you like (within the limit of 12 to 15 grams of net carbohydrate per meal and the 50 grams of total net carbs per day). You eat three meals, and you snack whenever you feel like it. The allowed-foods list for the first three days consists of meat, fish, eggs, most nuts and seeds, certain dairy products (including certain cheeses), and many vegetables.

Phase two, days four through seven, has a different goal: *promoting the intake of high levels of monounsaturated fats and shifting the balance of your fat intake away from saturated fats.* There is an appendix in *The GO-Diet* that lists the net carb content and the percentage of monounsaturated fat in about seventy-five different foods. When foods are low in monounsaturated fats, you just make up for it by adding more avocados, nuts, and olive oil.

Phase three is the rest of your life. Now you start concentrating on adding fiber and nutrients. The fiber comes not in the form of grain products like cereals (unless you want to use them as part of your 12- to 15-gram net carb per meal allowance, which will result in awfully small portions), but in the form of actual bran—wheat bran, oat bran, and, if you can find it, corn bran. Ground flaxseeds are also great. You can also use psyllium husks in cooking as a thickening agent or as a binder for meatballs and meatloaf. And there are actually a couple of very high-fiber commercial cereals that could be eaten as well (All-Bran and Fiber One come to mind). Your goal is to get 25 grams of fiber a day. (Most Americans get less than 10. Our Paleo ancestors probably got around 60. You do the math.)

One unique feature of the diet is the emphasis on *fermented milk products.* Drs. G and O are rightly concerned about yeast, which is hardly mentioned in some of the other programs, and feel it is very important to restore healthy bacteria to the gut by using cultured milk products like kefir, yogurt, and buttermilk. Even lactose-intolerant folks can usually tolerate them. These fermented products are high in "good" bacteria called *lactobacillus*. In addition to being extremely "gut-healthy," lactobacillus may also stimulate the immune system.

In the case of the fermented milk products—again, kefir, yogurt, and buttermilk—you do *not* count the carbohydrate content on the label. This is now fairly well accepted on the Internet support boards for low-carb dieters, even those not following the GO-Diet, and the explanation for it is credited to Drs. Goldberg and O'Mara. For those who are interested: the government standards for calculating "carbohydrate" content involve *measuring everything else that's in the food* (including water, ash, fats, and proteins) and then assuming that the rest is carbs. That's usually true. But to make fermented milk products, bacteria are implanted in the milk; these bacteria basically eat up all the carbohydrate milk sugar (lactose) and convert it into something called lactic acid, which is what curdles the milk and gives it its unique "fermented" taste. The process the government established counts the lactic acid as carbohydrate, but it's really not. Goldberg himself did the measurements in his lab and concluded that ½ cup of plain buttermilk, yogurt, or kefir yields only 2 grams of carbohydrate; 1 cup counts as 4 grams. The GO-Diet recommends at least 8 ounces of kefir, yogurt, or buttermilk per day. (The diet does *not* allow you to drink regular milk.)

Add to the above recommendations *at least* five servings of assorted vegetables a day, and you have the complete program. Among the excluded foods are milk, potatoes, sweet potatoes, beets, turnips, rice, corn, peas, beans (except green, wax, and pole), lentils, pasta, breads, bagels, cookies, cakes, most crackers, pretzels, and rice cakes.

The book contains a very good explanation of ketosis and an excellent debunking of the arguments against it. However, Drs. G and O don't recommend the use of ketone test strips (the usual home method of measuring whether the body is in ketosis). Goldberg and O'Mara point out that the strips—which are briefly dipped in a stream of urine—detect only two of the three main ketone bodies; the two that they do detect together produce only about a fifth of the total ketones produced. Because the third main ketone body (beta-hydroxybutyric acid, for those who care) is not detected by the strips, the strips may never turn color for some people, yet if you checked their blood levels, there would be plenty of ketones. Drs. G and O say they have seen lots of people test positive for urinary ketones who don't lose weight, as well as many people who are negative for ketones in the urine but drop weight like crazy. They advise their patients to save their money (the strips ain't cheap).

Drs. Goldberg and O'Mara did a preliminary twelve-week research study on their diet at a hospital in Chicago and found that the weight loss for the twenty-four subjects who completed the study ranged from a low of 4 pounds to a high of 45 pounds, with an average of about 20 pounds. That's not enormous, but it ain't bad, especially since you can eat an awful lot of delicious stuff on this program. Interestingly, calorie intake did not affect the results. True, the subject who lost the most weight ate an average of 1,200 calories a day, but the runner-up ate 2,600! And there was an average loss of 5 inches at the waist. Most frequently cited benefits by the participants were no bloating after a meal, better digestion, reduced use of antacids, abundant energy, fewer vague aches and pains, and a reduction of the role of food as central to their lives.

The GO-Diet as a Lifestyle: Who It Works for, Who Should Look Elsewhere

I think there's a big potential audience for this diet. A lot of people, despite very persuasive arguments to the contrary, still believe that fat, especially saturated fat, is deadly. This program avoids the controversy, advocating a generous intake of fat but from a source that just about everyone agrees is heart-healthy: monounsaturates. This diet should also appeal to people who don't want to count calories or limit food intake. And since it is so low in sugar, it should work well for sugar- or carb-addicted people.

But people who don't want to have to count *anything*—including carbohydrate grams and fat percentages—will probably not be happy with this program. It's also not a particularly fast way to lose weight.

JONNY'S LOWDOWN ★ ★ ★ ★ ☆

This is a great program. I think it's smart, edgy, and extremely healthy. Finding it was one of the pleasures of researching this book, as it is not nearly as well known as most of the other plans discussed. The authors are remarkably down-to-earth and refreshingly lacking in hype. The GO-Diet gets high points for the emphasis on fiber, which you don't see in a lot of programs, and for the inclusion of a source of "good" bacteria (the kefir, yogurt, or buttermilk). While I personally believe that saturated fats are not nearly as damaging as we have been led to believe—especially when they come from natural sources, are not "averaged in" with trans-fats, and are not accompanied by a huge load of sugar and carbohydrates—no one can fault the doctors for playing it safe with their emphasis on monounsaturated fats.

My only comment about the ease of this program has to do with the calculation of fat intake. I think trying to do the program literally, getting exactly 50 percent of your fat from monounsaturates, would be ridiculously cumbersome and difficult, though trying to approximate it by concentrating on high monounsaturated foods is certainly feasible—just don't get too obsessive about the numbers. And I would have liked to see a little more emphasis on omega-3s like fish and fish oils as well as exercise.

Books in the Series
The GO-Diet: The Goldberg-O'Mara Diet Plan
There is an audiotape available on the website.

About the Authors
Karen O'Mara, D.O., is a board-certified specialist in internal medicine and critical care who has been interested in nutrition and the effects of diet on health and illness for twenty years. Jack Goldberg, Ph.D., is a clinical biochemist and research scientist who discovered and patented the first commercial kit to test HDL cholesterol.

Website
The official website, www.go-diet.com, is exactly like the program—gentle, supportive, interactive, nurturing, friendly, and decidedly noncommercial. There's great information and practically nothing for sale except the book and an audiotape. The entire diet chapter from Goldberg and O'Mara's book is there, with permission to print and copy it in its entirety, as is a recipe section, info for type 2 diabetics from a paper published by the authors, a FAQ page, and a link to a support group and forum. There is also a very good BMI calculator. The site is so noncommercial that there is even a place where you can send a donation to support the site if you feel it has helped you.

The GO-Diet also has a support forum at http://clubs.yahoo.com/clubs/godiet.

THE HAMPTONS DIET

FRED PESCATORE, M.D.

WHAT IT IS IN A NUTSHELL

A lower-carb plan that's a twist on the Mediterranean diet: high in vegetables, fish, nuts, and omega-3 fats but favoring macadamia nut oil instead of olive oil. You choose from three plans—A, B, or C— depending on how much weight you would like to lose. Each plan has slightly different amounts of carbohydrate. All plans stress lean protein, nuts, vegetables, fish, and—you guessed it—macadamia nut oil.

About the Hamptons Diet

The Hamptons Diet starts with the premise that the low-fat, low-cholesterol message of the past couple of decades was—if not wholly wrong—terribly miscommunicated. No disagreement there: fat phobia gave rise to the ridiculous notion that we could consume as many fat-free foods as we wanted. By now practically everyone realizes that this silly philosophy led us into our current predicament: near-epidemic levels of obesity and diabetes. The low-fat, high-carb diet, particularly as practiced by people using tons of processed high-glycemic foods, produces increased levels of triglycerides, which increase the risk for coronary heart disease. And high-glycemic diets have been linked with diabetes and with several kinds of cancers.

So far, so good. Dr. Pescatore points to the fact that the American Heart Association diet—which recommends limiting total dietary fat to less than 30 percent of the diet and saturated fat to less than 10 percent— fails to lower triglycerides and actually lowers HDL (good cholesterol). In addition, the AHA diet has never consistently shown long-term improvement in any heart disease outcome. The original low-fat advice was also predicated on the simplistic idea that blood cholesterol was the whole picture when it came to cardiac risk. We now know that there are a host of measures that are far better predictors of heart disease than total cholesterol. These include triglycerides, HDL (good) cholesterol, LDL particle size, inflammatory markers like C-reactive protein, homocysteine, blood pressure, lipoprotein(a), and others, many of which respond quite poorly to a high-carb diet, particularly one high in sugars. And, as Dr. Walter

Willet recently proclaimed, research has shown that the percentage of fat in the diet—contrary to the advice of the last two decades—has shown absolutely no relationship to any major health outcome.

So why worry about fat at all? Having been the associate medical director of the Atkins Center for many years, Dr. Pescatore understands well that the demonization of all fat was a ridiculous idea. But rather than taking a stand for the wholehearted repeal of fat-phobia, the Hamptons Diet takes a more cautious approach. The author points to the benefits of the Mediterranean diet, an eating regimen that has long been touted as healthy by many nutritionists. This diet is high in fish, nuts, lean proteins, vegetables, and especially monounsaturated fat. The classic Mediterranean diet "does not regard all fat as bad," and, in fact, doesn't limit fat consumption at all. It does, however, specify which fats to eat and which to avoid (more on this in a moment).The primary monounsaturated fat in the Mediterranean diet is olive oil, which even fat phobics have conceded is a "heart-healthy" fat.

Dr. Pescatore has found an oil he feels is even better for you than olive oil, and this is the gimmick of the Hamptons Diet. Dr. Pescatore replaces olive oil with macadamia nut oil, an oil he claims has miraculous benefits for several reasons. First, you can use it in both hot and cold recipes. Second, it has a perfect ratio of omega-6 to omega-3 fatty acids (1:1). Third, it has a higher concentration of the healthy monounsaturates (omega-9 fats) than olive oil. And fourth, it has a high smoke point, which decreases the risk of trans-fatty acid formation. Dr. Pescatore's company, MacNut Oil, imports the macadamia nut oil he recommends in his resource section. That's not necessarily a bad thing—macadamia nut oil *is* a good food, and many of us sell products that we truly believe in and use ourselves—but it's worth disclosing.

There are six basic tenets of the Hamptons Diet:

1. Eat fish that is rich in omega-3 fats (for example, sardines, mackerel, salmon).
2. Eat nuts.
3. Do not eat trans-fats.
4. Do eat "healthful" fats (stay tuned). The author states: "In the Hamptons Diet, we use the most healthful oil—macadamia nut—and in the pure Mediterranean diet, olive oil is used.")
5. Consume ample quantities of vegetables and some fruits.
6. Consume moderate amounts of alcohol.

There are also three levels, or programs, somewhat cutely labeled the "A List," the "B List," and the "C List" in an amusing takeoff on the social stratification that is de rigueur in the diet's namesake hometown. The A program is for people who have more than 10 pounds to lose, and limits carb intake to 30 grams a day. There is also a long, detailed suggested list of A List–appropriate proteins, vegetables, fruits, spices, nuts, and nut butters. The B List is a transitional program for people who have fewer than 10 pounds to lose and are on their way to maintenance (the C List). On the B program, you consume between 40 and 60 grams of carbs (less for women), and can choose from another eight protein sources and an additional three dozen veggies. You can also now add some whole grains and fruits. And on the C program, which is for maintenance, you have an even wider range of grains and fruits to choose from, as the daily carb content goes up to 55 to 65 grams for women and 65 to 85 grams for men.

So why all the fuss about macadamia nut oil? Well, like olive oil, it contains an omega-9 fatty acid called oleic acid. Oleic acid, according to Dr. Pescatore, increases the incorporation of omega-3 fatty acids into the cell membrane, which is a good thing. He postulates that this might decrease the incidence of breast cancer, though he doesn't tell us how. We do know, however, that oleic acid has been shown to decrease total and LDL (bad) cholesterol, but, perhaps more important, it also lowers triglycerides and raises HDL (good) cholesterol. Dr. Pescatore takes the position that since we know that olive oil does these things, and since macadamia nut oil has even more of the active ingredient (omega-9 oleic acid) than olive oil does, it stands to reason that the cardiac and perhaps anticancer benefits might be even more pronounced in the Hamptons Diet than in the classic Mediterranean diet.

The Hamptons Diet, to its credit, does say that "some saturated fats are OK" and recommends, for example, eggs as a good source of "lean protein." Also to its credit, it makes the point that we need to eat much less of those omega-6 fats we were told were healthy in the days when low-fat was king—the polyunsaturated oils like grapeseed, corn, safflower, sunflower, soybean, and cottonseed. Kudos to Pescatore for making this point, often missed in other programs. I couldn't agree more.

The Hamptons Diet as a Lifestyle: Who It Works for, Who Should Look Elsewhere

This is a perfectly fine program for most people, though I suspect it's going to appeal more to people who have less than 20 pounds to lose. Its recipes and food lists are not for those on a strict budget—reading the menus makes me think of four-star restaurants and red velvet ropes. And it is clearly meant to be marketed to those who see themselves as part of the glamorous set, though that's more a statement about the marketing and the title. If you can afford the food and the exotic recipes appeal to you, and if you don't have a ton of weight to lose, go for it. Those who prefer a little more basic stuff or a little more structure might be put off.

JONNY'S LOWDOWN ★ ★ ★ ★ ★

Full disclosure: I like Fred Pescatore. He's a good guy. He means very well, he's knowledgeable, and, as medical director of the Atkins Center, he did a great deal of good by showing how to apply the principles of the Atkins approach to the treatment of children (his Feed Your Kids Well *remains my favorite book on children and diet). And it's hard to fault this program. The book has a definitive section on oils, is on the money on the issue of trans-fats, urges organic foods, and limits processed junk. What's not to like?*

The Hamptons Diet is clearly Dr. Pescatore's attempt to brand himself as an entity separate from his mentor Robert Atkins. I can understand this. My only real criticism of the Hamptons Diet is a personal one—I wish he had taken a stronger stand against those who deem all saturated fats the enemy. I guess I hold him to a higher standard than say, Dr. Agatston of South Beach fame. Unlike Agatston, Dr. Pescatore is a nutritionist, and a very good one at that; he has to know that if you followed all the principles in his book and still consumed saturated fats from healthy sources (a la Atkins for Life) you would be just fine. My guess is that he opted for a program that is more acceptable to the masses, who still believe that saturated fat is the worst thing you can eat.

The book is chock full of great recipes, the information is on track, the information on oils is outstanding, and the supplement program is well thought out.

About the Author

Fred Pescatore, M.D., is head of Partners in Integrative Medicine in New York. Previously, he was Associate Medical Director of the Atkins Center. Dr. Pescatore lectures across America and is actively involved in clinical research. He has written numerous papers and magazine articles in addition to three other books: *The Allergy and Asthma Cure, Thin for Good,* and *Feed Your Kids Well.* He is the president-elect of the International and American Association of Clinical Nutritionists and lives and works in New York, Dallas, and East Hampton.

Website

The site—www.hamptonsdiet.com—has feature articles on the Hamptons Diet, books by Dr. Pescatore, a basic how-to page for newbies, and a list of reasons that the authors feel the Hamptons Diet is superior to other programs. You can also subscribe to the newsletter. The official site for the company that imports Australian macadamia nut oil is www.macnutoil.com, and it's a good place to learn about (and purchase) this food, which can, truth be told, be used on a wide variety of low-carb plans, including Atkins.

THE LINDORA PROGRAM: LEAN FOR LIFE

CYNTHIA STAMPER GRAFF

WHAT IT IS IN A NUTSHELL

A six-week holistic weight loss program with a big emphasis on self-help, motivation, behavioral remodeling, and journaling. The first four weeks are for weight loss (calories and carbs are limited); the next two weeks are a period of "metabolic adjustment." You repeat the cycle until you reach your goal weight. After that, you go on the maintenance ("Lindora for Life") program.

About the Lindora Program

The Lindora program was started in 1971 by Dr. Marshall Stamper. The plan as detailed in the book *Lean for Life* is basically a do-it-yourself version of the program offered in the twenty-nine Lindora Medical Clinics in southern California. It's a very structured program with a tremendous self-help component. The emphasis is on retraining behaviors and on reconditioning how you think about food, weight, and goals in general. That's really the strong point of the program.

The diet part is as follows: days one through three are "prep days." The diet on the prep days looks like something you might find in virtually any woman's magazine at the supermarket. Sample instruction: "Your meals should include a protein, a salad with dressing, a potato or other starch, vegetables, fresh fruit, and milk." The plan does, however, emphasize protein-based snacks like cheese, nuts, and seeds. The idea is to use the prep period to gradually transition into the weight loss diet that's coming up for the next twenty-eight days. During the prep days, you can also have "craving-based foods" like pizza, and you're encouraged to use this period to satisfy any nagging cravings you may have before jumping in to the diet proper. During these three days, you also gather the stuff you're going to need for the next four weeks: ketone strips, a food scale, measuring cups, a weight scale, and so on. You also weigh and measure yourself and write down the results, and you do some mind-body visualization exercises.

After the initial prep days, it's time to start the four-week weight loss phase of the cycle. You begin with a "protein day." Actually, the first day of *every* week is a protein day, even in the maintenance phase. On the protein day, you have at least six protein servings and keep your carb intake in the range of 50 to 100 grams a day, or whatever it takes to get into ketosis (100 is most likely too high for the vast majority of people, and even 50 may be too high for some). You use the ketone sticks to monitor this. The "approved" protein choices are all pretty much low-fat selections (e.g., skim milk, low-fat cottage cheese, fat-free cold cuts, water-packed tuna). You can also choose from a million different Lean for Life products that the company sells and/or pick from a list of acceptable grocery store choices.

After completing the initial protein day, you go on to the weight loss plan for the rest of the week, then repeat that seven-day cycle for four weeks (one protein day, six "weight loss menu" days). The weight loss part of the week means three meals and three protein snacks a day, but you are still aiming for both ketosis and the reduction of cravings (by cutting out foods that tend to trigger them).

The basic weight loss menu consists of the following:

- protein six times a day (at all three meals plus three snacks)
- three fruits a day (or two fruits and one grain)
- two servings of vegetables a day

You can have fat-free salad dressing, any calorie-free beverage (including diet sodas and the like), powdered creamer for your coffee, and various spices.

After every twenty-eight-day weight loss module, you go on to a two-week "metabolic adjustment." The purpose of this period is to *gradually* increase the amount of food you eat and let your body's metabolism adjust to that increased amount without experiencing weight gain. The stated purpose of the metabolic adjustment is not to lose weight but to reset your body's thermostat to deal with the additional calories. (There's no science whatsoever to back this up.) The author reports that people resist this phase like crazy. Those who are losing want to keep losing and don't want to change what's working for them. Those who have arrived at their goal think they've crossed the finish line. But the Lindora folks claim that this period is absolutely necessary, because your body has learned, during the first twenty-eight days, to live on a lower number of calories. What you want to do now is "teach" your body to adapt to more food without actually storing fat. During this two-week metabolic adjustment, the first day of each week is still a protein-only day, but it's for focus, discipline, and of course weight control. You're not in ketosis during this fourteen-day period. The food choices are the same as they were during the first four weeks, but the portions are different, and on day eight you can add one more grain serving. Anytime you have a weight gain of 1½ pounds or more, you have a protein-only meal that evening. You keep repeating this until you're back on target, and you don't move on to the next level of food addition until your weight is back on track.

Once you're done with however many six-week cycles it takes you to get to your goal weight, you're ready for phase two, the Maintenance for Life program, which is a whole other book. Basically, the program continues to stress low-fat (what they call "lean foods") and higher protein. The lifelong daily maintenance menu is this:

- six protein servings a day (one at each meal and each snack)
- two vegetable servings a day
- three grain servings a day ("don't forget to choose low-fat crackers," the book exclaims!)
- three servings of fruit a day
- three servings of fat a day

The program tries to be all things to all people—it makes a valiant attempt at being both low-carb *and* politically correct, and tries not to offend anyone in the dietary pantheon. According to the book, during the weight loss phase you follow a "low-calorie, low-carbohydrate, low-fat, moderate-protein-structured eating plan."

The book has a section on "nine easy ways to reduce your fat intake" that could have been lifted from the pages of any popular magazine of the '80s. In truth, the entire sensibility of the book is that of a standard low-fat diet but with elevated protein intake. (All of the acceptable protein choices are low-fat.) Interestingly, on the list of "avoids" is hydrogenated fats "such as coffee creamers" (evidently they forgot that coffee creamers were on the *allowed* list a few pages earlier). Naturally, there is complete adherence to the politically correct mandate against animal fats of any kind. There's some very old-fashioned advice (such as limiting eggs if your cholesterol is high), and the list of approved cereals includes glycemic nightmares like Corn Flakes and Special K. Of course, there is not a word about aspartame or the controversy around artificial sweeteners.

At the same time, the program is edgy enough to take a stand on the subject of ketosis, which the program makes good use of. The author argues that people who experience the benign ketosis of the weight loss portion of the program lose weight more quickly than they would on traditional diets (undoubtedly true), which in turn increases their motivation to stick with the program until they achieve their goal (sure makes sense to me). Participants experience reduced hunger and fewer cravings, a very common effect on ketogenic diets. The book offers a short but accurate couple of paragraphs on why ketosis is perfectly safe, then lists the three situations in which one would not use a ketogenic diet (for a full explanation of ketosis, see chapter 5).

The Lindora folks recommend vitamin and mineral supplements (they sell their own, which is no surprise), essential fatty acids, potassium, and calcium—though they are way behind the curve on this one, failing to mention the importance of bone-supporting minerals like magnesium, manganese, and boron and vitamins like vitamin D, not to mention weight training!

Their recommendations on exercise are limited to walking. Most exercise specialists now feel that weight loss will not be achieved with walking alone, and nearly all recommend weight training as part of any program. Weight training is not discussed at all in this book.

The best part of the Lindora program is *not* the eating plan. It's what the book has to say about motivation, behavior modification, and self-help.

Journaling is essential to the Lindora program. Your journal is your "daily action plan." Every day there is a specific "mind-body" item that you focus on: it could be "recognizing rationalization," "the self-sabotage shuffle," "turning obstacles into opportunities," "values and vision," "visualizations," "affirming the positive," or any of a few dozen other such exercises, all of which are noted in your daily action plan. The book is filled with pithy little sayings—most of them are pretty good, actually—some by Stamper ("The most important words you'll ever hear are the ones you tell yourself"), some by Norman Vincent Peale ("Change your thoughts and you change your world"), and some that seem to be lifted directly from the reject pile of new-age greeting cards ("Regret is an appalling waste of energy; you can't build on it; it's only good for wallowing in").

Early on, the book lists what the Lindora program considers the "six essentials for success." These include being clear that your goal is to be lean for life (not just for the duration of the diet) and learning to recognize and eliminate your defensive barriers. Examples of barriers are denial and rationalization, such as "One little bit won't kill me," "I deserve this—I've been good all day," or my personal favorite, "I don't need to write down what I eat—I have a great memory."

There is a lot of work on learning to manage and control cravings. Lindora considers three main causes of cravings: *physical,* which includes insulin resistance and low serotonin levels as well as lack of exercise; *psychological,* about self-image; and *environmental,* meaning conditioned responses to triggers such as events, people, places, and emotions (an example of an environmental trigger and its associated eating behavior: movies and popcorn).

Lindora also focuses on relaxation techniques and the reduction of stress, pointing out that people who have difficulty managing stress have difficulty losing weight, and if they do lose, they regain. The program suggests tools to help individuals stop using food to self-medicate and manage stress.

Finally, there are "success strategies" for maintaining lifelong results: maintain a support system, continue exercising, maintain your daily action plan journal, weigh yourself every morning, eat three meals a day, do one protein day a week (to maintain a sense of awareness and control over your eating and to help curb the appetite), drink 80 ounces of calorie-free liquid daily, take vitamins, and do mental training exercises.

The Lindora Program as a Lifestyle: Who It Works for, Who Should Look Elsewhere

This is a program for people who really can commit to the whole self-help aspect of weight control. You can't just do the diet part of it and be successful. The program requires journaling, homework, and a lot of mindful, thoughtful activity. There is a ton of support available on the website, and if you live in southern California, the company encourages you to come to the Lindora centers on a regular basis. Lindora also sells a truckload of products and foods as part of the overall program. If this speaks to you, great. If it turns you off, look elsewhere. The diet itself is not for extremely carbohydrate-sensitive people.

JONNY'S LOWDOWN   ★ ★ ☆ ☆ ☆

The strength of this plan is clearly in its holistic approach and its motivational "we're all in this together" spirit. I've always been a fan of incorporating ways to increase consciousness about food into a program, and the program can't be faulted for its emphasis on self-

esteem, new habits, goal setting, and the mind-body connection. And because it takes such an aggressive approach to raising consciousness, I can easily see how it would be effective at retraining people to be aware of what they are eating and to be thoughtful and mindful about whether their eating habits are compatible with their goals of permanent weight management. So far, so good.

I'm not such a fan when it comes to the actual diet. You could certainly argue that it is realistic and allows a lot of stuff that other, sterner taskmasters banish, which makes it palatable for a lot of people. Maybe. But for me, it's a failed attempt to find the political middle ground, to satisfy the low-fat contingent, satisfy the low-calorie contingent, and, oh yes, throw some more protein into the mix. The emphasis on protein is a step in the right direction, but everything else about Lindora is very conventional and conservative. There are also far too few vegetables and way too many grains (in the maintenance program) for my liking.

I think this program has a place for people who want to really surrender to making the program a priority in their life for as long as it takes to get the job done; it will be very good for people who respond well to the self-help and psychological aspects. From a food point of view, there are many better diet systems and there are certainly a lot more sophisticated writers than Cynthia Stamper Graff when it comes to talking about food, hormones, and weight.

Books in the Series
Lean for Life Phase One: Weight Loss
Lean for Life Phase Two: Lifetime Solutions
Lean for Life Recipe Book

Best Book to Start With
Lean for Life Phase One: Weight Loss

About the Author
Cynthia Stamper Graff is the daughter of Dr. Marshall Stamper, who started the program, and she is president and CEO of Lindora, Inc. Graff is obviously a very successful businesswoman who has been instrumental in developing Lindora's atHome, atWork and online versions of the Lean for Life program. She has a degree in law.

Website

If you feel like you're visiting a homey mom-and-pop store when visiting some of the other low-carb sites, then visiting leanforlife.com will feel like you've just entered the Mall of America. This is a very slick, very professional, very well-run business that sells online versions of the program, telephone coaching, and a vast number of products (vitamins, food, books, etc.). For those who are interested, there is information on the many clinics in southern California where, depending on the program you choose, you get counseling two to five times a week, regular weigh-ins on a digital scale, medical supervision, and optional vitamin injections.

NEANDERTHIN

RAY AUDETTE

WHAT IT IS IN A NUTSHELL

The simplest of the low-carb diets to follow; also one of the most restrictive. You don't have to follow any formulas, compute any protein or carb allowances, look up any food counts, or figure out calories. Here's what you do.

Eat:
- *meats and fish*
- *fruits, especially berries*
- *vegetables*
- *nuts and seeds*

Do not eat:
- *grains*
- *beans*
- *potatoes*
- *dairy (especially milk)*
- *sugar*

About Neanderthin

The book has three premises.

1. A natural diet is best.
2. Nature is defined as the absence of technology.
3. Until the advent of agriculture, grains, beans, potatoes, milk, and refined sugar were not part of the human diet. So don't eat them.

Hence, no grains, beans, potatoes, milk, or refined sugar. Period.

The main theme of Neanderthin is that the root cause of numerous diseases of civilization (including obesity) is eating processed foods. More specifically, you should not eat foods that are inedible in their natural state and can only be eaten because they've been processed (chief among them: wheat, dairy, and sugar).

In the late 1970s, Ray Audette was suffering from rheumatoid arthritis (a crippling, painful autoimmune disease) that sidetracked his career in computers and threatened to destroy his health. Later, at the age of thirty-four, he was diagnosed with diabetes. He decided not to take these life sentences sitting down. He researched everything he could about the diseases and came up with a few basic observations and one major conclusion, which led to his development of the Neanderthin diet, another spin on "stone-age nutrition."

Observation number one: rheumatoid arthritis and diabetes are diseases of the autoimmune system—diseases in which the immune system wrongfully identifies something in its own body as foreign matter or an invader and proceeds to attack it. (He happens to be completely wrong about diabetes—it is *not* an autoimmune disease—but follow the argument anyway.) Observation number two: these diseases occur only within agricultural (or civilized) communities. (The more recently a population became agricultural, the more likely it is to have diabetic members.) Many of the foods that came into wide use during the agricultural era (such as wheat) aggravate these conditions. Audette looked at these two observations and made a decision: he would modify his own diet to emulate that of preagricultural (Paleolithic) peoples. He'd go "back to nature."

He decided to eat like a hunter-gatherer.

Obviously it worked, or he wouldn't have written this book. His blood sugar levels returned to normal almost immediately. He had more energy. His joints stopped hurting. He needed less sleep. He literally became a new man.

One who was on a mission.

The Neanderthin diet is pretty simple and follows one basic dietary guideline: eat only what you could eat if you were naked on the savanna with a sharp stick. It's a variation on the "eat only what you could hunt, fish, gather, or pluck" mantra. Forbidden foods are those that require technological intervention to make them edible. The book starts with a quote from the book of Genesis: "Do not eat the fruit of the tree of knowledge that makes the good the evil." Using the Greek translation of the phrase *tree of knowledge* and Hebrew translation of the words *good* and *evil*, he restates the quote this way: "Do not eat the fruit of the technology that makes the inedible the edible."

The appeal of the diet is that it's simple. Really simple. You don't count calories. You eat all you like from four basic food groups (meat/fish, nuts/seeds, fruits/berries, and vegetables). You don't reduce fat (except some saturated fats such as the skin of chicken). And you *do not* cheat. (One reason: the forbidden categories of foods have the innate ability to create cravings for themselves.) This is not a diet for the squeamish or the warm and fuzzy. When Audette says "forbidden fruits," he means business.

Audette suggests six steps to success in Paleo eating.

1. Make a commitment. Resolve that for some predetermined amount of time (three weeks would be great), you will not eat any grains, beans, potatoes, milk, or refined sugar. Period.
2. Rid your kitchen of the forbidden fruits: beans, grains, dairy products, potatoes, and sugar, as well as any products made from them.
3. Limit your carb intake. Fruits and vegetables are fine, of course, but he suggests choosing those that have a low-sugar content—pears, oranges, plums, and berries, for example, rather than bananas, mangoes, and dates. And he suggests raw fruits and vegetables over steamed, cooked, or canned ones.
4. Increase fat consumption, preferably from omega-3 fats, which are described in Audette's book in detail (see also chapter 4 of this book).
5 Drink a ton of water—eight glasses a day minimum, preferably 2 to 3 liters.
6. Increase physical activity. A Neander-fit program is included, with an emphasis on building muscle (rather than burning calories) and working at considerably less than full-out "no pain, no gain" intensity.

You also shouldn't drink alcohol, though he says that if you must, you can do damage control by drinking fruit-based alcohol such as wine or champagne.

Of the forbidden fruits—grains, beans, potatoes, dairy, and sugar—probably the least taboo are dairy products (not milk, though—just butter, yogurt, and cheese). Notice that all of these forbidden fruits are foods that require technological intervention to make them edible. When you find them in the wild in their original state, none of them can be eaten. (One could argue about the inclusion of milk here, as some hunter-gatherers—notably the Maasai in Africa—do drink the unprocessed milk of animals.) To critics who say that our physiology is perfectly able to handle "modern" foods, Audette answers that just because our physiology can handle a small dose of something doesn't mean it can deal with a large dose of the same thing without problems developing. For example, we have the enzymes needed to process alcohol in small amounts, but look what happens when we drink a lot. Maybe the same is true of foods like wheat, dairy, sugar, and other processed foods that nutritionist Robert Crayhon calls "ubiquifoods." At one time, these foods weren't in the human diet at all; now they have become so ubiquitous that they are the very *basis* of the modern diet. That's way too big an adjustment for our stone-age genes. And our bodies respond with the diseases of modern civilization, including obesity.

Audette comes down firmly on the side of the calorie debate that holds that weight gain is not simply a matter of quantity of calories but instead a matter of *quality*: "It cannot be overemphasized that it is not the calories or fat content that produces the weight gain, as has been traditionally proposed; instead, it is the alien proteins present in the forbidden fruits that cause an overweight condition."

A vegetarian diet, says Audette, is about as natural to humans as a diet of Cheerios is to a lion.

Neanderthin as a Lifestyle: Who It Works for, Who Should Look Elsewhere

This is a simple, take-no-prisoners approach. It will work well if you don't want a lot of rules or complicated calculations and don't want to have to weigh or measure or figure out how much of anything you're eating. People who want a really simple, black-and-white, "eat this but don't eat this" plan and are willing to put up with a fairly restrictive diet will like this program. What you give up in order to gain that simplicity is flexibility. There's almost no wiggle room on this diet, and if you're not comfortable with that, this program is not for you. Also remember that the focus of the book isn't primarily on weight loss; it's on health. Eating unlimited quantities of anything, even the best food on the planet, can stall or prevent weight loss. There's no discussion of what to do if that happens or how to modify the plan to account for calorie intake.

If you have a tremendous amount of weight to lose, you may find that a more structured plan works better, at least at the beginning stages.

JONNY'S LOWDOWN ★ ★ ★ ☆ ☆

The book is a little weak in making the connection between obesity and autoimmune diseases. While it's true that many immune system diseases (or "diseases of civilization") don't happen in hunter-gatherer societies when people eat a "native" diet devoid of processed foods, and while it's also true that you don't see much obesity in these same societies, it doesn't necessarily follow that obesity is an autoimmune disease (and, as mentioned earlier, diabetes certainly isn't). Audette points out that both obesity and autoimmune diseases respond well to Paleolithic nutrition, but this doesn't mean that they are the same thing—just that they have the same enemy.

That said, this book is a real delight. It has a terrific history of dieting, a very accessible history of Paleolithic nutrition, a great discussion of the anthropology of nutrition, a very good bibliography, and a great FAQ section. While it's a pretty strict diet, it's also very easy to follow—it doesn't require any complicated formulas or have phases, calculations, calorie counting, or even portion control. There's just one simple rule: if you could eat this food with a stick or a rock naked on the savanna, it's allowed. If you couldn't, it's forbidden. While some people may find that a pretty extreme position to take, it's also a pretty easy one to understand. And the health benefits are likely to be considerable.

Books in the Series
Neanderthin: Eat Like a Caveman to Achieve a Lean, Strong, Healthy Body

About the Author
Ray Audette is not a doctor or a nutritionist, just a very smart guy (and longtime Mensa member) who basically cured himself of two debilitating afflictions by using a low-carb Paleolithic diet and went on to write this book about his experiences and his research.

Website
The official website, www.neanderthin.com, is as simple and unpretentious as the book. It has a FAQ section, a copy of the introduction to the book (by Dr. Michael Eades, coauthor of *Protein Power*), booking info for Audette, a good section (with links) on Paleolithic nutrition, and some press clippings and articles about Audette from popular magazines.

THE PALEO DIET

LOREN CORDAIN, PH.D.

WHAT IT IS IN A NUTSHELL

All the lean meat, poultry, fish, and seafood you want, plus unlimited fruits and nonstarchy vegetables. No dairy, cereals, legumes, or processed foods.

About the Paleo Diet

The Paleo Diet is perhaps the most sophisticated example of the "stone-age" or "caveman" type of diet books (Neanderthin, page 104, is one example), and Dr. Loren Cordain is one of the best-known researchers in the field of what might be called "nutritional anthropology" or "Paleolithic nutrition." The general theory behind the Paleo Diet—and others like it—is this:

- Being fat comes primarily from eating a diet that is *completely unsuited* to our ancient genes and digestive system.
- The humans genus spent a couple of million years adapting to and functioning on a diet *entirely* different than the one we eat today.
- Our digestive systems—identical to those of our caveman ancestors—are simply unsuited for the staples of today's diet: dairy, refined sugar, fatty meat, and processed food.
- By returning to the diet that humans lived on for the vast majority of their time on earth, we can correct a great many of the problems in human health, including but not limited to obesity.

The argument for this position is pretty strong. DNA evidence shows that genetically, humans have hardly changed in the 2.5 million years the genus has been on the planet. The human genome has changed less than 0.02 percent (1/50th of 1 percent) in forty thousand years. Most of the diseases of modern civilization—including cancer, obesity, diabetes, and heart disease—have happened at the same time that we've experienced a sea change in our diet, and the modern diet is completely different from the one humans have lived on for the overwhelming bulk of our time on the planet.

Through fossil records and research on contemporary hunter-gatherer societies, we have a pretty good idea of what Paleolithic peoples ate—and it didn't look like anything you'd find at Burger King.

Consider the diet of our Paleo ancestors, before the invention of modern foods: they ate no dairy (how easy would it be to milk a wild animal?) and no cereal grains; they didn't salt their food; the only sweetener they used was honey, which they ate rarely (when they could find it); wild animal foods dominated their diet (so protein intake was high and carb intake was low); and since all carbs came from wild fruits and non-starchy vegetables, fiber was very high.

Beginning to get the picture?

On the other hand, the average American diet contains:

• 31 percent calories from cereals
• 14 percent calories from dairy
• 8 percent calories from beverages, especially sodas and fruit juices
• 4 percent calories from oils and dressings, especially processed oils and omega-6s
• 4 percent calories from sweets like candy, cookies, and cake

That means 61 percent of calories in a modern diet come from foods that were largely unknown before the adoption of agriculture (a drop in the time bucket as far as evolution is concerned), and *most* of them weren't even available until a couple of hundred years ago, when food processing became the norm. The remaining 39 percent of our calories come from animal foods, but ones that are very different from those of our cavemen ancestors. The animal foods the average American is likely to consume are mostly hot dogs, fatty ground beef, bacon, and highly processed deli meats. (When looked at in this way, is it any wonder there are studies linking "meat" consumption in industrial societies to a number of health issues? Maybe meat as a category has gotten a bum rap and it's the *kind* of meats we eat that's the problem!)

Cordain claims that a return to a diet of our ancestors—what has been described elsewhere as eating what you could hunt, fish, gather, grow, or pluck—is the answer not only to obesity and overweight, but to a multitude of other health problems. Though it seems like he stresses protein as the most important component in the diet, in actuality he makes it clear that protein *alone*—without fat or the alkalizing influence of tons of vegetables and fruits—is a big problem. Add those and the problem disappears: "There is no such thing as too much protein as long as you are eating plenty of fresh fruits and vegetables," Cordain says. And he is pretty flexible about the possible balance among them, pointing out that some hunter-gatherer societies that survived into the twentieth century lived healthy lives free of chronic disease while getting 97 percent of their calories from animal foods (the Inuit of Alaska), while others got the majority of their calories (65 percent) from plant foods (the !Kung of Africa). Most Paleo societies fall somewhere between these two extremes. *No* Paleo peoples, however, ate refined sugar.

On the Paleo Diet, fully 50 to 55 percent of your calories come from lean meats, organ meats, poultry, fish, and seafood. The rest come from vegetables (except for starchy ones like potatoes and yams) and "healthy" fats (more about these in Jonny's Lowdown). It's simple and easy. There is no calorie counting, no protein gram counting, no fat gram counting, and no carb gram counting. By staying within these guidelines, Cordain claims you will:

- have built-in protection against overeating because protein (and fiber) naturally feels more satiating
- enjoy the increased metabolic activity (and increased calorie burning) that protein provides (see chapter 2 for studies that show this)
- control insulin and reduce insulin resistance, making weight loss a breeze

The Paleo Diet itself allows "cheating." There are three levels of commitment, with level one allowing you three "open" (read: cheat) meals a week, level two permitting two such meals, and level three only one.

Many people not previously familiar with the material in chapter 2 of this book will find Cordain's passionate argument against grains surprising, as we have been so conditioned to think of grains, especially whole grains, as wonderful foods. Cordain is particularly expert on this subject, having written the seminal paper "Cereal Grains: Humanity's Double-Edged Sword",[7] and what he has to say on the subject is worth considering even if you don't adopt this particular dietary program.

The Problem with Grains

Here's the synopsis: the agricultural revolution began about ten thousand years ago in the Middle East. Dwindling food resources—especially wild game—and rising populations gave birth to the need for smarter, more efficient ways for people to support themselves and their families. Some enterprising people figured out how to sow and harvest wild wheat seeds. Then they tried barley. Then legumes. Livestock—sheep, goats, and pigs—wasn't far behind. Later, cattle. Domesticated farm animals were milkable. Over time, there was a complete change in the diet of most of humanity.

Without the agricultural revolution, we would not have civilization as we know it. Our ability to farm—to domesticate animals for dairy products, to raise cattle, and especially to grow and cultivate grains—was responsible for allowing us to live in denser conditions and encouraged towns and cities to develop. It allowed us to become independent from our original food source—hunted game.

But this new lifestyle came with a price. Early farmers were shorter in stature than their forebears had been. Examination of their bones and teeth showed more infectious diseases and shorter life spans. Egyptian mummies frequently reveal obese bodies. There were more cases of osteoporosis, rickets, and vitamin and mineral deficiency diseases, in large measure because of cereal-based diets (whole grains and legumes contain "antinutrients," pyridoxine glucosides and phytates, that respectively block absorption of B vitamins in the intestines and chemically bind iron, zinc, copper, and calcium and block their absorption). And the skulls of those living on modern foods revealed teeth filled with cavities and jaws that were misshapen and too small for the teeth (Dr. Weston Price's seminal 1939 book, *Nutrition and Physical Degeneration*, contains many pictures that dramatically illustrate this phenomenon).

Then came fermentation and salting. Grains were fed to livestock, making them fatter but also changing the quality of their meat and their fat. (Interesting, isn't it, that grains are the food of choice for fattening livestock and yet are still recommended by the dietary establishment as the foundation food of a weight loss program!) Meat was preserved by pickling, salting, and smoking. Two hundred years ago, things got even worse. We now had ways to refine sugar and flour and to can foods, almost always with the addition or creation of trans-fats, sugar, refined oils high in omega-6s, and high-fructose corn syrup, not to mention additives, preservatives, emulsifiers, and other toxins.

As Cordain says, imagine Paleo man with a Twinkie or a pizza. He wouldn't even recognize them as food.

Cordain is one of the few writers to talk about something called the acid-base balance, a very hot subject in nutrition these days. Briefly, it goes like this: everything reports to the kidneys as either an acid or an alkaline.

When there is too much acid, the body needs to neutralize it with alkaline substances like calcium. Meats are one of the top five acid-producing foods—but the other four—grains, legumes, cheese, and salt—were rarely or never eaten by our Paleo ancestors, who buffered the acid load of their meat with plenty of fruits and vegetables. The main "buffering" compound in the body is calcium, and the main storehouse for calcium is the bones; this is how high-protein diets got their (false) reputation for causing bone loss. Cordain correctly points out that loss of calcium does *not* happen when there are plenty of fruits and vegetables in the diet, and especially when other acid-producing foods (like cereal grains and dairy) are absent.

The Paleo Diet as a Lifestyle: Who It Works for, Who Should Look Elsewhere

The straightforward simplicity of the Paleo Diet—all you want of *these* foods, none at all of *those*—makes it pretty easy to follow and a good choice for those who are put off by counting grams, calories, and carbohydrates, figuring out protein allowances, or computing food blocks. But that same lack of rigidity makes it a poor choice for those who need more structure. And although it restricts nearly all of the usual problem foods for carbohydrate addicts, the unlimited fruit could easily be a problem for those who are insulin-resistant. In addition, since it is not primarily a weight loss diet, it may be frustrating for those whose main focus for the immediate future is on losing fat.

JONNY'S LOWDOWN ★ ★ ★ ☆ ☆

The Paleo Diet is a frustrating program to rate. On one hand, you have to give credit to a no-grain diet that eliminates sugar, dairy, and trans-fats and recommends tons of vegetables. How bad can that be? Most people—especially those who eat the typical American diet—are going to reap such enormous benefits from this program that I almost want to give it five stars just for effort.

On the other hand, there are some major problems. For one thing, Cordain completely buys into the cholesterol–heart disease hypothesis; I believe that this hypothesis, in its current form, is less than a decade away from being dumped on the pile of scientific flotsam and jetsam. He also accepts the dogma that all saturated fats are bad, largely because they raise cholesterol (some do; many don't; and ultimately it may not matter much). Cordain puts eggs on the "avoid" list for their cholesterol content (something we now know is completely irrelevant, since dietary cholesterol has virtually no impact on serum cholesterol) and warns against such natural traditional fats as butter and cream, which he puts in the same category as such trans-fat nightmares as nonfat dairy creamer and frozen yogurt. He recommends canola oil (I don't agree, see page 228). He puts sweet potatoes—a "good" starch by almost anyone's standards—in the same class as french fries and tapioca pudding. He makes the fairly incredible statement that "fruit won't make you fat on this diet even in unlimited amounts." And he completely misrepresents other low-carb diets, saying that they call for complete restriction of all carbohydrates to "between 30 and 100 grams a day," which, according to Cordain, means that "fruits and vegetables are largely off-limits"—a statement that is not only demonstrably false but inconsistent; 100 grams of usable carbs a day buys you an awful lot of broccoli!

That said, he's a good guy and a sincere and responsible scholar, and his overall recommendations will propel a person eating the average American diet light-years ahead in his quest for good health. Done with care, Cordain's diet may also make you lose weight.

Books in the Series
The Paleo Diet

About the Author
Loren Cordain, Ph.D., is one of the world's most renowned scientists researching the original human diet. Generally recognized as the leading expert on Paleolithic nutrition, he is a professor in the Health and Exercise Science Department at Colorado State University. Cordain recently published a groundbreaking paper showing the relationship between acne and the Western diet.

Website
The official home for Loren Cordain, thepaleodiet.com, provides great links to published research about the Paleo Diet, as well as a great FAQ

page. Another site, paleodiet.com, is even more varied and contains thought-provoking papers on a variety of topics related to what the hunter-gatherers ate, including discussions of the link between grains and autoimmune diseases, the calcium question, trans-fats, and the advantages of the "original" diet. There is also a site, paleofood.com, devoted to recipes using mainly meat, fish, fruit, vegetables, nuts, and berries. The vast majority of recipes are completely grain-free, bean-free, potato-free, dairy-free, and sugar-free.

PROTEIN POWER

MICHAEL EADES, M.D., AND MARY DAN EADES, M.D.

WHAT IT IS IN A NUTSHELL

A three-phase plan in which you:

- *Eat no less than a minimum calculated amount of protein per day (you are free to eat more but not less)*
- *Eat no more than a maximum amount of carbohydrate per day (you are free to eat less but not more)*

The maximum amount of carbohydrates depends on which phase of the diet you are in. Phase one is intervention and allows up to 30 grams of carbohydrate a day; phase two is transition and allows up to 55 grams; phase three is the maintenance phase, and the amount of carbs will vary according to the individual.

About Protein Power

In the Eades plan, you first determine your protein needs through an easy-to-follow series of steps.

1. Measure your wrist, then your waist.
2. Refer to a chart to estimate your body fat from these measurements.
3. Now you calculate your total number of fat pounds. For example, if you're 200 pounds with 20 percent body fat, you would have 40 fat pounds.
4. Subtract the number of fat pounds from your total weight to get the number of lean body weight pounds (muscle, bone, and the like). Using the above example, you would subtract 40 pounds from 200 and wind up with a lean body weight of 160 pounds.
5. Multiply your lean body weight by an "activity factor" to get your minimum daily protein needs (in grams). The activity factor ranges from 0.5 for someone who is completely sedentary to 0.9 for a competitive athlete. For example, if the 200-pound guy with 40 fat pounds and 160 lean pounds were sedentary, he'd multiply 160 by 0.5 for a total of 80 grams of protein per day minimum.

Knowing your lean body weight also allows you to calculate a realistic weight goal, which is done using the worksheets and very easy formulas.

Note: In *The Protein Power Lifeplan*, the authors have simplified the process even more. You don't even have to take your wrist or waist measurements, compute your lean body mass, or multiply by an activity factor. There's a simple table in which you look for your height and weight, and the table tells you immediately what your minimum protein requirement is. It couldn't be easier. It's not as refined and accurate as the method in the original *Protein Power*, but it will give you a decent estimate of your minimum requirement and is good for people who just don't want to do the calculations. (My personal opinion: the calculations are easy.)

Once you know your minimum daily protein needs, you simply decide what phase of the diet you're going to be on. Phase one, intervention, is for those who have a lot of fat to lose and/or who want to correct a health problem. In phase one, you take in 30 grams or less of carbohydrate a day (in *Protein Power Lifeplan*, this number is amended to 40) plus, of course, *at least* your minimum protein requirement. Phase two is the one to go with if you want to lose a little fat, recompose your body (i.e., change the ratio of fat to muscle or, as people often say, "tone up"), or improve your general health. In phase two, the maximum carb allowance is upped to 55 grams a day, in addition, of course, to the protein allowance determined above. You can eat *more* than your minimum protein requirement but not less, and you can eat *less* than your maximum carb allotment but not more. The rest of the diet comes from fat.

Nearly everyone will fall into one of four categories of minimum protein requirement—less than 60 grams a day, between 60 and 80 grams a day, between 80 and 100 grams a day, or between 100 and 120 grams a day. You find the category you belong to and then refer to the corresponding chart. The chart will tell you exactly what protein foods in what amounts you can have *per meal and snack*. For example, if you're in the 80- to 100-gram category, you should be getting about 34 grams of protein per meal. The chart shows you exactly how to make any combination you can think of from meat, fish, poultry, eggs, hard cheeses, soft cheeses, curd cheeses, or tofu to get the right amount of protein per meal.

Like nearly all the diet or lifestyle plans discussed in this book, Protein Power is all about controlling and balancing insulin. The Eades have a clever way of determining the actual insulin-raising (or active) carbohydrate content of foods. Even though fiber is not metabolically active, it's technically counted as a carbohydrate on food labels and the like. But it doesn't raise insulin at all, since it's not even digested. So the Eades have come up with a formula in which you subtract the fiber from the total carb content of a food to get what they call the effective carbohydrate content, or ECC. That's the only number you have to pay attention to when counting your carbohydrate grams. For example, 1 cup of fresh raspberries has 14 grams of carbohydrate but 6 grams of fiber, so you'd subtract the 6 grams of fiber from the 14 grams of total carbohydrate to get a mere 8 grams of ECC, and only those 8 grams would count toward your carbohydrate allowance for the day. (This is now standard operating procedure for most low-carb diets, some of which call the number effective carbs, some net carbs.)

The book has charts of the ECC for a huge number of foods, so you don't have to figure them out for yourself. You use these charts to put together your daily carbohydrate allowance (or, if a food is not listed in the chart, you can easily compute it yourself from the label's listing of total carbs and total fiber). Counting only effective carbs, you could easily have 1 cup of broccoli, 1 cup of cabbage, 3 celery ribs, 1 cup of green beans, 1 cup of lettuce, ½ cup of mushrooms, 1 cup of zucchini, 1 cup of spinach, and 1 cup of raspberries in one day on phase one. Even though the total carb content of these foods is about 44 grams, 16 of them are fiber—subtracting the 16 from the 44 (all done for you in the charts) leaves you with only 28 grams of usable (effective) carbohydrate, well under the cutoff for phase one and not even close to the cutoff for phase two.

Calories are barely mentioned in Protein Power. The idea is that calories are self-regulating if you are eating the foods that put you in correct metabolic balance (an idea that runs throughout many low-carb diet plans). The Eadeses do warn you that since you may not be as hungry on a low-carb plan as you were before, you can easily *under*eat, so it's important to be sure that your calories don't fall below 850 to 1,000 a day. (The 850 figure seems really, *really* low—nearly every other weight loss expert, including myself, uses 1,000 to 1,250 as the bare minimum, and some even suggest not dropping below 1,250. If the food eaten produces a hormonally balanced state and the calories are coming from good stuff, most women will drop weight on 1,250 calories and most men on 1,500.)

On the other hand, especially in *The Protein Power Lifeplan*, the authors explain that if you're doing everything right—i.e., eating the minimum protein requirement and not exceeding the maximum carb allotment—and you're *still* not losing weight, you might be consuming too many calories, especially calories from fat. Nuts seem to be a frequent culprit: since nuts are only fat and protein, many low-carbers munch on these with abandon because they have very little effect on insulin. But while a 1-ounce portion (which is pretty small!) may have only 160 calories and a few grams of carbs at most, three to four portions can add an awful lot of calories (and carb grams) to a diet plan and could effectively slow down or stop weight loss altogether. As with most low-carb plans, the message here is: though calories are not the whole story by a long shot, they still matter, so don't ignore them.

Phase three is the maintenance phase, which is what you stay on once you've reached your goal. To get there, you add 10 grams of carbohydrate to your daily allotment in phase two, and stay there and stabilize for about five to seven days. Then you add another 10 grams. You continue in this way until you find the amount of carbs you can take in and still keep your weight stable. The Eadeses have found that *most* people will stabilize when they've reached the point at which the number of carb grams equals the number of protein grams, but they discuss the exceptions to this general rule and tell you what to do if you don't fit the template.

The maintenance phase is pretty cool. There is really no food you can't have "in some quantity at some time." The trick is knowing what you're doing. As the authors put it, there are foods that are "so rich in sugars and starches, such potent unbalancers of your metabolic hormones, that you cannot have unlimited amounts of them anytime you want unless you are willing to accept the consequences of that action." They even have recovery guidelines for those times when you throw caution to the wind, and have a "nutritional vacation," such as on birthdays, holidays, and the like. You simply return to phase one for three days (or until you have lost any of the weight you might have gained), move to phase two for the rest of the week, and then return to your maintenance level of carb consumption.

The thing about *The Protein Power Lifeplan*, and to a lesser extent the original book, is that it is about so much more than just a diet. There is absolutely first-rate information about cholesterol and the "cholesterol hoax," plus wonderful explanations of how insulin works in the body and its relationship to heart disease, high blood pressure, diabetes, and obesity. There is a terrific exposition on the Paleolithic diet. And in *Lifeplan*, the authors go into even more detail on all of these topics, plus they include discussions of antioxidants, leaky gut syndrome and autoimmune responses, sugar, iron overload, magnesium, brain health, and a further expansion of the nutritional plan.

Lifeplan also has a cool concept. It suggests three levels of "commitment" to health: the purist, the dilettante, and the hedonist. All of these approaches share the same requirements for protein, the same need for high-quality fat, the same prohibition on trans-fatty acids, and the same limitations of carbohydrate grams (depending on what phase you're in). (Even at the lowest level of commitment, the hedonist, you're still *way* better off than you would be following the standard American diet or, for that matter, the standard high-carb, low-fat diet.) All of the levels should theoretically give the same weight loss results. The difference is in overall health benefits.

The purist regimen is really restrictive and most resembles Ray Audette's Neanderthin plan. Purists eat *no* cereal grains or products made from them (à la *The No-Grain Diet* of Joseph Mercola). They eat *no* dairy or legumes (such as beans). They eat *only* organic fruits and vegetables and *only* natural meat and poultry—no processed foods, no sugars (except occasionally honey), no artificial sweeteners, no caffeine, and no alcohol. It's probably the healthiest diet in the world to follow, but also next to impossible for most folks. However, for people with serious health issues, it may mean the difference between life and death.

Next up is the dilettante. You aim for organic foods whenever possible but are not obsessive about it. You still avoid some grains (wheat, for example) but can eat others (like oats and rice). You eliminate high-fructose corn syrup but can have some other sweeteners, even table sugar (in very limited amounts), and the prohibition against alcohol and caffeine is lifted. This is the program the Eades themselves follow.

Finally, there is the hedonist, where everything goes, within the limits of your carbohydrate allowance. You still have to keep to the basic parameters of the program but you can fulfill those requirements with just about any foods you wish. Obviously, the high-carb content of some foods, such as potatoes, may make it impossible to fit portions of those foods into the phase one plan, when carbs are limited to 7 to 10 grams per meal and snack. But once you're on phase two or three, you can eat anything you want as long as you don't exceed the maximum number of carbs for the day.

Protein Power as a Lifestyle:
Who It Works for, Who Should Look Elsewhere

This is a great plan if you have a lot of weight to lose or if you have any of the health conditions discussed in the book. In its maintenance phase, it's a great plan to follow, period. But you've got to be willing to do a little figuring. You can't eyeball portions on the first two phases (which you can do on the Zone or even on phase three of this plan). You've got to be exact about carb gram content and about meeting your minimum protein needs. The calculations to figure out your protein needs could conceivably put some folks off (although it's a nonissue in *Lifeplan*). Having to check ECC for every food might be a pain in the butt for some, and could be a real problem if you eat out often, unless you get really familiar with the carb content of a lot of foods. If you're willing to put in the effort, it's totally worth it. If you're not into counting, measuring, and keeping really clear records (in your mind, if not on paper), this is going to be a hard plan for you, and you might be better off with a simpler formula.

JONNY'S LOWDOWN ★ ★ ★ ★ ★

It's hard to find anything wrong with this plan and the concepts and theories behind it. In some ways it's like the Zone with an induction phase, which may be why Barry Sears, whose Zone diet is way higher in carbs and lower in fat, is still able to endorse it (phase three, the maintenance phase of Protein Power, is not far from Zone-like eating). The only credible argument I've heard against this type of plan is from endocrinologist Dr. Diana Schwarzbein, whose dietary regimen is not considered high-protein but is definitely still on the lower-carb side of the fence (see "The Schwarzbein Principle" on page 127). Her concern is that too much protein without enough carbo- hydrate will raise the hormone cortisol, which has a whole other set of problems attached to it. It's a fair objection, and only time and additional research will clarify these hazy areas. In the meantime, I'm continuing to recommend The Protein Power Lifeplan *as a basic text- book to all my clients who just want to live a healthy lifestyle and manage their weight. It's hard to find anything commercially avail- able that's more comprehensive.*

Books in the Series

Protein Power: The High-Protein, Low-Carbohydrate Way to Lose Weight, Lower Cholesterol and Blood Pressure, and Restore Your Health—in Just Weeks!

The Protein Power Lifeplan is a new comprehensive blueprint for optimal health.

The 30-Day Low-Carb Diet Solution A simple thirty-day what-to-eat plan based on Protein Power; a kind of "Protein Power for Dummies."

The Low-Carb Comfort Food Cookbook is just what it says it is!

Best Book to Start With

It's a toss-up between *Protein Power* and *The Protein Power Lifeplan*. *Protein Power* is the original and is the most detailed in terms of the weight loss plan. *Lifeplan* is like a textbook on how to live a healthy life. It has a ton of stuff about cholesterol, heart disease, stress, brain aging, and the like, and it reviews the nutritional concepts in the original book.

About the Authors

The Eadeses are homey, folksy, personally engaging, and utterly brilliant doctors who have been working in the field of weight loss and nutritional medicine for fifteen years. Both are from Arkansas (Michael grew up across the street from President Clinton) and got their medical degrees from the University of Arkansas. They founded the Colorado Center for Metabolic Medicine, now known as the Rosedale Center for Metabolic Medicine. The Eadeses are a kinder, gentler Robert Atkins. They are very strong, powerfully knowledgeable folks with a couple dozen years of experience between them in metabolic medicine, and they come to conclusions that are not all that different from those made by Atkins: limiting carbs is the key to health, fat is not the enemy, and eating meat and other traditional protein sources does not necessarily mean you're going to hell.

Website

The official website for Michael and Mary Dan Eades is eatprotein.com. Here, you will find a bookstore, a nutrition products store, a community weight loss bulletin board, a lot of good articles, recipes, and a terrific FAQ section.

For followers of Protein Power, www.dvdmon.com/pp is a must. It's run by Levi Wallach, a low-carber for several years who is a moderator for the Protein Power bulletin board and the author of the widely distributed free primer about the Protein Power eating plan titled "Protein Power in a Nutshell."

THE SCARSDALE DIET

HERMAN TARNOWER, M.D.

WHAT IT IS IN A NUTSHELL

A low-calorie, low-fat, low-carbohydrate, high-protein diet that speci-fies exactly what you can and cannot eat with very little room for flexibility. You go on the basic diet for two weeks; then you go on the slightly relaxed "lifetime keep slim program" for two weeks. If you still have weight to lose, you repeat the cycle. Forbidden are sugar, full-fat dairy products, cakes, pies, cookies, candy, chocolate, potatoes, rice, sweet potatoes, yams, beans, avocados, spaghetti, macaroni, flour-based products, fatty meats, peanut butter, butter, margarine, oils, and any kind of fat used in cooking.

About the Scarsdale Diet

Even by diet book standards, the Scarsdale diet made laughable claims, promising a pound a day of weight loss, totaling as much as 20 pounds or more in two weeks. Tarnower also claimed that the diet worked for everyone, from teenagers to octogenarians, and that *90 percent* of them maintained their desired weight.

The diet consisted of two two-week segments: the basic diet and the maintenance diet, or "keep slim program." The idea is that you would do the basic diet for two weeks and then switch to the maintenance version. If, after four weeks, you still had weight to lose, you went back to the orig-inal program and repeated the two-week/two-week cycle. The first two weeks were rigidly specific, with every one of the twenty-one meals per week dictated by the book. Tarnower was a cantankerous control freak who insisted that the diet be followed strictly, with absolutely no variation per-mitted. During the maintenance phase, the rules were slightly—though *only* slightly—relaxed; you could make certain substitutions, could add one alcoholic drink a day, and could use nuts "sparingly."

Tarnower devoted a section in the book to "The Mystery of Diet Chemistry," but he was either remarkably uninformed on the subject or just downright stupid. He explained that "a carefully designed combina-tion of foods can increase the fat-burning process in the human system" and that the Scarsdale diet provided just such a combination of foods, making it possible to lose an average of a pound or more each day. He attributed this to the metabolic state called ketosis (see chapter 5), which figures prominently in the Atkins diet; however, Tarnower showed little understanding of how it worked. Here's what he said: "If you are producing [ketones,] it is a sign that your body is burning off fat at an accelerated rate; you are enjoying Fast Fat Metabolism." Of course, this statement ignores the fact that the body is producing ketones at all times and that the production of ketones is a normal state of metabolism. Perhaps Tarnower was confusing the mere *production of ketones* with the *dietary ketosis* that Atkins addressed, but the problem was that it would have been completely impossible to get into dietary ketosis on the Scarsdale diet, as you will see in a minute. The "Mystery of Diet Chemistry" section—which ran all of about two pages—mentioned nothing about insulin.

The diet itself was about 1,000 calories *or less* per day and averaged 43 percent protein, 23 percent fat, and 35 percent carbs. With those numbers, a dieter would be taking in 88 grams of carbohydrate a day, which by the standards of the American diet certainly qualifies as relatively low-carb, but would prevent virtually anyone from reaching the state of ketosis that Tarnower seemed to think necessary. Tarnower subscribed to the calorie theory wholeheartedly, made no mention of the possibility of metabolic variances among people, and believed completely in the diet-heart hypotheses, which holds that both fat and cholesterol in the diet cause heart disease, so he kept both as low as possible. He also believed that fat made you fat, another reason he advocated cutting fat consumption way down and forbade any oils, butter, dairy, animal fat, or avocados. The diet then can be seen as a hodgepodge of low-fat, low-carbohydrate, and low-calorie thinking.

Breakfast was the same each day: half a grapefruit, black coffee or tea, and one slice of protein bread with no topping. (Tarnower gave the recipe for the "protein" bread, though there is absolutely nothing in it that would distinguish it as a "high-protein" bread. It's made of flour, water, yeast, and seasoning.) Twice a week for lunch, you ate all the fruit you wanted, period (plus the requisite black coffee, which seemed to be a part of every meal). The rest of the meals were some combination of protein and vegetables. There was absolutely no sugar, potatoes, pasta, flour-based foods (other than his "protein bread"), full-fat dairy, or desserts. You were permitted to eat carrots and celery in any amount you wished, as often as you liked.

In its heyday, the Scarsdale diet got a lot of media attention, including an article in *The New York Times* by Georgia Dullea headlined "If It's Friday, It Must Be Spinach and Cheese." In that article she enthused: "The Scarsdale Diet: This is where the losers live, the real losers. This is the home of the famous 14-day Scarsdale diet. . . . Weight losses of up to 20 pounds in two weeks are reported here. Rarely do dieters feel hungry or cranky. . . . The Scarsdale Diet is spreading. . . . Requests are coming from as far away as California and Mexico. Now London is ringing up about the Scarsdale Diet. . . . Everywhere you go people are talking about [it]."

Tarnower was something of a paternalistic jerk, given to statements like "Let's face it—most overweight people *love to eat*. The very obese are often gluttonous." One of his readers wrote to him with the following question: "When I diet, I get cranky and my husband says, 'I like you better fat than cranky.' Have you any suggestions?" Tarnower wrote back, "You should be able to diet without getting cranky. Your husband, I am sure, would like to have you attractive, lean, and pleasant!" Tarnower was ultimately shot to death in 1980 by his former lover, school headmistress Jean Harris, who, it was rumored, had run out of the amphetamines he prescribed for her.

JONNY'S LOWDOWN   Zero Stars

This diet is a complete waste of time, and is only mentioned here because it is still in print and still has a following. This is the kind of book that gives low-carbing a bad name. It is based on no real knowledge of the hormonal response to food, tries to be all things to all people (low-fat, low-calorie, and low-carb), limits calories to an almost dangerous level, and on top of all that is unrealistically rigid. The only thing it brings to the table—done so much better by others—is a limitation on sugar, starch, and flour.

Books in the Series

The Complete Scarsdale Medical Diet: Plus Dr. Tarnower's Lifetime Keep-Slim Program

About the Author

Herman Tarnower was a cardiologist and internist who was honorary president and chairman of the board of the Westchester Heart Association. He had been a clinical professor of medicine at New York Medical College, an attending cardiologist at White Plains Hospital in New York, and a consulting cardiologist at St. Agnes Hospital in White Plains.

Website

There is no official Scarsdale diet website, but occasional support sites can be found by searching the Internet.

THE SCHWARZBEIN PRINCIPLE

DIANA SCHWARZBEIN, M.D.

WHAT IT IS IN A NUTSHELL

A program designed not specifically for weight loss but for metabolic healing, which, when successful, results in weight loss. Schwarzbein says, "You need to get healthy to lose weight, not lose weight to get healthy." In her second book in the series, The Schwarzbein Principle II, *you compute your protein requirement and your maximum carbohydrate allowance for each meal and snack, then construct your menu accordingly.*

About the Schwarzbein Principle

Let me start by saying this: if you are a dedicated low-carber, the original *Schwarzbein Principle* should be in your library, regardless of whether you choose to follow the program or not. It's as good a basic reference book on hormonal health, the need for good fats, the arguments against a low-fat diet, and the relationship of hormones to health and aging as we're likely to see. If you're not yet familiar with the case against the low-fat diet and the concept of eating plenty of good fats (which include saturates!) and protein, this is a great place to start. If these concepts are old-hat to you and you want to actually try the program, the second book, *The Schwarzbein Principle II*, is the place to begin. The original is the overview and will give you the basics; *Schwarzbein II* is a more fully realized eating plan.

The Schwarzbein Principle can be summed up as follows:

- All systems of the human body are connected.
- One imbalance creates another imbalance.
- Eating too many man-made carbohydrates is the number one reason for hormonal imbalances.
- Poor eating and lifestyle habits—not genetics—cause diseases of aging.

The actual eating plan depends on where you fit in a matrix of four metabolic types. What type you are depends on the operating health of two of the major hormonal systems in your body: your *insulin metabolism* and your *adrenal metabolism*. Most people reading *Living the Low-Carb Life* understand by now the concept of insulin resistance and the role elevated insulin levels play in weight gain. We saw in chapter 2 just how this mechanism operates, and it is the underlying concept in every one of the diet plans discussed in this book. What has *not* been emphasized in any of the plans so far is adrenal health.

The adrenal glands are responsible for the secretion of two critical hormones: *cortisol* and *adrenaline*. These are also known as *stress hormones*—they are involved in the "fight or flight" response. Cortisol is a major hormone. It keeps your blood pressure from dropping too low, and you need it in every cell of your body—without it, you would die. Adrenaline is another major hormone; it keeps your heart beating. Adrenaline is the primitive hormone that saved our butts from being eaten when confronted with a saber-toothed tiger on the savanna. That's why cortisol and adrenaline are called the "fight or flight" hormones—in response to stress (like a life-threatening emergency), they prepare you for either picking up a club to fight off a bear or running like hell for the nearest tree.

These hormones served our Paleolithic ancestors well as a kind of "turbo" system for emergency response. The problem is that our current lifestyle causes them to charge around our systems far more than is strictly necessary. They are our constant companions. Our poor, overworked adrenals respond to daily stresses and secrete them when we're stuck in traffic, when we have a report due, when we get into a fight with the hotel clerk, when the telemarketer interrupts our dinner, and when we have a fight with our boyfriend/girlfriend/husband/wife/son/daughter/boss. And just like our poor pancreas eventually can "burn out" from the constant demand put on it to produce enough insulin to deal with a chronically high-carbohydrate diet, so can our poor adrenals eventually reach a similarly exhausted state. This is what Schwarzbein and others call *adrenal burnout*. It is hardly uncommon.

So if we're interested only in weight loss, why should we care about our adrenals?

Well, first off, the adrenal hormone cortisol, like all hormones in the body, sends a message. Several, actually. One is to break down muscle for fuel. If you break down muscle, you do two things: you lower your metabolic rate (since muscle is where the fat and calories are burned) and you reduce the number of muscle cells that are able to accept sugar, leading to more sugar being stored as fat and eventually more insulin resistance. Cortisol also sends a message to the brain to "refuel" for emergency, leading almost inevitably to stress eating.

Since cortisol is involved in breaking down the bodily proteins—both functional and structural—eventually, if levels of cortisol remain high, the body will do something to protect itself against breaking down too much. Can you guess what hormone it sends in as reinforcement? *Insulin.* Too much cortisol eventually triggers insulin, the storage hormone, to counter the catabolic (breaking-down) processes in an attempt to rebuild the ship. If this happens frequently enough, you will eventually have high levels of insulin and will become insulin-resistant. Remember that adrenaline helps your body *use up* your biochemicals; insulin helps your body *rebuild them*— including the fat stores! Hence, chronically high cortisol can wind up being a cause of insulin resistance.

It gets worse. Chronic oversecretion of the stress hormone cortisol will cause you to use up serotonin. Less serotonin almost always goes hand in hand with cravings, especially for sugar and carbohydrate. Those cravings, a kind of biochemical "mandate," can be irresistible even for people with amazing willpower. Give into the cravings—as most people will—and the cycle continues. You use up serotonin anytime your cortisol and adrenaline levels get too high—when you don't sleep, when you are stressed, and when you overuse stimulants (including refined sugar, nicotine, and caffeine). This is one reason why stress management figures so prominently in the Schwarzbein program.

In the Schwarzbein Principle, you first determine which of four metabolic categories you fit into:

1. insulin-sensitive with healthy adrenals
2. insulin-sensitive with burned-out adrenals
3. insulin-resistant with healthy adrenals
4. insulin-resistant with burned-out adrenals

These four categories represent varying degrees of metabolic damage and require very different eating plans for healing. The underlying thinking here is that you *must* heal your metabolism before you can begin to lose weight. The program consists of five elements:

1. nutrition
2. stress management
3. cross-training exercise (usually of a low-intensity level)
4. eliminating stimulants and drugs
5. hormone replacement therapy, if needed

All five elements don't have to be done at once. The transition into metabolic health is gradual and gentle and takes place in stages.

You first determine your protein needs using a very simple formula. Those with healthy adrenals do not have to monitor protein; they can "listen to their bodies," though guidelines are given for those who want them. The formula and guidelines give *minimum* protein needs and should be divided among the three meals (and usually two snacks) that you will eat every day. You can eat more protein if you want, but not less. Then you determine your carbohydrate allowance, which is also divided into three meals and two snacks. You do not count calories, and you do not measure or count fat.

Carbohydrate allowances range from a low of 15 grams per meal and 7½ grams per snack (60 grams per day) to a high of 45 grams per meal and 20 grams per snack (175 grams per day), though the high end of the range is only for the rare person who is insulin-sensitive with healthy adrenals and is very, very active. There are meal plans given for 15, 20, 25, 30, 35, and 40 grams of carbs per meal. There are vegetarian versions of all meal plans, and there are even low-saturated-fat versions of most of the meal plans for those very special cases where saturated fat has to be limited (Schwarzbein does not normally limit saturated fat).

Carbs—though much more limited than in standard diets—are not eliminated and, in Schwarzbein's view, are essential to the success of the program. The reason is this: if you eat too *many* carbs (and too much food), your insulin levels will rise too high and you will become insulin-resistant if you aren't already; if you already are, too many carbs will certainly make matters worse. But if you don't eat *enough* carbs, you will raise adrenaline and cortisol too high, using up your precious biochemicals and eventually becoming insulin-resistant anyway.

The Schwarzbein Principle as a Lifestyle: Who It Works for, Who Should Look Elsewhere

People who flock from all over the country to Diana Schwarzbein's practice in Santa Barbara, California, are frequently people at the end of their rope—they have tried every diet, damaged their metabolisms, and turned their hormonal balance on its ear. She has an amazing success rate, but you clearly have to be patient. This is not a diet for weight loss; it is a program for metabolic healing, and in many cases you have to be prepared to actually gain weight before you begin to lose. In addition, the careful

computing of grams of carbohydrate per meal and snack doesn't appeal
to everyone. If you're willing to be patient and are looking at the long-
term picture, you've probably come to the right place. If you need more
immediate results, if you're concerned only with weight loss, if you can't
deal with counting carbs, or if you don't feel you've damaged your metabolism all that much, this might not be the best place to start.

JONNY'S LOWDOWN ★ ★ ★ ★ ☆

*You simply cannot say enough good things about Diana Schwarzbein.
She truly is a giant in the field and one of the most knowledgeable
cutting-edge endocrinologists in the country. Interestingly, many of
the people I interviewed for this book started with more basic plans
like Atkins and then, when they got closer to maintenance, moved to
the Schwarzbein Principle. As an overall plan for health, this is five-
star material. But as a weight loss diet—which it was never intended
to be—it may not be the ideal entry-level plan, as it requires a good
deal of patience and a lot of commitment.*

Books in the Series
*The Schwarzbein Principle: The Truth About Losing Weight, Being Healthy, and
Feeling Younger*
*The Schwarzbein Principle II—The Transition: A Regeneration Process to
Prevent and Reverse Accelerated Aging*
The Schwarzbein Principle Cookbook
The Schwarzbein Principle Vegetarian Cookbook

Best Book to Start With
The Schwarzbein Principle II: The Transition (unless you're unfamiliar with
the whole lower-carb, higher-fat concept, in which case you couldn't do
better than the original *Schwarzbein Principle*)

About the Author
Diana Schwarzbein, M.D., is a leading authority on metabolic healing
and hormonal health. She founded the Endocrinology Institute of Santa
Barbara, where she specializes in metabolism, diabetes, osteoporosis,
menopause, and thyroid conditions. She is a frequent and very in-demand
speaker at workshops and conferences, such as the prestigious and cutting-
edge annual nutrition conference Boulderfest.

Website

At schwarzbeinprinciple.com, you can order a package of metabolic tests, complete with a full interpretation. The site has personal experiences, a book and vitamin store, and a great FAQ section with clips from Schwarzbein's appearances on various television shows, where you can actually hear the answers to frequent questions.

SOMERSIZING

SUZANNE SOMERS

WHAT IT IS IN A NUTSHELL

A version of food combining. You eat full-fat foods like butter, cream, eggs, and red meat, plus whole-grain carbs, fruit, and vegetables, but only in certain combinations. No calorie counting or carb measuring.

About Somersizing

The basic premise of Somersizing is that foods fall into four groups, which Suzanne Somers defines as protein/fats, veggies, carbs, and fruits. There is a fifth group called "funky foods," which you can't eat at all, at least during level one, the weight loss phase. Funky foods are sugar, white flour, caffeine, alcohol, beets, carrots, white rice, corn, potatoes, sweet potatoes, parsnips, yams, pumpkin, several kinds of squash, and bananas.

The foods in the four Somersizing food groups have to be combined in specific ways. Protein/fats can be eaten together or in combination with vegetables, but not with carbohydrates. Carbohydrates can be eaten with vegetables, but not with protein/fats. Fruits need to be eaten alone.

It's a lovely system. The problem is that it has absolutely no basis in fact and doesn't even make sense on an intuitive level. While Somers gives a good if very amateurish explanation of insulin, the glycemic index of food, and the connection of insulin to weight gain, she doesn't seem to understand that combining protein, fat, or both with carbohydrate is precisely what is most likely to blunt the insulin response (or the glycemic effect of the meal).

She also doesn't understand the glycemic load. The glycemic load, a much more telling measure of a food's ability to raise blood sugar than the somewhat old-fashioned glycemic index, is based on the glycemic index times the amount of actual carbohydrate in a usual-size portion of the food. While carrots do have a high glycemic index, they have a glycemic *load* of three on a scale that goes from zero to the high twenties. Beets have a glycemic load of five. There's no need to eliminate either one. (For more on the difference between the glycemic index and the glycemic load, see page 247.)

Then there are the "combo" foods that she suggests you leave out (at least during level one) because they contain mixtures of protein and carbohydrates. These foods include nuts, olives, avocados, and a few others. Here's what she says about nuts: "They are a protein, they *do* have fat, and they are rich in carbohydrates. That makes them a no-no for Somersizing purposes." Evidently she has never looked at a food count book. Nuts are primarily a fat, they *do* have some protein, and they have almost *no* usable or effective carbohydrate.* Example: an ounce of almonds has 6 grams of carbs, of which 3 are fiber, leaving only 3 grams of effective carbohydrate mixed with its 14 grams of fat. Pecans have only 1 usable gram of carbohydrate mixed with its 21 grams of fat. Olives have *no* grams of carbohydrate (they're on her combo list for God only knows what reason). And the carb content of an entire avocado—which is not exactly one portion—is only 5 grams. These foods are all almost entirely fat (good fat, of course), but are considered "funky" because they have trace amounts of carbs mixed in (except for the olives, which have none). Therefore, according to Somers, you can't eat these foods while losing weight. But you *can* eat whole-grain pastas and cereals, which are far more "mixed" foods than nuts or avocados! Fettuccine contains 40 grams of carbs but 8 grams of protein; spaghetti has 7 to 10 grams of protein with its 40 grams of carbs; and whole-grain oatmeal contains about 6 grams of protein with its 27 grams of carbohydrate. If you're going to forbid nuts because they break the "no carbs mixed with protein" rule, why on earth would you permit foods like these that have even an even *greater* mix?

She is right that we are better off frying in saturated fats like butter or lard than in unsaturated oil like corn, safflower, or canola. And let's give her credit for some good statements, such as:

- "Sadly, people are eliminating saturated fats like eggs, cheese, butter, and red meat, thinking they are the culprit for raised cholesterol and heart disease when in actuality raised insulin levels and trans-fats are the problem."
- "Get back to eating real fats like butter, cream, and eggs."
- "Have no fear of the egg. Embrace it. It is one of earth's most perfect foods. And please, eat the yolk. The yolk contains the essential fats we need to thrive."

---

*To get the "effective" (or "net") carb content of a food, you simply look at the label and subtract the number of grams of fiber from the total number of carbohydrates. What's left is the net amount of carbs, which is all you need to count. For a fuller discussion of net/effective carbs, see page 229.

All good stuff, especially the point about eating real, natural fats. Finally, she gets points—or at least one star—for her constant emphasis on eliminating refined foods: "There is nothing healthy about replacing real foods with fat-free products that have no nutritional benefit."

Somersizing as a Lifestyle: Who It Works for, Who Should Look Elsewhere

Well, obviously this plan works for some people, because her books are filled with before-and-after pictures of her fans, and her website is crowded with enthusiastic "Somersizers." My guess is that even with Somersizing's convoluted biochemistry, its emphasis on real foods is a vast improvement over the standard American diet, so if that's what you've been eating and you switch to this, you're probably going to benefit. The real appeal is that you can eat all these rich foods and don't have to "cut out" carbs. If you don't mind doing the voodoo nutrition of figuring out what goes with what, you could try this diet—it certainly won't harm you. If you are insulin-resistant, sugar-sensitive, or carb-addicted, the pasta, cereals, and such—whole-grain or not—are not going to be welcome, and you should look elsewhere.

JONNY'S LOWDOWN   ★ ★ ☆ ☆

It's hard to dislike Suzanne Somers. She's smart, gorgeous, and a tremendous businesswoman (witness her ability to sell millions of dollars worth of the useless Thighmaster), and she has an uncanny ability to inspire Oprah-like devotion in her fans. What she is not: a nutritionist. To read these books is to profoundly understand the meaning of the phrase "a little knowledge is a dangerous thing."

So is this book totally worthless?

No. Not totally. It's a small step in the right direction, but it's a few dollars short and a few weeks late. She makes the familiar arguments against low-calorie, low-fat diets (good). She is good on the subject of trans-fats.

But just when you're thinking it might be safe to go back in the water, here comes a statement like this: "A single potato is so high in starch it provides us with more energy than most people need in a day." All at once, can everybody say "gibberish"? I'm no defender of potatoes, but this statement is beyond the pale. And her hawking of her special sweetener, SomerSweet, as a "miracle" because it's made of fructose and "has little effect on insulin" doesn't exactly inspire confidence. Fructose is actually linked to insulin resistance (through a mechanism other than raising blood sugar), and it also raises triglycerides—a serious risk factor for heart disease. (For more on triglycerides, see page 42) The Drs. Eades called fructose "potentially the most dangerous and damaging of all the sugars."[8] Some miracle.

I doubt this diet would work for everyone because the carbs are not low enough to produce an appetite-blunting effect, and the basically unlimited calories of the rich foods allowed—in the presence of what are potentially higher insulin levels than she anticipates—are not a recipe for weight loss success. It might work for people who have been eating really, really badly on a diet composed completely of processed fast foods—the switch to whole foods alone might be more hunger-satisfying, definitely more healthy, and possibly enough to stimulate weight loss.

One more thing: Somers has enlisted Dr. Diana Schwarzbein to write the introduction, and quotes her frequently. Dr. Schwarzbein is one of the best and brightest endocrinologists in the country, and her own program, the Schwarzbein Principle, is reviewed on page 142. But let's be clear: with all due respect to Dr. Schwarzbein, whom I know, have studied with, and have worked with, this program is no Schwarzbein Principle—it's not even Schwarzbein Principle Lite. I suspect that Schwarzbein likes Somers and endorses her because of her emphasis on eating real food. Beyond that, don't let the Schwarzbein name fool you into thinking there's any real science or meat to this program. There's not.

I gave this plan two stars purely for the emphasis on real food.

Books in the Series

Suzanne Somers' Fast and Easy: Lose Weight the Somersize Way with Quick, Delicious Meals for the Entire Family!

Suzanne Somers' Eat, Cheat, and Melt the Fat Away

Eat Great, Lose Weight

Suzanne Somers' Get Skinny on Fabulous Food

Somersize Desserts

Somersizing (video, 1996)

Best Book to Start With

It doesn't make much difference. *Eat Great, Lose Weight* was the first, but all of the books recap the program and differ only in the recipes section. As good as any is *Suzanne Somers' Eat, Cheat, and Melt the Fat Away.*

About the Author

Suzanne Somers is a former star of *Three's Company* and has had a highly successful second career as a marketer of fitness, beauty, and health products. She's also well known as a pitchwoman on Home Shopping Network, where she sells, among other things, jewelry.

Website

If you're a fan, you'll love suzannesomers.com; if you're not, you'll be nauseated. She pitches all of her products and has a beauty section, a lifestyle section, a fitness section (where she sells the godawful Thighmaster, among other things), a community with transcripts of chats, a motivational section with little Hallmark card–type sayings, and, of course, a Somersizing section, where she sells the rapidly expanding catalog of books in the series. The site is Oprah Lite.

THE SOUTH BEACH DIET

ARTHUR AGATSTON, M.D.

WHAT IT IS IN A NUTSHELL

*A three-phase diet plan. For the first two weeks you cut out com-
pletely: bread, rice, potatoes, pasta, baked goods, fruit, sugar, and
alcohol. During the second phase, you add back just enough carbs to
let you continue to lose weight. In the third phase, when you've
reached your goal weight, you can add back still more carbs from
any category of food you like.*

About the South Beach Diet

The South Beach diet is very . . . *friendly.* Written by a cardiologist, it has
the benefit of a terrific marketing campaign, sports a great-looking cover,
and borrows the cachet of a sleek, sexy, very "in" area of Miami known for
its celebrities, models, and generally very good-looking people. That gets
your attention. More important is the fact that the information deserves it.

According to the author, Arthur Agatston, the South Beach Diet was
designed *not* with weight loss as its main goal but to improve the heart
health of his patients "by changing their blood chemistry." Agatston says
his heart patients—and his diabetics ones—lost weight "like crazy" ("10,
20, 30, even 50 pounds within months"), much of it from their midsec-
tions. The diet caught on and wound up featured on the local ABC affil-
iate station in a segment in which Miami Beach residents who wanted to
lose weight were put on the diet and then followed around for a month.
The station, WPLG, scored big with the feature, and it became an annual
"South Beach Diet challenge" for three years. Eventually, the South Beach
diet became known nationally, and was enthusiastically endorsed by a
wide range of people, including former president Bill Clinton.

Here's how it works. For the first fourteen days, you are on a decidedly low-carb regimen in which you cut out all bread, rice, potatoes,
pasta, baked goods, dairy, fruit, sugar, and alcohol. Eggs are unlimited.
You can have most kinds of cheese (except for Brie, Edam, and full-fat
cheese), certain sugar-free desserts, and a couple of kinds of nuts. You
can also drink coffee. According to Agatston, you will lose between 8 and

13 pounds in the first two weeks, and most of that will come off your mid-section.

In phase two, you reintroduce fruit, certain cereals, bran muffins, pasta, whole-grain breads, and other starches, albeit in small amounts. On this phase, you continue to lose weight at the reasonable rate of 1 to 2 pounds a week. When you get to your goal, you go on phase three, which is your lifetime-maintenance "forever" plan. At this point, you can eat anything—there are no restrictions on what kind of carbs you can take in, which, of course, makes it very attractive for some people. Regarding these "foods you love," the author says, "You won't be able to have all of them, all the time. You'll learn to enjoy them a little differently than before—maybe a little less enthusiastically. But you will enjoy them again."

Agatston starts with the same basic premise as the low-carb theorists: high amounts of insulin are responsible for weight gain, and limiting carbs stabilizes both blood sugar and insulin. He explains, "The equation behind most obesity is simple: the faster the sugar and starches you eat are processed and absorbed into your bloodstream, the fatter you get." He suggests eating foods and combinations of foods (i.e., proteins and fats with minimal carbs) that cause *gradual* rather than *sharp* increases in blood sugar. He makes distinctions between good carbs (low-glycemic, whole-grain) and bad (processed, sugary, high in starch). So far, so good.

The author is a cardiologist and takes a traditional approach to "good fats" and "bad fats." Though one could dispute his wholesale damnation of saturated fats, one could also argue that his condemnation of them is likely to make him more acceptable to the medical establishment, which is a good thing, as his thinking on the subjects of carb consumption, blood sugar, insulin, and weight gain is right on the money. And while he and I might have a friendly disagreement over saturated fats, we concur that trans-fats are the worst, and Agatston hammers this important point home time and again. And no one is going to object to his inclusion of plenty of good marine fats like fish oils.

The popularity of the diet is probably due to how realistic it is. ("It's important for people to like the food they eat. Eating is meant to bring pleasure even when you're trying to lose weight. That's a sensible way to think about food and it's one of the basic principles of the South Beach Diet.") Agatston has some great recipes for desserts, like a tiramisu made from ricotta cheese and cocoa powder, as well as some good side dishes, "mashed potatoes" made from cauliflower. But the most appealing part of the diet may be the fact that after the initial Atkins-like spartan regimen, you can add back just about any carbs you want, as long as you keep the portions small and continue to lose weight; when you get to your goal, you can eat anything you want as long as you don't gain.

This could be a problem for some people. Such unstructured eating looks great on paper and works great for many, but it can be a slippery slope for others. Start by adding one slice of bread or one piece of chocolate cake, and for many people, the ballgame is over. It's like letting an alcoholic have one drink. But if you can follow his advice and stick to the moderate portion doctrine, you'll allow those "favorite foods" to become occasional treats rather than mainstays of your diet. In this scenario, you'll love the foods you're eating, you won't feel overly restricted, and the health benefits you receive are likely to be enormous. This is truly healthy, realistic, controlled-carb eating for the masses.

The South Beach Diet as a Lifestyle: Who It Works for, Who Should Look Elsewhere

People who want to have their cake and eat it, *literally*, will love this plan. Because it makes a lot of concessions to "real-life" eating habits and, after the weight loss period, does not restrict any food whatsoever, it's bound to have a ton of appeal. And if you are the kind of person who can do moderation, it's a great diet, providing plenty of protein, good fats, vegetables, and just enough carbohydrates to keep the demons at bay. However, this liberal way of doing things is potentially problematic for people who like specified amounts and clear instructions and want to know exactly what they can and can't eat. If you fall into this category, you might be better off either staying on the first phase a bit longer or starting with a more structured plan and graduating to South Beach later on.

JONNY'S LOWDOWN	★ ★ ★ ★ ★

This is a terrific book. Although some of my colleagues have criticized it for "not being anything new," (one internet pundit called it "Atkins for the first two weeks and then the Zone"), I'm not sure this criticism is fair. Sure, much of the information on insulin and weight control has been out there for a while—but those of us who have been preaching it have remained outside the mainstream.

The genius of Agatston is that he has taken this information and made it extremely user-friendly and accessible, and has done so while making sure not to alienate his more conservative colleagues in the medical profession. This makes it much more likely that his important message will actually be heard. The friendly tone, accessibility, and overall permissiveness of the plan practically guarantees that its intelligent, lower-carb message will reach thousands of people who might have ignored the more "militant" platforms. For that we owe Agatston a lot of thanks. Adopting some form of the South Beach diet would represent a giant step forward for most Americans, and because it is presented in such an unintimidating way, it's more likely that people will adopt it.

Books in the Series

The South Beach Diet: The Delicious, Doctor-Designed, Foolproof Plan for Fast and Healthy Weight Loss
The South Beach Diet Cookbook
The South Beach Diet Good Fats/Good Carbs Guide

About the Author

Arthur Agatston, M.D., is a specialist in noninvasive cardiac imaging—the technology that produces sophisticated pictures of the heart and the coronary blood vessels. In CT (computerized tomography) scanning all over the world, the measure of coronary calcium is called the Agatston Score, and the protocol for calcium screening is often referred to as the Agatston Method. He maintains an active, full-time cardiology practice (both clinical and research) in Miami, Florida, and has served on committees of the American College of Cardiology and the Society of Atherosclerosis Imaging; for the latter, he is a member of the founding board of directors.

Website

The official website, southbeachdiet.com, encourages you to join up (it costs $29.95 for six weeks). For this you get a weight tracker (you type in your weight and chart your progress), a meal planner and scheduler, an online journal where you can record your thoughts and feelings, and access to message boards where you can post and ask questions of the experts, including Agatston. The "free" part of the site is basically an advertisement for the paid part and offers no other information of note.

SUGAR BUSTERS!

H. LEIGHTON STEWARD, M.S., MORRISON BETHEA, M.D., SAMUEL ANDREWS, M.D., AND LUIS BALART, M.D.

WHAT IT IS IN A NUTSHELL

Lower-carb for dummies—technically, it's not a low-carb diet at all. A basic plan that essentially focuses on reducing or eliminating sugar from the diet. No counting of calories, carbs, protein, or fat.

About Sugar Busters!

Sugar Busters! was the brainchild of a Fortune 500 CEO and three respected New Orleans doctors—a cardiovascular surgeon, an endocrinologist, and a gastroenterologist—whose success with this way of eating led to the publication of the book. Legend has it that it was originally a self-published manuscript that circulated, got enormous attention, and eventually landed the authors a real book deal.

The four basic premises of Sugar Busters! are really simple.

1. Too much insulin wreaks havoc on our bodies and is a huge player in the weight loss game.
2. Sugar produces insulin.
3. Sugar is toxic.
4. If you reduce sugar with the Sugar Busters! diet, you will control insulin.

Like many of the authors discussed in this book, the authors of *Sugar Busters!* subscribe to the theory that calories are not as important as the type of foods eaten. They cite a study from the *American Journal of Clinical Nutrition* that concluded that calorie intake alone is *not* sufficient to predict weight gain or loss in any given individual.[9] They also subscribe to the theory that it is not dietary fat that makes you fat so much as it is dietary sugar. (By now you understand the reason: excess carbohydrates feed the production mill for triglycerides, the form of fat that is stored in the fat tissues.)

Not only does dietary sugar get converted into fat, but as you remember from chapter 2, lots of sugar and carbs in the diet produce increased levels of insulin, the hormone that creates fat storage *and* blocks fat burning (technically called lipolysis). The authors say, quite correctly, that "we cannot survive without insulin, *but* we can survive a lot better without *too much* insulin." That's a darn good quote. Dietary sugar is now recognized as an independent risk factor for cardiovascular disease, largely through the mechanism of its effect on insulin secretion. Insulin also causes retention of salt (increasing blood pressure) and a thickening of the arterial walls (see chapter 2 for details). The authors state that it also causes enlargement of the left ventricle, which is the chamber involved in 99 percent of heart attacks, and that it causes the development of plaque in or on the walls of blood vessels.

Glucagon, the sister hormone of insulin, also produced by the pancreas, has the opposite effect of insulin. It tells the body to break down fat. It is a "releasing" hormone, not a "storing" hormone. Glucagon tends to rise after a higher-protein meal and is inhibited by high levels of insulin.

So it is no surprise that the stated purpose of the Sugar Busters! diet is this: *controlling insulin by controlling sugar.* To eliminate or reduce the sugars that are so detrimental to your health and your waistline, the authors rely heavily on the *glycemic index,* a measure of how quickly blood sugar is raised in response to a food (more on this in Jonny's Lowdown). The authors state that knowledge of the glycemic index is key to understanding the Sugar Busters! diet concept. There is a list of acceptable and unacceptable foods, based largely on the glycemic index. (The list of acceptable foods is way larger than that of many of the plans in this book.)

So far, so good. The authors recommend a diet composed of natural, unrefined sugars; whole, unprocessed grains; vegetables; fruits; lean meats; fiber; and alcohol, in moderation. There are a few dozen fruits that are allowed, as are whole-grain breads and pastas, virtually all dairy products, lots of vegetables, and of course meats, fowl, and fish. There is no counting of carbs, calories, fat grams, or protein, but the authors do recommend cutting saturated fats. Foods to avoid include potatoes, white rice, all kinds of corn, carrots, beets, white bread, and of course sugar. The authors state that if you follow their recommendations, you will wind up with a diet of about 40 percent carbohydrates (of the low-glycemic variety), 30 percent protein, and 30 percent fat (exactly what Barry Sears recommends in *The Zone,* though the authors do not credit him).

They also recommend not eating after 8 P.M. and eating multiple (three) meals, because they believe several small meals produce less overall insulin secretion than one or two large meals. They believe portion control is key and state that if you place proper servings on the plate, counting grams is not necessary.

Other than offering general rules of what to stay away from, there is no specific "diet," though they offer a sample fourteen-day meal plan and many recipes.

Sugar Busters! as a Lifestyle: Who It Works for, Who Should Look Elsewhere

Sugar Busters! is not really a diet and is very loosely constructed. As an alternative to the standard American diet, it's a move in the right direction. The basic concept—less white sugar and fewer foods that contain it—is a good one, though awfully simple, and not necessarily one that by itself will produce results in metabolically resistant people. If you need more structure, or if you are very carb-sensitive or carb-addicted, this is not the best place to start.

JONNY'S LOWDOWN ★ ★ ☆ ☆ ☆

It's funny—when the first Sugar Busters! book came out, the conventional nutrition establishment (dietitians, etc.) attacked it for blaming sugar and insulin for overweight instead of putting the blame where it "belonged"—on calories. We on the "left wing" didn't think very highly of the book because it didn't go far enough. It's filled with some half-baked concepts, such as the idea that fructose is a "good" sugar because it doesn't raise blood sugar a lot (ignoring the fact that it raises triglycerides more than any other sugar and actually raises insulin through a different means). The book doesn't—even in the newer edition—make any distinction between the glycemic index and the glycemic load, a difference that readers of this book will understand is very important (see page 247). It makes a big deal about carrots but allows fruit juice and "whole-grain pasta" (let me know if you can find a real-life example of the latter). The first sample meal on day one is "orange juice, 1 package instant oatmeal with skim milk, Equal and coffee," which is ridiculous from a glycemic and insulin-control point of view. But with that said, the authors are very clear that they tried to design their way of eating for compliance, not cheating. For most of America, it's a step forward. People who are knowledgeable about carb intake, insulin resistance, chronic weight problems, and the like will probably find this program far too lenient and somewhat unsophisticated. The stars are awarded for effort.

Books in the Series
The New Sugar Busters! Cut Sugar to Trim Fat
Sugar Busters! for Kids
Sugar Busters! Quick & Easy Cookbook
Sugar Busters! Shopper's Guide

Best Book to Start With
The New Sugar Busters! Cut Sugar to Trim Fat by H. Leighton Steward, Morrison Bethea, M.D., Samuel Andrews, M.D., and Luis Balart, M.D.

About the Authors
H. Leighton Steward has an M.S. and is the CEO of a Fortune 500 energy company. Morrison Bethea, M.D., is a cardiac surgeon and a diplomat of the American Board of Thoracic Surgery. Samuel Andrews, M.D., is a practicing endocrinologist and a clinical associate professor of medicine at Louisiana State University. Luis Balart, M.D., is a gastroenterologist at Tenet's Memorial Medical Center in New Orleans and clinical associate professor of medicine at Louisiana State.

Website
The official site, sugarbusters.com, contains a brief explanation of the Sugar Busters! concept, info about the authors, ordering info, details about the books, a FAQ page, and a nice reader's forum called "Sweet Talk."

THE ZONE

BARRY SEARS, PH.D.

WHAT IT IS IN A NUTSHELL

An eating plan consisting of 40 percent carbohydrates, 30 percent protein, and 30 percent fat. Zone orthodoxy calls for eating five times a day—three meals and two snacks, each of which should contain the 40/30/30 distribution.

About the Zone

Tell Barry Sears, creator of the Zone, that his eating plan is a high-protein diet, and you're likely to be met with either an icy stare or a frustrated sigh, depending on his mood. Most often, you'll get a resigned explanation that you sense (correctly) he's given a thousand times. "The Zone," he says patiently, "is *not* a high-protein diet. It is a protein-*adequate* diet. The amount of protein recommended on the Zone is very similar to what Americans are currently consuming. The amount of fruits and vegetables that are recommended on the Zone diet is nearly three times the amounts recommended by the U.S. government, even though the amount of total carbohydrates is lower."

He's got a point. This just might be the most misunderstood and falsely maligned popular dietary approach of all time, considering the fact that it has probably had the most influence on changing the dietary tenor of the times, especially in altering the prevailing attitude about fat as the demon behind obesity and disease. Let's go over just what the Zone is and what it isn't.

The Zone is not a high-protein diet, despite the fact that critics—who seem never to have read the book—continue to refer to it as such, especially in popular magazines. The amount of protein on the Zone diet could hardly be considered high (except by the intransigent right-wing of the dietary establishment, the American Dietetic Association). On a 1,500 calorie diet, 30 percent protein—the amount recommended by Sears—works out to 112 grams of protein (roughly 16 ounces) a day. That's about 4 ounces per meal and 2 ounces per snack for the average man, nowhere near an excessive amount.

The Zone is also not a low-carb diet. Do the math—you're always eating slightly more carbohydrates at every meal than you are eating protein or fat. In fact, 40 percent of your meal is carbohydrates, yielding, with the same 1,500 calorie intake, 150 grams of carbs a day. Just for comparison, Atkins allows 20 grams per day on the induction phase of his program. The Zone allows more than seven times that amount. The Zone diet gets most of its carbohydrates from fruits and vegetables and uses the starchy carbohydrates—breads, pastas, rice, cereal, and the like—sparingly, almost, says Sears, "as condiments."

The Zone was never meant solely as a weight loss diet. It was designed to reduce heart disease through the control of inflammation, and its success and popularity surprised Sears as much as anyone. The fact that so many people lose weight and feel terrific on it, and that it has been adopted by a number of celebrities, put it in the public arena and made Sears either a hero or a monster, depending on what academic pundit you listen to.

The Theory Behind the Zone: A Short Lesson in Nutritional Endocrinology

Think of your body and its organs, glands, hormones, and other chemical compounds as one huge biological Internet, where messages (sometimes conflicting ones) are constantly being sent out, received, interpreted, misinterpreted, and acted upon. Hormones are particularly potent messengers; when you receive a message from a hormone in your biological e-mailbox, you pay attention. Insulin is a hormone—a major one. It's secreted by the pancreas in response to the increased blood sugar that you get after you ingest food (particularly carbohydrates). Insulin is intimately tied to levels of blood sugar. If you eat a Snickers bar, your blood sugar rises and the pancreas says, *"Uh oh, dude ate a Snickers; let's get to work."* It secretes some insulin. The job of that insulin is to bring the blood sugar back down into the normal range. It does this by "escorting" the sugar out of the bloodstream and into the cells. According to Sears, excess insulin is the culprit behind skyrocketing rates of obesity, a premise he shares with all low-carb diet writers.

There are two basic ways to raise insulin levels. One is to eat too many carbohydrates. The other is to eat too much food. Americans do both.

The "Zone" actually refers to an *optimal range* of insulin levels. The diet claims to keep insulin levels from rising too high by replacing some of the carbs in the typical American diet with fat (which has no effect on insulin) and protein (which has some effect but not as much as carbs). The balance among carbs, protein, and fat at each meal and snack is designed to prevent blood sugar levels (or insulin levels) from going too high (or too low). This, combined with the fact that the diet is not too high in calories, is responsible for the weight loss effects on the diet.

The *health* effects of the diet are caused by a different, though related, pathway. Remember that the Zone diet was birthed in the midst of a high-carb, low-fat diet mania. All of us in the field of nutrition were seeing clients who had virtually cut fat out of their diets (and almost always replaced it with carbohydrates). They thought they were eating healthily. It was not unusual in those days (and even now, for that matter) to see a woman eating a bagel and orange juice for breakfast, a salad for lunch, a nonfat frozen yogurt for an afternoon snack, and pasta for dinner, then wondering why she wasn't losing weight. The Zone almost single-handedly put the argument for inclusion of good fats in the diet back on the table. And it is through the inclusion of this fat that the Zone diet is thought to have one of its most significant health effects.

Here's how it works. The body makes an entire class of "superhormones" called eicosanoids out of the "raw materials" of essential fats. Eicosanoids are made by every one of the 60 trillion cells in your body. They don't circulate in the body—they're made in a cell, they do their action in the nearby vicinity, and then they self-destruct, all within a matter of seconds, like those little tapes they used to give Peter Graves on *Mission: Impossible*—so they are virtually undectable in the bloodstream. But their importance on human health is incalculable. The 1982 Nobel Prize in Medicine was awarded for eicosanoid research. Your doctor may not know much about eicosanoids, but he or she has undoubtedly heard of prostaglandins. Prostaglandins are eicosanoids made by the prostate gland and were one of the first groups of eicosanoids to be studied.

The type of fat you eat influences the kinds of eicosanoids you make. Eicosanoids come in many "flavors" and types, but for our purposes we'll identify two major classes: the "good" and the "bad." The good are responsible for preventing blood clots, reducing pain, and causing dilation (opening) of the blood vessels, among other things. The bad are responsible for promoting blood clots, promoting pain, and causing constriction (closing) of the blood vessels. The point is not to get rid of *all* the bad ones, but to have a balance between the good and the bad. (For example, if you didn't have eicosanoids that promoted blood clots, you would bleed to death from a minor wound.) Aspirin works by knocking out *all* eicosanoid production for a while, which is a little like killing a fly with a sledgehammer. Corticosteroids do the same thing. The fat included in the Zone diet specifically fosters the creation of good eicosanoids and an optimum balance between the good and the bad.

The insulin connection is this: insulin stimulates the key enzyme involved in producing *arachidonic acid,* which is the "building material" of the bad eicosanoids. So by controlling insulin levels with the Zone diet, you not only lose weight, you also reduce many of the symptoms and health risks that come from an imbalance of good and bad eicosanoids. The promise of the Zone is that controlling insulin will result in increased fat loss, decreased likelihood of cardiovascular disease, and greater physical and mental performance. By controlling eicosanoids, you will have decreased inflammation and increased blood flow, which will help improve virtually every chronic disease condition and improve physical performance.

So What Can You Eat?

A lot. The best protein choices on the plan are skinless chicken, turkey, all kinds of fish, very lean cuts of meat, low-fat dairy products, egg whites, tofu, and soy meat substitutes. For carbohydrates, Sears likes all vegetables except corn and carrots and all fruits except bananas and raisins. The heavy starches like pasta, bread, cereals, rice, and the like are used very, very sparingly. For fats, use olive oil, almonds, avocados, and fish oil.

It's really simple to make a Zone meal, actually, and doesn't require a lot of complicated calculations. All you have to do is divide your plate into thirds. On one-third of the plate, put some low-fat protein—a typical portion would fit in the palm of your hand and be about the thickness of a deck of cards. Then fill the other two-thirds of the plate with vegetables and fruits. Once in a great while, part of that two-thirds can consist of pasta or rice, but again more as a condiment than a main dish. Add a dash of fat, and you have the basic Zone meal.

The Zone as a Lifestyle: Who It Works for, Who Should Look Elsewhere

The one criticism you hear about the Zone from the average person is that it is difficult to follow. Technically, if you're trying for the exact proportions of 40/30/30, that's correct. The fact is that you really *don't* have to achieve Zone-perfect proportions to get the beneficial effects—an approximation works perfectly well—but the lack of precision may be a problem for people who like their diets very exact and specific. Some people find that thinking about food in terms of Zone "blocks" is cumbersome. If you happen to love doing the math, and the computations of grams, calories, and so on is something you eat for breakfast, this is the perfect diet for you.

This is a great program if you are not overweight but just want a healthy way of eating that will in all likelihood reduce your risk for a number of unpleasant diseases and conditions. If you are only moderately overweight and believe you are not insulin-resistant (i.e., do not have a particular problem with carbohydrates), it's a great way to eat, but you will have to watch calories. If you are very overweight or very sedentary—or both—this program is probably too high in carbohydrates for you, and you might be better off using one of the more carb-limited programs (such as Protein Power or Atkins), at least to begin with.

The other thing to consider in choosing this program as a lifestyle is whether or not you can tolerate this level of carbohydrate. If you are carb-addicted, getting 40 percent of your calories from carbs may seem outrageously high. The program *does* allow things that trigger carb cravings—like bread and even pasta, albeit in small amounts—but for some people, small amounts are too much. Remember, it *is* entirely possible to create Zone-perfect meals using only vegetables and fruits as carbohydrate sources, and if you're able to live with that, you will do fine.

JONNY'S LOWDOWN ★ ★ ★ ★ ★

It's hard to underestimate Dr. Sears' contribution to the current nutritional zeitgeist. He almost single-handedly forced the dietary establishment to reevaluate the prohibition on fats. I have a few minor disagreements—I don't believe saturated fats from natural sources like butter and eggs are a problem, and I also don't agree with his position that supplements aren't necessary if you are eating correctly (a position, to be fair, that he has modified considerably in recent years). That said, the Zone template of 40 percent carbs, 30 percent protein, and 30 percent fat is darn close to ideal as a starting point for a healthy diet. I'm a huge believer in biochemical individuality and not in the "one size fits all" diet mentality, but we still need a basic template from which to individualize our diets; the Zone is as good a basic template as exists anywhere. Some people may need less carbohydrates; some may even need more. But the 40/30/30 plan beats the USDA Food Pyramid as a place from which to begin constructing an individual diet plan.

Books in the Series

The Zone

Mastering the Zone is a complete Zone cookbook.

A Week in the Zone gives the basics of the plan and instructions for how to apply them to eating out, fast-food restaurants, and other real-life situations. This is very easy to understand, is written for the general reader, and has a great list of Zone-friendly snacks.

The Soy Zone shows how to apply the Zone principles to a vegetarian diet.

The Anti-Aging Zone is a hard-to-find but excellent book that shows you how to create a Zone lifestyle that slows the aging process by including such things as exercise and meditation. It also discusses how controlling insulin can extend your life and improve your health.

The Omega Rx Zone is a good recap of the principles of the Zone diet, as well as an argument for the profound benefits of fish oil, which he calls "as close to a medical miracle as anything we're likely to see in this century."

What to Eat in the Zone: The Quick and Easy, Mix-and-Match Counter for Staying in the Zone is a guide to how to put together Zone meals.

Zone Meal in Seconds: 150 Fast and Delicious Recipes for Breakfast, Lunch, and Dinner is Sears' latest, and guides readers through the latest Zone dietary guidelines, together with 150 tasty Zone recipes.

Best Book to Start With

A Week in the Zone, which is a kind of "Zone for Dummies." *Into the Zone* started the franchise and contains the most detailed explanations of how the Zone works, but it was originally written for cardiologists, so be prepared for some technical stuff.

About the Author

Barry Sears, president of Sears Labs, is a biochemist with a Ph.D. in biological chemistry from Indiana University. He was a National Institutes of Health Fellow at the University of Virginia Medical School, a researcher at the Boston University School of Medicine, and a staff scientist at MIT. Since 1982, he has been studying the use of food to alter hormonal response.

Website

The official site for up-to-date Zone information direct from the source is drsears.com. It contains FAQs, Zone research, forums, a Q&A section with Sears, and even a "Critics Corner," in which Sears responds to various articles or news stories that are critical of his program.

A Note on the Zone Food Delivery Programs

Various companies have sprung up around the country that produce Zone meals and snacks and deliver them to your door on a daily basis. Most of these companies are not affiliated with Sears, nor does he endorse their products. The average cost per day of the service is about $35–$42. Some companies are local only; some are national. The only Zone meal delivery system that is actually endorsed by Sears is Zone Cuisine, a company that currently delivers food only in the metropolitan New York region. For more information, visit zonecuisine.com.

CHAPTER 4

Supplements and Diet Drugs

The modern farmer treats the plant but the true farmer treats the soil.

—John Hernandez, M.D.

L et me guess. You'd like me to cut right to the chase and answer the question "Are there pills that can make me lose weight?"

Well, the short answer is "Not by themselves." To produce an effect, virtually any drug on the market has to be used as part of an overall program of calorie reduction, lifestyle change, and behavior modification. If there were a drug you could take that would make weight drop off without your having to do anything at all or change anything about the way you eat or exercise, people would be lining up for miles to get it.

But there isn't.

There are some drugs that *have* been shown to make a difference in weight loss programs for the obese. How *much* of a difference is a whole other matter.

Normally, I wouldn't spend a lot of time discussing the drug options for weight loss for four reasons: (1) I don't think they produce enough weight loss to make much of a difference to most people; (2) they are very, very expensive; (3) my own personal orientation to drugs is "The less, the better"; and (4) the risks frequently outweigh the benefits. But there is a special reason for taking the time to go over the pros and cons of each of the drugs covered here (including some that doctors rarely use much anymore). That special reason can be summed up in two words: the Internet.

I get at least three e-mail spams a day offering all sorts of drugs—including every one of the "diet" drugs mentioned here. All are easily available from online pharmacies without a prescription. It's easy to see how people might be tempted to buy them, especially when they read the merchandising and advertising on these drugs, which often say things like "77 percent of obese patients lost a significant amount of weight" (Meridia). The aggressive marketing and easy availability of these drugs make it mandatory that we take a closer look at just what it is they actually do (and *don't* do).

What you should know about me before reading further (full-disclosure department): my position, as someone involved in nutritional and natural medicine for more than a decade, is that the fewer drugs you take, the better. That's not to say there aren't medications that can change people's lives; obviously there are, and obviously they have a place in treatment. It's just that I would like to see nutritional and lifestyle modifications used as often as possible, with drugs used as a last resort rather than a first-choice intervention. And if you *do* use drugs—and there are doctors who use them with some success—then they *must* be part of an overall program that involves lifestyle and behavioral changes.

Are You a Candidate for Medication?

As of 1999, $321 million was spent on medications for obesity, a figure that will undoubtedly grow as the obesity epidemic continues and newer drugs come to market.[1] The medications for obesity currently approved by the FDA are very specifically limited for use in adults with a body mass index (BMI) of 27 or more who *also* have obesity-related medical conditions, or for adults with a BMI of 30 or more who do not have obesity-related medical conditions.[2,3] (To compute your BMI easily, go to the website listed in Resources.) In other words, if you just want to tone up or lose 10 pounds, these meds are *not for you*. You should also know that only two of the following medications, Meridia and Xenical, have been approved by the FDA for long-term use. The others are approved for "a few weeks," which is widely interpreted to mean up to three months. That doesn't mean they aren't safe for longer use—just that long-term use of these drugs has never been studied. Nor does it mean that doctors don't prescribe them for longer than three months—they do. It's called "off-label" use, and it's done all the time. In fact, the prevailing opinion of many bariatric physicians (those who specialize in treating obesity) is that obesity is a chronic disease just like diabetes and that it needs to be treated (with medication if necessary) indefinitely. They frequently say something to the effect of: "You wouldn't expect someone being treated with medication for high blood pressure to have their blood pressure under control if they go off their meds, would you? It's the same thing with obesity." In fact, the sad truth is that the biggest problem with obesity meds is that people gain the weight back—or at least a lot of it—once they go off the pills. Dr. George Bray, a recognized leader in the field of obesity treatment, says, "Obesity is a chronic illness—medication has to be used long-term."

Now that you know that these drugs work only for as long as you take them, if you buy them off the Internet and self-medicate indefinitely by using stimulant pharmaceuticals that have never been tested for long-term use, you are essentially playing Russian roulette with your health.

Weight loss drugs fall into roughly two categories and work by different mechanisms. The first category is appetite suppressants. The second might be called "digestive inhibitors." All of the following except for Xenical, which is a digestive inhibitor, are appetite suppressants. And all, except for Meridia and Xenical, are approved for short-term use only. Some innovative physicians are treating obesity and overweight with drugs that are not conventionally used for weight loss but seem to produce it as a side effect. We'll talk about those later.

Appetite Suppressants

All of the appetite suppressants are called noradrenergic drugs, which means that they do their work by causing the release of two chemicals, norepinephrine and epinephrine. The release of those chemicals causes you to feel less hungry or not hungry at all. Obviously, if you're not fighting hunger, it's a lot easier to eat less. The most common side effect of the appetite suppressants is jitters—people sometimes feel wired and have a sense that their heart is beating faster, as if they drank a whole pot of coffee. Some people, by the way, like this feeling. They feel they have more "energy." Some people hate it. The feeling usually goes away in time.

The consumer version of the *Physicians' Desk Reference*, or *PDR*, says that you should take these drugs only for a "short time," and when you build up a tolerance for them, you should stop using them. It specifically warns *not* to compensate for the tolerance by upping the dose. Doctors differ in their experience of the "tolerance" aspects. Some feel that in small dosages, patients can stay on these indefinitely and keep getting results. Others cycle the treatment. Dr. Anton Steiner, director of the Tri State Medical Clinic in Los Angeles, has had good results using pharmacology as part of his treatment of obese patients, and will frequently keep patients on these medications for periods of up to nine months. When tolerance to the lower dosages is reached, he will up the dosage periodically until the maximum dose is reached and then put the patient on a "drug holiday." But he is adamant about using drugs as *part* of an overall program of lifestyle change: he feels extended use gives the patient more time to learn a new lifestyle, get guidance and support for that lifestyle, and build confidence that he or she can maintain it.

Dr. Jay Piatek of the Piatek Institute in Indianapolis is one of the doctors who believe that obese and overweight patients frequently have brain chemistry issues that make it particularly difficult for them to adhere to a change in lifestyle, especially when it comes to eating behavior. He sees pharmaceuticals as a way of helping his patients modify their brain chemistry so that it is easier for them to stay on a diet, resist compulsions to eat, and feel good about themselves while changing their behavior. Piatek has been using the antiseizure drugs topiramate (Topamax) and zonisamide (Zonegran) and has had very good results, especially when they're used in combination with a stimulant such as phentermine. He also uses nutritional supplements and behavior modification as part of an overall program of lifestyle change. His book *The Obesity Conspiracy* discusses his treatment protocol in more detail.

> *The drugs my doctor prescribed helped me get to a point where I could really look at my life, reorder my priorities, and change my relationship to food. Now it's time to think about getting off them.*
> —Patty MacV.

With the exception of Steiner and Piatek, virtually every holistic, integrative, or nutritionally based doctor I spoke to recoiled in horror at the mention of diet drugs. The most frequently cited objections were dependency, adrenal stress and burnout (the drugs are, after all, stimulants), and the fact that you have to keep taking them in order to keep the weight off. Dr. Diana Schwarzbein points out that all stimulants (including coffee) can lead to insulin resistance, which is precisely what you don't want if you're trying to lose weight! Stimulants do this by increasing adrenaline, which eventually produces a "backlash" of insulin production to prevent the breakdown of too many structural and functional proteins in the body.

Considering all those negatives, the gains are pretty unimpressive. When you do the math—which we'll look at in a moment—you see that the best any of these drugs can do is *maybe* add 1½ pounds per month to your weight loss efforts, and very few of them can even do that. That's less than ½ pound a week, and that's only for the highest dosages in the most successful studies. More typically the results are 1 pound a *month*, or ¼ pound per week. A big portion of this weight is regained when you stop taking the meds.

To this I'd like to add that the drug industry doesn't exactly have a stellar record when it comes to obesity treatments. Take a look at this chart, adapted from Bray's *Contemporary Diagnosis and Management of Obesity.*

DISASTERS WITH DRUG TREATMENTS FOR OBESITY AND WEIGHT LOSS		
Year	**Drug**	**Outcome**
1893	thyroid	hyperthyroidism
1933	dinitrophenol	cataracts, neuropathy
1937	amphetamine	addiction
1967	"rainbow pills" (digitalis, diuretics)	death
1971	aminorex	pulmonary hypertension
1997	phen-fen (phentermine + fenfluramine/ phentermine + dexfenfluramine)	valvular insufficiency
2000	phenylpropanolamine (Dexatrim, etc.) (ingredient voluntarily withdrawn from market)	stroke

George Bray, *Contemporary Diagnosis and Management of Obesity* (Newtown, Penn.: Handbooks in Health Care Co., 1998).

Get my drift?

Following is an examination of the main appetite suppressants on the market.

Phentermine

This is number one on the Hit Parade of appetite suppressants. It's a schedule 4 drug, which means that the government considers that it has *some* potential for abuse, even though virtually all doctors who prescribe it believe it has none. One of the ingredients in phen-fen, this is the part of the combo that was *not* associated with the valvular problems attached to its partner, fenfluramine. Fenfluramine was pulled off the market, but phentermine remains. It works in an entirely different way from fenfluramine, which increased serotonin release in the brain (serotonin, you may remember, is the "feel-good" neurotransmitter involved in appetite and behavior control). The trade names for phentermine are Adipex-P and Fastin. There's also a resin-based phentermine called Ionamin. Typically, these three drugs *may* produce a couple of pounds of additional weight loss *a month* when compared with a placebo, but frequently they produce less. None of them is cheap.

Phendimetrazine

Phendimetrazine is a schedule 3 drug, which means that the government thinks it has higher potential for abuse than a schedule 4 drug. Phendimetrazine has been around since the 1960s, but very few doctors use it anymore. Again, the best you'll get is ½ pound a week more weight loss than with a placebo, and that's on a good week. There have been reports of problems (ischemic stroke, a fatality) going back to at least 1988. One of its trade names is Bontril. You can find it on the Internet for $89 a month.

Diethylpropion

This schedule 4 drug is sold under the trade name Tenuate. It's another appetite suppressant that few docs are using these days, but it is hawked on my friendly local Internet pharmacy for $99 per month.

Benzphetamine

A schedule 3 controlled substance, benzphetamine is closely related to amphetamine and has a high potential for abuse. The brand name commonly seen is Didrex. It's highly addictive and very expensive. One Internet site sells it for $99 a month. Avoid it like the plague.

All of these medications except phentermine are somewhat old-fashioned and are rarely used these days. Phentermine, however, remains very popular.

Phen-Pro refers to the combination of phentermine and Prozac, a combo that some docs experimented with after phen-fen was taken off the market. Phen-Pro isn't used much anymore, but many doctors *have* noticed that phentermine in combination with a mild antidepressant is a winning combination. The combinations most often cited are phentermine with Lexapro and phentermine with Celexa.

Sibutramine (Meridia)

Sibutramine is one of the two drugs approved by the FDA for long-term use. It was originally studied as an antidepressant but performed very poorly. However, during the studies on depression, it was found to cause a mild amount of weight loss—between 2.2 and 4.4 pounds during the course of the studies.[5] It works by a slightly different mechanism than the appetite suppressants like phentermine. It's called an SNRI because it is both a **s**erotonin *and* **n**orepinephrine **r**euptake **i**nhibitor. The norepinephrine is responsible for the appetite suppression. Sibutramine works directly on the centers in the brain that tell you you're satisfied. According to Dr. Anton Steiner, you are satisfied sooner when you take sibutramine—one might think of it as a kind of "portion control" pill.

Sibutramine has also been said to "raise metabolism" because it stimulates brown fat metabolism. Brown fat is a particular kind of metabolically active fat that actually causes the body to burn calories. Everyone got very excited about this thermogenic effect because in lab studies with rodents, there *was* a 30 percent increase in metabolism; however, with humans, it's an entirely different story. It *may* stimulate brown fat metabolism, but only by about 2 to 4 percent and for less than twenty-four hours.[5]

So how good is sibutramine? The major clinical study that brought this drug onto the radar screen was called the STORM trial—Sibutramine Trial of Obesity Reduction and Maintenance.[6] The researchers—and the marketers of the drug, sold as Meridia—proudly proclaimed that 77 percent of the people taking it lost a significant amount of weight. Sounds good, right? But let's look at what really happened.

The initial trial lasted six months, but the overall study continued for two years. Eight European centers recruited 605 obese patients and put them on sibutramine *combined with* a reduced-calorie diet (reduced by 600 calories per day). Of those patients, 467 (77 percent) lost 5 percent of their body weight. So far, so good. But what happened afterward? Those 467 patients stayed on the program for another eighteen months. Of these, 115 were taken off the medication and put into a placebo group—they regained weight. The remaining 352 were kept on the meds. Out of that 352, 148 dropped out. Now we've got 204 patients left on the meds. Of these 204, 115 were not able to maintain 80 percent or more of their original weight loss, but 89 people were.

If you look at the number who were left on the meds (352) versus the number who were able to maintain 80 percent of their weight loss (89), you're left with—at the end of two years—*a 25 percent success rate*. Big deal. And that, remember, is just for the people who *remained* on medication for two years, not for the people who didn't. Impressive? Not very.

It's interesting that the people who so solemnly proclaim that this medication was a success due to its first six months are the very same ones who trashed recent studies of the Atkins diet in the *New England Journal of Medicine*[7,8] because, in *one* of the studies, the low-carbers (along with everyone else in the study) regained weight *after* the first six months, just like the people in the sibutramine study did.

And how much weight loss are we talking about here, anyway? In the STORM trial, the original average weight loss was a respectable 24 pounds over the first six months (although some people lost much less). That's about a pound a week—not too shabby. But after the full two years, the average weight loss in the sibutramine group—those who remained in the study, that is—was only 12 pounds more than the placebo group, an average of ½ pound a month. In another one-year trial, patients treated with sibutramine lost between ½ pound and ⁹⁄₁₀ pound *per month* more than the placebo group, depending on what dosage they were given, 10 or 15 milligrams.[9] And in other studies,[10,11] weight loss after one year averaged about 1 pound a month for the folks on 10 milligrams a day, up to a big 1½ pounds a month (or ³⁄₁₀ of a pound a week) for those taking 30 milligrams a day. A review of all studies lasting thirty-six to fifty-two weeks found an average weight loss of about ¼ pound a week.[12]

Not much of a bargain, considering the price.

On a typical Internet pharmacy site at the time of this writing, a month's supply of the 10-milligram dose of Meridia was running $189 a month. A month's supply of the 15-milligram dose would set you back $239. That's almost $8 a day for *at best* ½ pound a week (at worst ½ pound a *month*) more than you could do with a placebo.

Oh, one more thing. Sibutramine was taken off the market in Italy after 50 adverse events and 2 deaths from cardiovascular causes were reported in that country. In the United Kingdom, there were 215 reports of 411 adverse reactions (including 95 serious ones and 2 deaths). Between February 1998 and September 2001, the FDA in the United States received reports of 397 adverse events, including 143 cardiac arrhythmias and 29 deaths (19 of them due to cardiovascular causes). Ten of those deaths involved people under fifty years of age, and three involved women under thirty.[13]

Are we having fun yet?

Orlistat (Xenical)

Marketed under the trade name Xenical, orlistat is the only member of the second category of weight loss drugs, a category that could be called "digestive inhibitors." And it's the only drug other than sibutramine (Meridia) currently approved for long-term use. Xenical works by blocking some of the fat that you eat from being digested and assimilated. It does this by blocking up to 75 percent of the digestive enzyme lipase—which breaks down fat—resulting in as much as 30 percent of the fat you eat not going to your hips. What should be immediately apparent is that it does nothing for the fat that is *already* on your hips. People lose weight on Xenical—especially in conjunction with a lower-calorie diet—because it essentially lowers caloric intake automatically. If you, for example, were eating 2,000 calories a day and 30 percent of them were from fat, you would normally be taking in 600 fat calories. By taking Xenical with a fatty meal, you are now essentially taking in only 400 calories from fat. Stick to that plan for a week and you'd be consuming 1,400 calories less a week, which adds up to . . . about $\frac{4}{10}$ pound a week.

The first big study to put Xenical on the map was a two-year European study.[14] During the first year, participants were put on a lower-calorie diet, and during the second year they adhered to a maintenance diet. The Xenical group lost between 2 and 3 percent more weight than the placebo group. In a second two-year European trial, obese patients were put on a reduced-calorie diet (reduced from their regular intake by 600 calories a day) and given 120 milligrams of Xenical three times a day.[15] At the end of the year, they had lost about 9 pounds more than the placebo group (about ¾ pound a month). A similar design was used in a two-year study in the United States that produced an average of a mere ½ pound *a month* more in the Xenical group than in the placebo group.[16]

Does it get any better? Not much. Another study showed that 120 milligrams three times a day produced weight loss of no more than ⅓ to ½ pound per week greater than placebo, and another showed 6.6 pounds greater than with placebo over the course of a *year* (basically ½ pound a month).[17]

Xenical has a great safety profile, but there's a catch. Because the drug keeps some fat from being absorbed, it can have a bunch of very unpleasant side effects, euphemistically grouped under the term *anal leakage*. Typical symptoms: flatus with discharge, oily spotting, fecal urgency, fatty/oily stools, oily diarrhea, fecal incontinence, and increased defecation and spotting. When you're laying out anywhere from $169 to $259 a month for that extra ½ pound of weight loss, don't forget to stock up on Depends.

New on the Horizon: Starch Blockers

Starch blockers are a recent addition to the ever-expanding list of over-the-counter potions sold for weight loss. Introduced in the 1970s, starch blockers were found to be ineffective and were taken off the market in 1982. But the new breed of starch blocker—appropriately named Phase 2—has a lot of promise. Made from a refined, potent extract of white kidney beans, the starch blocker binds to an enzyme called amylase, preventing it from breaking starch down into sugar. The company that makes Phase 2, which is the ingredient in most commercial formulas you'll find at the store, claims that when you take it immediately before a starch-heavy meal, up to 66 percent of the starch in the meal is blocked from absorption.

The studies on Phase 2 have not been published and were commissioned by the manufacturer of the starch blocker, so we need to wait and see about the long-term efficacy of this product. The plus side: it lets you do a low-carb diet and occasionally have some pasta or other high-carb dish. The negative side: the amount of starch you *do* absorb may still be too much for some very sugar-sensitive people, and the illusion that you can now eat these foods "safely" may be a really slippery slope for carb, sugar, and grain addicts. Finally, not absorbing most of the calories doesn't mean that you're protected from the effects of compounds in some starches that may be allergenic (such as gluten). With very careful use, these products might have a place, but I'll have to wait and see before recommending them.

Over the Counter, but Not for Long: Ephedra

Virtually all of the commercial dietary "miracle" products—TrimSpa, Metabolife, Ripped Fuel, Xenadrine, and the rest—work by two pathways: suppressing appetite and increasing metabolic rate (called thermogenesis, which is the production of heat from food). They do so with varying degrees of success. The active ingredient in all of them is—or at least used to be—ephedra. A ton of information has come down the pike recently about ephedra, much of it inflammatory and a great deal of it inaccurate.

When ephedra has been used in supervised weight loss research studies, it's been given in the dosage of 60 milligrams per day in three divided dosages of 20 milligrams, each combined with 200 milligrams of caffeine. In any supervised study using this dose, ephedra has not shown itself to be dangerous, and the side effect of "the jitters" was usually pretty well tolerated.[18,19] It is not—I repeat, *not*—for people with high blood pressure *or* for people who are sensitive to ephedrine or caffeine *or* for people who have any kind of heart, kidney, or liver problems *or* for people taking any medication, including over-the-counter meds (unless you check with your doctor).

Ephedra works by stimulating brown fat metabolism, thereby increasing the bodily production of heat (upping your metabolism *slightly*), and by suppressing your appetite. The possible side effects are very annoying and include nervousness, insomnia, and possibly dizziness. The benefits in the way of fat loss are very mild but do exist. Ephedra can definitely raise your blood pressure and may interact with other medications.

One of the problems with ephedra is that people are using amounts that are way higher than the recommended dosage, which is generally about 25 milligrams. Ephedra products with as much as 250 milligrams per tablet are available at every mall. Many people take it for "energy" or as a party drug, and many high school and college athletes take it because they think it will enhance athletic performance. Probably more than a few of them don't pay any attention to the conditions under which you should never take the stuff.

There are many nutritionally oriented health practitioners who are fans of ephedra when it's used properly (though they are certainly a minority), notably Dr. Shari Lieberman, author of *The Real Vitamin and Mineral Book*, and Dr. C. Leigh Broadhurst. But it probably doesn't matter anymore. "Its time is over," says Broadhurst. There's just too much bad publicity and public outcry about it, and it will almost certainly be taken off the market soon. The new ephedra-free diet pills have simply replaced ephedra with bitter orange, which has many of the same "fat-burning/appetite-suppressing" effects but doesn't yet have the bad rap. (See below for more about bitter orange.)

If ephedra *does* manage to dodge the bullet and stay on the market—and you decide to try it—make sure that you do not fit into any of the categories mentioned above, and *never* take more than the recommended dosage. When all is said and done, it is still an adrenal stimulant—a kind of legal speed, if you will—and it's hard to believe that longtime use can have any beneficial effects on your health.

The bottom line is this: medications don't *cause* you to lose weight. They *may*—and this is a big "may"—make it easier for you to choose better foods, such as proteins over carbohydrates, and they may help you to keep portions under control. Medications may help you follow a lifestyle plan, and you have to be willing to see them in that light. Steiner summed it up best: "Pills don't work alone. *Programs*, however, do."

Supplements

Memorize this: there are no supplements you can take for weight loss that will cause the pounds to just melt off without you having to do anything at all.

That doesn't mean there aren't supplements you need to take. There are. What supplements *can* do is correct deficiencies and help with metabolic issues that might be *standing in the way* of your losing weight. In that sense, they are essential to your overall program.

Normalizing blood sugar and insulin response is one of the most important keys to weight loss for many—if not most—people. Making a positive impact on the blood sugar–insulin continuum is the main purpose of the low-carb diets discussed in this book. Other conditions that get in the way of weight loss are low energy and fatigue, nutrient deficiencies, adrenal stress, yeast overgrowth, thyroid problems, depression, sleep disorders, food cravings, and even an overtaxed liver. Proper supplements can make a serious positive impact on many, if not all, of these conditions.

Some of the supplements discussed here will help with blood sugar control; others with energy, liver health, or relaxation and sleep; and still others with cravings or appetite. Some will do double duty, helping a number of conditions simultaneously. Remember that improving one or more of these things can have a *profound* effect on your ability to follow a program, but there isn't a one that you can simply take and watch the weight drop off. (If there were, I would probably be selling it and writing this book from a villa on the beach in St. Martin. Then again, as my father used to say, *if my grandmother had wheels, she'd be a wagon.*)

One more note: virtually no supplement—vitamin, mineral, or herb—does just one thing in the body. Most work synergistically and on a number of different pathways, doing good all over the place. A full discussion of the benefits and purposes of, say, vitamin C or vitamin E would fill a small book (for those interested, there are several excellent books on supplements listed in Resources). So understand that, for the purposes of *Living the Low-Carb Life*, I'm just going to discuss the aspects of the following supplements that affect weight loss and closely related issues. That should not be taken to mean that these fellows don't do a heck of a lot more than the things we're talking about, just that this discussion is intentionally narrowed to the scope of this book.

> *Whenever a doctor tells me that there is "no good research" on vitamin supplements, I know he has never bothered to do a literature search on pubmed.*
> —Constantine X.

At the bare minimum, a high-quality multivitamin and mineral formula should be part of everyone's health regimen, even before considering any of the supplements discussed below. People eating grain-based diets can easily suffer from mineral depletions (see "The Problem with Grains" on page 126), and so can people on low-carb diets, especially in the introductory phases. Mineral depletions can decrease activity in the energy-production cycles of the body, effectively slowing down your metabolism.[20] You want to make sure you've covered that base right at the beginning.

The Number One Supplement for Weight Control: It's Going to Surprise You

It's not expensive, it's not exotic, and it's not sexy, but it works like a charm. It's plain, old-fashioned fiber. More than a dozen clinical studies have used dietary fiber supplements for weight loss, most with positive outcomes.[21] When you take the fiber supplement with water before meals, the water-soluble fiber binds to water in the stomach, making you feel full and less likely to overeat. It also suppresses hunger.[22] Fiber supplements have also been shown to enhance blood sugar control and insulin effects and even to reduce the number of calories (adding up to about 3 to 18 pounds a year) that the body absorbs.[23] And a study in the prestigious *New England Journal of Medicine* found that a diet with 50 grams of fiber per day lowered insulin levels in the blood.[24]

One of the most impressive studies of all followed 2,900 healthy subjects for ten years and looked at the relationship between fiber, cardiovascular disease, weight, and insulin. The results were spectacular. Fiber was inversely associated with insulin levels and weight *and* low fiber intake turned out to be a better predictor of heart disease than saturated-fat consumption! The subjects who consumed the most fiber gained less weight over the course of the ten years than who consumed the least.[25]

Guar gum seems to be one of the most effective fiber supplements, but other studies have used glucomannan, which can be taken in pill form. If you choose this form, make sure to buy the capsules rather than the tablets, since you don't want the fiber coming in contact with water until it gets into your stomach. Another way of adding fiber is with a powdered supplement like psyllium husks, flaxseeds, or even the old standby, sugar-free Metamucil. Some of my personal favorite fiber supplements are Cellulose Fiber by Vital Nutrients, Superseed by Garden of Life, or plain ground flaxseed. In addition, fiber has a ton of other wide-ranging positive effects on the body, like helping to prevent certain kinds of cancer and lowering cholesterol and triglycerides.

Americans currently get a paltry amount of fiber in their diets, estimated at 10 grams a day. Most health organizations like the American Cancer Society recommend about 30 grams, and our caveman ancestors got much more (maybe around 50 or 60 grams). You can—and should—add fiber by eating as many fibrous vegetables and fruits as you can, but it's doubtful you'll get enough to have the kind of therapeutic effect I'm talking about. So eat those vegetables, but supplement your intake as well. Incidentally, all the grain foods and cereals we've been taught are a great source of fiber are actually fiber lightweights. Most commercial breads have a couple of grams at best, and most cereals have embarrassingly low amounts. The only two commercial cereals worth talking about when it comes to fiber are All-Bran and Fiber One, both of which have around 10 grams per serving. Nice.

Oh, one more thing. I have a theory that I'll share with you. In those few studies where a high-carbohydrate, low-fat diet has been shown to help with weight loss or improve blood lipid profiles, usually in controlled conditions like a clinic or other supervised setting, I believe that what created the benefit was *not* the low-fat diet but the fact that the researchers gave their subjects high-fiber foods. I believe it was the fiber that made the difference, as most of those studies substituted high-fiber carbohydrates for the ones the subjects had normally been eating. One of the reasons the GO-Diet got such a high rating in this book is that it is one of the few programs that truly emphasizes fiber as a constituent of weight loss and health.

A Supplements Overview

The supplements discussed in the following pages are the ones that have the strongest credentials for use in a weight loss program. In most cases they have a sizable amount of research to back up their use, or they have been used successfully in clinical practice by responsible and thoughtful practitioners for a long enough time to warrant their inclusion in the discussion, or both. (Clinical observation should never be ignored. Remember that there was no good scientific research on aspirin until very recently—for decades it has been used simply because it has been observed to work.)

There are also a few supplements that I have listed under the category *of possible use*, which will be discussed briefly at the end of the chapter. These supplements have some research behind them, but in my opinion the jury is still out—the research is either not yet strong enough, the clinical evidence not solid enough, or the results have been mixed. These supplements, however, bear watching and may turn out to be very useful.

Finally, there are three products I do not recommend at this time for reasons that I will discuss at the end of the chapter.

Supplements of possible use:
• gymnema sylvestre
• hydroxycitrate
• banaba leaf extract (corosolic acid)

Supplements not recommended at this time:
• CLA
• flaxseed oil (for men)
• vanadium (vanadyl sulfate) *except* under a health practitioner's supervision

The chart on page 184 shows the influence of various supplements on areas of concern to people on low-carb (or other) weight loss programs.

Supplement	Impacts blood sugar control	Impacts energy and fatigue	Impacts PMS	Impacts adrenal health	Impacts cravings/appetite control/mood	Stimulates metabolism/burns fat	Impacts liver health
B complex		X		X		X	
B₅				X			
B₆			X		X		
C		X		X	X		
E	X						
omega-3s	possibly			X	X	X	
GLA			X			X	
magnesium	X		X		X		
alpha lipoic acid	X						X
chromium	X						
high-dose biotin	X						
carnitine		X		X		X	
CoQ10		X				X (3)	
green tea (EGCG)						X	
ginseng	X	X					
5-HTP					X (1)		
bitter orange						X	
glutamine					X		
neptune krill oil			X				
vanadyl sulfate	X (2)						

1. 5-HTP is one of the few supplements that has been shown to have an effect on weight loss by itself.
2. Vanadyl sulfate is recommended only under a physician's supervision.
3. See discussion of CoQ10 on page 195.

B Complex

I put the majority of my clients on B vitamins. Energizing for many people, B vitamins are necessary for metabolizing carbohydrates, fats, and proteins, and your need for them increases significantly when you are under stress. A lot of people just plain feel better on them. Certain members of the B vitamin family, like B₅, B₆, choline, and inositol, have special importance to people on weight loss programs. Choline is important in the transport and metabolism of fats, while inositol is important for the uptake of fatty acids by the cells. Both have been shown to alleviate, prevent, or improve fatty liver. They are usually included in a B complex formula; "fat-burning formulas" may have increased amounts.

B_5 (Pantothenic Acid)

B_5 is "mother's little helper" for the adrenal glands. It is used in the production of stress hormones, and some studies have shown that supplemental pantothenic acid can help us resist or withstand stress in general.[26] If you are under stress or your adrenals are in danger of being burnt out or exhausted, you most certainly need this supplement. I recommend taking it separately from the B complex, which you should take in addition. A good amount is 250 milligrams twice a day.

B_6

Vitamin B_6 is one of the most important supplements you can take, and if you are a woman, it's *especially* important. It helps convert estradiol, a very active form of estrogen, into estriol, a very benign form. Birth control pills deplete the body of B_6, and supplementing can help relieve the depression that sometimes accompanies use of birth control pills.[27] This may be because, for both women and men, B_6 is necessary to convert tryptophan into serotonin, as well as for the synthesis of dopamine and norepinephrine, all neurotransmitters that affect weight and appetite. Remember that low serotonin states are almost always associated with carbohydrate cravings.

In addition, in some (but not all) animal studies, vitamin B_6 deficient rats that were fed a high-protein (70 percent protein) diet developed fatty liver. A low intake of B_6 can impair glucose tolerance.[28] And in a low-carbohydrate diet, the body makes needed glucose from noncarbohydrate sources (like protein), a process called gluconeogenesis (see chapter 2 for a full explanation of this process). During gluconeogenesis, B_6 levels are depleted from muscle, another reason for supplementing with B_6 while on a low-carb diet.[29] As with B_5, I recommend that if you do supplement with B_6, you take it at a different time than you take your B complex vitamin. A good amount is 50 milligrams once a day, as long as you are also taking your B complex.

Vitamin C

Vitamin C basically helps almost everything. When you have high blood sugar, vitamin C can't travel into the cells.[30] While by itself vitamin C probably does not promote weight loss, it is depleted by stress—understandable, since it is found in very high levels in the adrenals and the brain[31]—and, like vitamin B$_6$, is necessary for making serotonin.[32] If stress or depression contribute to your weight issues, you should definitely be supplementing with vitamin C, 1,000 to 2,000 milligrams per day.

Vitamin E

Vitamin E has a demonstrable effect on insulin resistance.[33–35] According to diabetes expert Dr. Richard Bernstein, vitamin E in dosages of up to 1,200 IUs a day has also been shown to reduce glycosylation, one of the most destructive and aging effects of high blood sugar (see chapter 2 and "Alpha Lipoic Acid" below). Bernstein recommends 400 to 1,200 IUs a day to many of his patients. Note that the most commonly sold vitamin E is alpha-tocopherol, but this is only one of eight different components in vitamin E, and there's a lot of evidence that just taking alpha-tocopherol by itself does not give you the maximum benefit. You should look for a combination of alpha-tocopherol and gamma-tocopherol, or even gamma-tocopherol alone. You should also look for a vitamin E supplement that contains tocotrienols, another set of very important heart-healthy compounds in the vitamin E family. Natural vitamin E is unquestionably more effective than any of the synthetic kinds.

The studies that showed benefit for insulin metabolism used 900 IUs. Vitamin E is generally sold in 400 IU capsules. If you're using vitamin E for its general protective effect, add at least 400 IUs to your daily regimen, preferably 800. If you're using it for its therapeutic effects on blood sugar metabolism, take at least 800 IUs.

Omega-3s

Along with magnesium and alpha lipoic acid, omega-3s are the supplements I recommend for just about everybody. The impact of omega-3s on so many areas of human health are so enormous that it would require a whole book to fully explain them (and several have been published, notably *The Omega Rx Zone* by Dr. Barry Sears and *The Omega-3 Connection* by Dr. Andrew Stoll). For our purposes, let's talk about blood sugar regulation and insulin resistance. The evidence that omega-3 fats increase insulin sensitivity and help with blood sugar regulation is not perfect—some studies show that they have no effect,[36] and a couple show that they do.[37, 38]

But virtually every clinician, including myself, who uses nutritional supplements with clients recommends omega-3s, though because of their numerous overlapping positive effects on the body, it's difficult to say just what their specific role is in terms of blood sugar and insulin. Nonetheless, the clinical evidence for their use is overwhelmingly positive. Dr. Shari Lieberman, author of *The Real Vitamin and Mineral Book*, says it's hard to say whether omega-3s have a specific blood sugar–lowering effect, though they *probably* do, but she points out that they *definitely* lower C-reactive protein, a measure of inflammation and a risk factor for heart disease that is often elevated in diabetics. "Personally, I think they protect the cells in the pancreas," she says. Dr. David Leonardi of the Leonardi Medical Institute for Vitality and Longevity in Denver, Colorado, uses omega-3s routinely with his diabetic patients precisely for the anti-inflammatory effects. "Diabetes is a disease of inflammation, among other things," he says. Omega-3s also reduce triglycerides and increase good cholesterol. Omega-3s are the first of the fatty acids to be depleted when you lose fat, so the need for supplementation increases even more when you're on a weight loss program.

There has been some controversy about how to supplement with omega-3s. There are basically three omega-3 fatty acids we are interested in: ALA (alpha linolenic acid)—which is found in flaxseeds—and EPA (eicosapentaenoic acid) and DHA (docosahexaenoic acid), both of which are found in fish. EPA and DHA are the most important, and the body is *supposed* to make them from ALA. Unfortunately, it doesn't always do this successfully—only about 20 percent of ALA eventually winds up as EPA and DHA. This has led many clinicians, myself included, to favor supplementing with fish oil—since it contains ready-made EPA and DHA—and to just forget about the "parent molecule" of ALA found in flaxseed oil. Others—like Ann Louise Gittleman, author of *The Fat Flush Plan*—argue that even though only a small percentage of ALA actually gets transformed successfully into EPA and DHA, ALA has valuable properties of its own (including anti-inflammatory ones) and for that reason should be used in *conjunction* with fish oil.

The controversy has heated up with the publication of a number of studies that show an unexpected correlation between increased ALA consumption in men and prostate cancer, which is why I do not recommend flaxseed *oil* for men at this time.[39–41] There are a couple of possible explanations for the unusual prostate cancer finding. One is that the men were not taking antioxidants, which would protect the fragile oil from becoming damaged. A second is that the source of the ALA was rancid or oxidized. Although there is ALA in flaxseeds themselves, the chances of the oil *in the seeds* becoming rancid or oxidized is next to zero.

> ### When I take supplements I know I'm doing something really good for myself, and that helps me focus on the other things I need to be doing for my health, like eating right and exercising every day. It seems to all go together.
>
> —Maryanne DiC.

I think that given our current knowledge, the best recommendation is to take fish oil supplements on a regular basis, and for both men and women to feel free to add ground flaxseeds to everything they eat, including protein shakes. (There is no good reason for women not to take flaxseed oil if they like.) You could also opt for cod liver oil, an amazing source of EPA and DHA, but if you live where there's a lot of sun in the summer, you might want to choose another supplement during the sunny months. Cod liver oil contains high amounts of vitamin D, and you could get too much if you took cod liver oil *and* went into the sun on a regular basis.

GLA (Gamma Linolenic Acid)

If you're taking omega-3s, which I hope you are, some GLA (at least 80 milligrams) should be taken daily to balance them. GLA may also help with weight loss. GLA is gamma linolenic acid, an extremely important omega-6 fatty acid that the body makes in the presence of an enzyme (delta-6-desaturase) that is *inhibited* by insulin as well as by trans-fatty acids. Hence, most people don't get enough GLA. It's important to our discussion because it stimulates brown adipose tissue—which translates to less body fat accumulation and more fat burning.[42] Ann Louise Gittleman has said for years that she has seen clients break weight plateaus just by adding GLA. Robert Atkins reported on one study in which half the overweight people lost weight just by taking 400 milligrams per day of GLA.[43] While I doubt that GLA by itself will do anything much, I don't doubt that together with a lower-carb, moderate-calorie diet and a program like those discussed in this book, it will move things along.

For women with PMS, GLA is just about a necessity. It has been used for decades as a treatment for PMS and is an essential part of the "PMS cocktail" I recommend in my practice with great success: GLA, magnesium, B$_6$, and neptune krill oil. Since cravings and carb binges are often part of PMS, improving PMS symptoms becomes a big part of successful weight loss for most women. With the PMS cocktail, you should see results within three menstrual cycles.

The usual sources for GLA are evening primrose oil and borage oil, but I much prefer that you get the actual pure GLA supplement. Although there are typically a couple hundred milligrams of GLA in each 1,000-milligram evening primrose oil capsule, which is good, the rest of the oil is vegetable oil, which you don't want or need. So it makes far more sense to simply take straight GLA.

Magnesium

I consider magnesium one of the most important supplements you can take and recommend it to virtually all of my clients, especially if there is any chance of blood sugar problems or insulin resistance. The minimum amount is 400 milligrams daily, and I prefer 800 milligrams.

The connection between magnesium and insulin was pointed out recently in a superb lecture at the annual Boulderfest Nutrition Conference by diabetes expert Dr. Ron Rosedale of the Rosedale Center for Metabolic Medicine.[44] Insulin stores magnesium, and when and if your cells become resistant to insulin, you're not going to store magnesium very well. Magnesium is also necessary for the *action* of insulin, so the more magnesium you lose, the more insulin-resistant you become. The more insulin-resistant you become, the more magnesium you lose. It's a nasty little circle. And since, among other things, magnesium relaxes muscles, when you lose it, your blood vessels constrict and you may have higher blood pressure and reduced energy.

Not a good scenario.

The importance of magnesium to heart health and bone health have been written about extensively, so if for some reason you're not already taking it for those reasons, then take it for its effect on your blood sugar (which in turn influences the amount of insulin your body secretes and therefore impacts weight loss). Magnesium is absolutely essential for managing blood sugar, and magnesium deficiency correlates with insulin resistance.[45] (Even the American Diabetes Association admits "strong associations . . . between magnesium deficiency and insulin resistance.") Many nutritionists estimate that as much as 80 percent of the population doesn't get enough magnesium (and it could easily be more). As an added benefit, magnesium supplementation can bring down LDL ("bad") cholesterol and bring up HDL ("good") cholesterol,[46-47] not exactly a bad "side effect"!

Alpha Lipoic Acid

If there is a supplement other than fish oil that I feel safe recommending for just about everyone, it is alpha lipoic acid. Aside from its impact on blood sugar, insulin sensitivity, and liver health, this superstar nutrient does "double whammy" magic by acting as a powerful antioxidant on its own and by protecting other antioxidants such as vitamins C and E, making it a powerful antiaging nutrient.

While alpha lipoic acid is not specifically a nutrient for weight loss, it can help with two areas that can stall your weight loss progress. The first is insulin resistance. Alpha lipoic acid has been shown to improve insulin sensitivity,[48-49] and if for no other reason than that, it belongs in the program of anyone who has a lot of weight to lose.

Along those same lines, some of the most impressive research with alpha lipoic acid has been done on diabetic neuropathy, the peripheral pain most diabetics feel in their extremities. Glucose (sugar) *causes* neuropathy. It does this by a nasty little process called glycation, which is when excess sugar literally sticks to protein in the blood, gumming up the works, impairing signals to nerves, making circulation difficult (especially in the tiny capillaries in the eyes and toes), and creating the aptly named AGES (**a**dvanced **g**lycolated **e**nd-products). (For a full discussion of glycation, see chapter 2.) Alpha lipoic acid is, among other things, an antiglycation agent; hence, we can assume it does good things to elevated levels of blood sugar.

Another way alpha lipoic acid may help weight loss is with its protective effect on the liver. The liver is the body's main fat-processing factory, and if there's a traffic jam there, fat burning is not going to be optimal. Fatty liver—a condition many very overweight people have—and/or an excess of medications, toxins, pollutants, and the like that have to be detoxified by the liver can definitely slow things up. Alpha lipoic acid is a powerful liver protector. In one spellbinding report by Dr. Burt Berkson, an emergency treatment with alpha lipoic acid played a central role in saving the lives of two young patients whose deaths from mushroom poisoning/liver toxicity would have been a virtual certainty. Berkson has also reported on a successful treatment for the serious liver disease hepatitis C that uses alpha lipoic acid, selenium, and milk thistle.[50]

For overall health and protection, I recommend 50 to 100 milligrams of alpha lipoic acid daily as a supplement, but for effects on blood sugar, insulin, and the liver, I suggest at least 600 milligrams per day. The only "downside" to alpha lipoic acid is that it is relatively expensive.

Chromium

I recommend chromium for anyone I suspect has problems with blood sugar and/or insulin resistance or who is chronically unable to lose weight. Chromium is insulin's helpmate: it makes insulin do its job of getting sugar out of the bloodstream and into the cells more effectively. We've already seen how high levels of insulin contribute to both weight gain and the inability to lose fat. If your body doesn't need to overproduce insulin, you will have a more favorable and balanced hormonal environment for both health and weight loss.

Indeed, chromium as a supplement has been tested in a number of studies, specifically for its weight loss properties and its muscle-building properties. The studies are conflicting. By itself, chromium probably does not "cause" you to lose weight. But by having a positive effect on blood sugar via its ability to increase the effectiveness of insulin, it is automatically helping to control one of the biggest obstacles to weight loss. Dr. Harry Preuss, one of the most distinguished and respected chromium researchers in the world, summed it up this way: "If you have a properly functioning glucose and insulin system, the tendency is to lose fat and build muscle." In fact, one of the most impressive studies of chromium was done by Preuss himself on twenty-eight overweight African-American women. Two groups took part in a modest diet and exercise program; one group was given niacin-bound chromium (200 micrograms three times a day), and the other was given a placebo. The women getting the chromium had a significant loss of fat and a sparing of muscle.[51]

Other studies have also demonstrated chromium's positive effects. In one study, 1,000 micrograms a day of chromium given to type 2 diabetics produced a beneficial effect on glucose, insulin, cholesterol, and hemoglobin A1c levels (an important measure for diabetes).[52] Another study showed that while chromium supplementation didn't have an effect on everyone, it had a significant positive effect on fasting insulin levels in those subjects who had high fasting levels to begin with (fasting insulin is measured by a blood test performed when you have not had anything to eat or drink except water for at least eight hours). High fasting insulin levels are a sign that there's too much insulin in the system and a good indication that there are blood sugar problems.[53]

But is chromium safe?

Here's the deal. There has been a lot of media attention recently on the supposed link of chromium picolinate to DNA damage and precancerous conditions. Indeed, a number of somewhat disturbing studies have come out that have raised eyebrows.[54–56] However, there are two things you should know.

One, the studies are all focused on the possible—I repeat, *possible*—damaging effects of picolinic acid, i.e., the "picolinate" part of chromium picolinate. These studies do *not* cast any doubt whatsoever on the safety of chromium itself, which has been shown time and again to be one of the safest nutrients you can take.[57, 58] Doses of chromium that are about three hundred times the currently recommended daily dietary intake have been found safe in animals.[59]

Two, not everyone agrees that these studies are meaningful. Shari Lieberman, a certified nutrition specialist and author of *The Real Vitamin and Mineral Book*, calls them "junk science." She says, "Show me where the amount of picolinate used in those hamster cell studies has any bearing whatsoever on what a human being would consume if they took chromium picolinate in the ranges we're recommending." Dr. C. Leigh Broadhurst, who worked with Dr. Richard Anderson on the development of chromium picolinate at the USDA, agrees. Others are more cautious. "I'm about 99.9 percent sure that chromium picolinate is safe," says Dr. Harry Preuss. "But if there's even a glimmer of doubt, and it's something you're going to be taking for years, why not stick with a form of chromium where there's no question whatsoever about the safety?"

So, what to do? Should you take chromium if you are struggling with weight, blood sugar, and insulin resistance issues? *Absolutely*. And if you want to be absolutely 100 percent on the safe side, choose a form other than picolinate. Three that come to mind are chromium polynicotinate (niacin-bound chromium, available, for example, in a brand called Chrome-Mate), GTF chromium, or chromium arginate (inexpensive, reliable, and available from Designs for Health; see Resources).

The recommended dose for chromium is 200 micrograms three times a day, though it is frequently used in dosages up to 1,000 micrograms with no negative effects. Chromium in general is not well absorbed. It should be taken on an empty stomach, preferably about twenty minutes or so before a meal.

High-Dose Biotin

Biotin is associated in the public's mind with shiny hair, clear skin, and healthy nails, but when used in megadoses (one hundred or more times the amount found in your typical B complex), it can be very effective for lowering blood sugar. It enhances insulin sensitivity and increases the activity of an enzyme called glucokinase, which is responsible for helping the liver use sugar.[60] One study that used 9 milligrams a day of biotin produced significant decreases in fasting blood sugar levels in type 2 diabetics,[61] and another did the same by using 8 to 16 grams a day.[62] Dr. David Leonardi treats a large number of diabetics at the Leonardi Medical Institute for Vitality and Longevity in Denver, Colorado, and frequently sees excellent results in those patients taking 15 milligrams a day. And it was recently suggested that high-dose biotin taken with chromium may be a viable treatment for insulin resistance.[63]

Carnitine

Carnitine, also known (and referred to interchangeably) as L-carnitine, is a very interesting nutrient with a fascinating pedigree. I frequently recommend it for weight loss clients in the dosage of 1 to 2 grams a day. However, you're unlikely to get the full weight loss benefits from it unless you use it in the form and dosages described at the end of this section and in conjunction with a low-carb, reduced-calorie diet. And there are many other terrific things that carnitine does for the overweight patient that you should know about, while we're at it.

Carnitine is a spectacular nutrient because of its demonstrably positive therapeutic value for the heart,[64, 65] because it increases energy and combats fatigue, and because it has been shown repeatedly to lower triglycerides as well as lipoprotein(a), a serious risk factor for heart disease.[66] In one trial, people with diabetes were given carnitine, and both their cholesterol and their triglycerides dropped 25 to 39 percent in just ten days.[67] From the basic raw material of carnitine, the body naturally makes acetyl-L-carnitine, a particular form of carnitine that is enormously protective for the brain. Relative to our concerns here, carnitine improves insulin sensitivity in insulin-resistant diabetics and helps with glucose uptake in nondiabetic patients.[68]

But although this amino acid–like nutrient has a reputation as a weight loss aid, until recently study after disappointing study failed to show an effect on weight loss or body composition. There were some studies that indicated otherwise,[69] but they were few and far between. Many clinicians believe that while carnitine is amazing for a number of applications, its use as a weight loss supplement is questionable.

Many others, however, do not agree. Some of the greatest clinicians in America routinely use it, have seen terrific results with it, and sing its praises from the rooftops. Their experience with it can't be ignored. Atkins routinely recommended from 2 to 5 grams (sometimes more) for patients at his clinic. Patrick Quillin, Ph.D., R.D., called carnitine a "'wonder nutrient' that could make weight reduction just a bit easier."[70] And one of the country's most revered nutritionists and educators, Robert Crayhon of the Crayhon Research Institute, calls it "the best nutrient there is for promoting weight loss." He even wrote a book about it called *The Carnitine Miracle*.

So what's the deal? It is well established that carnitine is *absolutely necessary* for "fat burning." There's no disagreement about what it does in the body—carnitine is the "escort" for fat on its journey into the little "furnaces" of the cell (the mitochondria), where it is burned for fuel. The only question is whether carnitine supplementation actually increases the amount of fat "burned."

It's beginning to look like it does. An extremely impressive study with normal subjects demonstrated that supplemental carnitine actually *increased* fat burning, even in subjects *without* carnitine deficiencies.[71] Some recent animal studies showed that supplemental carnitine significantly increased weight loss[72] and reduced fat gain.[73]

Here's what you should keep in mind about carnitine.

- Carnitine works best with a lower-carb diet (insulin blunts its action).
- Carnitine needs to be taken in the tartrate form.
- The amount of carnitine *usually* included in commercial "fat-burning" formulas is completely meaningless and ineffective; if you're going to give carnitine a fair trial, you need to use meaningful doses (see below).
- The main source of carnitine is animal foods. If you're a vegetarian, it's a virtual certainty that you should be supplementing with carnitine, especially if you're trying to lose weight. If your main source of protein is soy, be aware that unless it's fortified, it's lacking in methionine, one of the two amino acids from which the body makes its own carnitine.

- Carnitine lowers cortisol levels (and can therefore be helpful for adrenal health),[74] and adrenal activity affects weight gain and loss.

Carnitine *alone* cannot promote weight loss. But in combination with diet, it can and will decrease body fat and body weight, probably more than diet alone would. Carnitine in conjunction with a low-carb diet and an exercise program makes a winning combination. If you are a vegetarian, there's no question that you should use it, and if your plan calls for ketosis, you should definitely use it as well, since when carnitine is deficient, conversion of fat to ketones is impaired.[75]

Plan to use no less than 1 gram, preferably 2 grams or more, and remember to get the tartrate form. A great time to take it is on an empty stomach before working out. The best carnitine is the tartrate form marketed by both Designs for Health and Crayhon Research. The powder makes higher doses very easy and palatable (it tastes like lemony Tang). One teaspoon equals 2,800 milligrams (2.8 grams). Be aware that it's expensive.

CoQ10 (Coenzyme Q10)

CoQ10 is not a weight loss supplement per se but is vitally important in the production of energy, and if you are low or deficient in it, it may keep you from losing weight.[76] CoQ10 is short for coenzyme Q10. Technically, it's not a vitamin (because it's synthesized in the cells), but it acts like a vitamin in the body because it is involved in so many metabolic functions. It is found in high concentrations in the heart (also in the kidneys, liver, and pancreas) and is considered a very important nutrient for heart health largely because of its importance in the creation of molecules of energy (known as ATP) that are required in large amounts by the heart.[77] It can also decrease blood sugar in diabetics. CoQ10 is frequently depleted by medications, especially statin drugs. (If you're on a statin, you should definitely be on CoQ10.)

If energy and fatigue are an issue for you, I often recommend the "energy cocktail" of carnitine, CoQ10, and ginseng. Remember, however, that lack of energy is often due to lifestyle—not enough high-quality sleep, the wrong diet, and adrenal burnout. You need to address those issues and not take the "cocktail" as a substitute for doing something about them.

Green Tea (EGCG)

Dr. Shari Lieberman, author of *The Real Vitamin and Mineral Book*, considers the active compound in green tea to be one of the best weight loss supplements available, and I agree.

Compounds in green tea can raise your metabolism. The particular compound responsible for the increase in fat-burning ability is called EGCG (epigallocatechin gallate), and it works by increasing the production of noradrenaline, which turns up your metabolism.[78] EGCG also stimulates brown fat metabolism, thus increasing thermogenesis.[79] Green tea extracts have been shown to increase fat burning as well as metabolic rate (the amount of calories you burn) for up to twenty-four hours.[80, 81] In animal studies, they have been shown to have a mild antiobesity effect,[82] and if that were not enough, the EGCG in green tea has recently been shown to enhance insulin activity.[83]

You'd need to drink five or more cups of the tea a day to get the amount of EGCG required to produce an effect, so high-quality supplements are probably the way to go.

Ginseng

Ginseng is what is known as an adaptagen, which means it can help you restore equilibrium to something that is out of balance. In that sense, it's like the thermostat on your central air conditioning/heating unit—if the room is too hot, the thermostat tells the unit to cool things off, but if the room's too cold, the thermostat signals the unit to warm things up.

Ginseng is traditionally used for energy, especially during times of stress or fatigue, but recent evidence has shown that it is amazing for helping to regulate blood sugar, and may possibly be of value in weight loss as well. In one study, it elevated mood and reduced fasting blood sugar.[84] In two animal studies, it improved glucose tolerance while the animals lost weight,[85] and in another it produced a significant amount of weight loss, an increase in calories expended, and a reduction in the amount of calories consumed. It also decreased cholesterol![86]

This may be why Asian ginseng is commonly used in traditional Chinese medicine to treat diabetes. In animal research, it has been shown to increase the number of insulin receptors,[87] and recent studies showed that even nondiabetics taking American ginseng before eating had less elevated blood sugar readings after they ate.[88]

Siberian ginseng might be worth a try if you're fatigued, or try American ginseng if you're concerned about your blood sugar. Alternatively, you can get the more stimulating Panax type, also known as Chinese or Korean ginseng.

5-HTP

This supplement (a metabolite of the amino acid tryptophan) has been found to have an effect on weight loss in several impressive studies, even sometimes without dietary changes.[89] 5-HTP (5-hydroxytryptophan) is the immediate precursor to serotonin and has been found very useful as an antidepressant. It's thought to exert its influence over eating behavior by affecting serotonin. Studies have shown that 5-HTP decreases food intake (predominately carbohydrates) and promotes weight loss.[90, 91] If you're currently taking antidepressants, make sure to check with your doctor before adding 5-HTP to your supplement regimen. I recommend always including B_6 along with your 5-HTP, since B_6 is needed for the conversion to serotonin.

Bitter Orange

Bitter orange (citrus aurantium) is the ingredient found in most of the new "ephedra-free" diet pills. It's an herb that contains the active ingredient synephrine. Synephrine is chemically very similar to ephedrine and pseudoephedrine and has similar effects in terms of providing an energy boost, suppressing the appetite, and increasing metabolic rate and caloric expenditure. By stimulating specific adrenergic receptors, synephrine is thought to stimulate fat metabolism without the negative cardiovascular side effects experienced by some people with ephedra, also called ma huang.

Bitter orange usually contains about 1 to 6 percent synephrine, but some manufacturers boost the content to as much as 30 percent.[92] It does have a thermogenic (fat-burning) effect[93]; in animal studies, synephrine caused weight loss but also increased the risk of cardiovascular problems.[94]

Bitter orange can also increase the side effects of many medications, including (but not limited to) Xanax, Zocor, Sudafed, Buspar, Celexa, Zoloft, Allegra, prednisone, Meridia, Viagra, and a number of blood pressure medications.[95] Do *not* take bitter orange if you have high blood pressure or are pregnant.

The bottom line is this: bitter orange is a stimulant, and the same cautions about other stimulants (like ephedra) apply. You should be just as careful with "ephedra-free" pills containing bitter orange as you would be with ephedra.

Glutamine

Glutamine is your secret weapon against carbohydrate cravings. I use it all the time with my clients—I have them combine a couple of grams of the powder with a little heavy cream and xylitol for sweetener. This has a remarkable ability to curb the urge for something sweet.

Glutamine's usefulness as a craving buster was first discovered when it was shown that about 12 grams of glutamine curbed alcohol cravings.[96] Its effect on sugar cravings was acknowledged by a research director at the National Institute of Health as far back as 1986.[97] Atkins routinely used it with his patients to combat the compulsion to eat sugar.[98] Dr. Ron Rosedale explains that glutamine acts as a brain fuel, so it can help eliminate carbohydrate cravings while you are in that "transition" period.[99] Glutamine (also known as L-glutamine) comes in capsules or powders, but I prefer the powder for its versatility and fast-acting ability.

Neptune Krill Oil

Neptune krill oil (NKO) is a relatively new supplement that shows tremendous promise in the treatment of PMS. It's basically a fish oil, a low-temperature extract of the abundant Antarctic krill (*Euphausia superba*). Reportedly, it has an ORAC value (antioxidant rating) of 378—more than three hundred times that of vitamins A and E and forty-eight times greater than most fish oils. A recent study evaluated the effectiveness of NKO for the management of PMS in an outpatient clinic. In seventy patients, a significant improvement was found after three menstrual cycles. The authors concluded that NKO can significantly reduce the emotional symptoms of premenstrual syndrome.[100] The dosage is 3 grams a day. You can also take NKO together with the three products I have been successfully using for PMS with my clients for years: B_6, magnesium, and GLA.

Possibly Helpful

Gymnema Sylvestre

Gymnema sylvestre is an herb with an interesting double relationship to sugar. In Sanskrit, *gymnema* means "sugar destroyer." If you place it on the tongue, it blocks the sensation of sweetness! But if you take it internally, it seems to help control blood sugar levels, at least in diabetics. It may well turn out to have a place in the supplement regimen of those trying to control blood sugar and increase insulin sensitivity.

Hydroxycitrate (Hydroxycitric Acid)

Hydroxycitric acid, an extract from the plant *Garcinia cambogia*, is often sold and promoted as a weight loss aid. In animal studies, it suppressed appetite and encouraged weight loss, and it has also been suggested that hydroxycitric acid interferes with the body's ability to produce and store fat. But a lot of human studies have been very disappointing. It does, however, have its supporters, among them vitamin expert Dr. Shari Lieberman, who argues that some of the disappointing studies were badly designed. As far as I'm concerned, the jury is out on this one. I haven't personally seen much success with it, but I'm willing to be proven wrong.

Banaba Leaf Extract (Corosolic Acid)

Banaba leaf extract contains a compound called corosolic acid, which has been used for centuries as an aid to weight loss and blood sugar control. Corosolic acid is used routinely in the weight loss protocol of Dr. Alan Schwartz, medical director of the Holistic Resource Center in Agoura Hills, California, and it is now beginning to get some attention nationally for its ability to lower blood sugar when taken in the range of about 48 milligrams a day. A very thorough discussion of the actions of corosolic acid and the research so far can be found in the September 2000 issue of *Life Extension*, the magazine of the Life Extension Foundation. The article is also available online: lef.org.

Not Recommended at This Time

CLA (Conjugated Linoleic Acid)

There have been some very promising studies on CLA, a fatty acid found in beef, lamb, and dairy products. A substantial amount of research has shown it to reduce the incidence and size of tumors[101, 102] and, in some research, the amount of body fat on both animals and humans. However, as of this writing, some disturbing studies have appeared showing that CLA supplementation increased insulin resistance in obese men[103] as well as C-reactive protein, a risk factor for heart disease.[104] Two recent articles suggested that, in view of the fact that the benefit in the positive CLA studies wasn't that spectacular to begin with and that supplementation might increase the risk factors for diabetes and heart disease, it shouldn't be recommended at the present time.[105–107] I agree.

Flaxseed Oil (for Men)

Although flaxseeds are a great source of one of the omega-3 fats (alpha linolenic acid, probably the least important of the three omega-3s we care about), several recent disturbing studies have found a small but surprising relationship between alpha linolenic acid intake and prostate cancer in men.[108–110] Though there may well turn out to be an explanation for this, until we know more, I don't recommend flaxseed oil for men, though it's fine for women. I do, however, strongly recommend that both men and women supplement with fish oil, the source of the two most important omega-3 fatty acids, which have been linked to nothing but terrific health benefits.

Vanadium (Vanadyl Sulfate)

Vanadium has long been used by many clinicians to help improve blood sugar control. In one of the few studies in which it was tested alone, at relatively high dosages it improved glycemic control, lowered fasting blood sugar, and incidentally lowered LDL cholesterol by an average of 12 mg/dl.[111] The problem with vanadium is that the dosages given to get these results are very, very high relative to what we usually get in the diet, and no one is completely sure what constitutes a toxic dose. It's probably going to turn out to be a great addition to the arsenal, but right now I believe it should be used only by people who have insulin disorders and only under the supervision of a nutrition-trained physician.

CHAPTER 5

The Five Biggest Myths About Low-Carb Diets

T he five issues I cover in this chapter are definitely the subject of frequently asked questions. "So," you may be thinking, "why not talk about them in the FAQ chapter?" Well, these particular questions are so significant to the low-carb dieter and the answers require so much detail and exposition that I felt they deserved a chapter of their own.

Over the years, there have been many criticisms leveled at low-carbohydrate diets. Some of these have been repeated so often that they are now taken as gospel, even though they have never been closely examined (they will be here). Some are based on complete misunderstandings of biochemistry and physiology, and some on an astonishing distortion or misreading of the program being criticized. (One supposedly reputable health information website recently criticized the Zone on the basis of the "fact" that "the Zone diet contains less than 1,000 calories," which is simply untrue.)

In reading dozens of critiques of low-carbohydrate diets, I discovered that there are five issues that come up repeatedly. This chapter addresses all five. Since you may well hear some of these criticisms from well-meaning people, including your doctor, I have compiled a number of reference studies on the What's New?/For Your Doctor page on JonnyBowden.com, which I will update regularly. I urge you to share this information with your health-care practitioner if he or she has any concerns related to the issues in this chapter. Of course, if your doctor has specific concerns that apply to you individually, you should always follow his or her guidance.

MYTH #1: Low-Carbohydrate Diets Induce Ketosis, a Dangerous Metabolic State

Bear with me while I tell you a story. Follow this, and you will understand more about ketosis than half the doctors in America.

Back in the 1990s, a lot of restaurants in New York City served a delicious fish that nobody would order. In fact, the presence of this fish on the menu caused more than a little distress in some circles and led to some heated exchanges between customers and restaurant managers. Animal rights activists—who were frequently baby boomers with enough disposable income to keep the restaurants afloat—were the most vitriolic in their condemnation of the establishments that served this fish, but the outcry from "regular" folks was not much more muted.

The fish was dolphin.

You can, I'm sure, see the problem.

No one wanted to patronize an establishment that was so heartless as to serve up Flipper for the gastronomical whims of its customers.

Quite understandable.

Problem was: "dolphin" *isn't* "Flipper."

Dolphins were, and are, quite ordinary but tasty fish that look exactly like fish and bear not even a passing resemblance to the bottle-nosed dolphins that delight us at Sea World and with whom they happen, by some weird taxonomical screwup, to share the same name. In fact, they aren't even the same *species* (one being, of course, a fish, while the other is a mammal). Plus, the dolphin (fish) does not perform adorable tricks and does not appear to have much rapport with the average human being.

But go tell that to the table for four in the back where the kid is crying and the parents are threatening to never come back to this restaurant, ever.

Waiters explained, probably as many times as they had to say, "Hi, I'm Jason and I'll be your server for today," that dolphin was not *dolphin*. Yes, they did in fact share the same name, but one was a *fish* and one was the lovable *marine mammal*, and the dish on the menu, sir, was not Flipper.

Didn't matter.

No matter how many times this conversation was repeated in restaurants throughout the city, and probably throughout the country (though I can personally attest only to the number of times I heard it in New York City), it fell on deaf ears.

So restaurant owners did a smart thing.

They changed the name of the fish.
"Dolphin" now became known as "mahi-mahi."
End of problem.
Which brings us to ketosis.

Ketosis: Friend or Foe?

It is very difficult to read about—or write about—low-carbohydrate dieting without dealing with the term *ketosis*. If you've been around low-carb diets at all—if you've experimented with them, talked about them to your friends, read about them, read *warnings* about them—you've surely heard of ketosis. You've probably heard that it's some kind of metabolic state that accompanies these diets and that you should avoid it—and those "high-protein" fad diets that produce it—at all costs. Several years ago, in a column at iVillage, I wrote the following, which is still true today:

> Ketosis is so misunderstood and maligned that I really feel it's worthwhile to go into it in some detail. For those of you who are new to this, ketosis is something that happens in the body when you eat very, very few carbohydrates. Since there's very little sugar coming in, *your body burns fat for fuel almost exclusively*—this is called "being in ketosis." Many popular diet programs have made use of this "metabolic advantage," most famously the Atkins program, and dietitians (and doctors) have been screaming about how dangerous it is ever since, although they can never seem to tell us why. It's been popular among dieters because, among other things, even the most metabolically resistant people usually lose weight on a ketogenic diet, and many people, after an initial adjustment from a sugar-burning to a fat-burning metabolism, feel great, with increased energy and a noticeable sense of well-being.

Atkins himself wrote rhapsodically of ketosis in the first and second editions of his *New Diet Revolution*, calling it "one of life's charmed gifts. . . . As delightful as sex and sunshine, and it has fewer drawbacks than either of them." It was Atkins who gave ketosis the nickname "the metabolic advantage."

So how can something so harmless and benevolent (and so conducive to weight loss) be widely considered one of the most dangerous states the body can be in? (If you doubt that this is the prevailing opinion, try asking your mainstream doctor what he or she thinks of it. Or ask a dietitian.)

The reason is quite simple, actually. For the better part of thirty years, mainstream medicine, dietitians, and most of the critics of the low-carb diet have *completely confused two conditions*, as different from each other as the dolphin (fish) and the dolphin (Flipper). One of those conditions is ordinary, benign, dietary ketosis, of which we're speaking here. The other is a life-threatening condition called diabetic ketoacidosis (more on this in a minute). Getting the mainstream to understand the difference has been harder than getting the kid at the table to understand that the restaurant really isn't serving cooked Flipper.

Atkins, in the last edition of *New Diet Revolution*, pretty much gave up the thirty-year fight to get the medical establishment to understand the difference and stopped using the term *ketosis*. He switched to the term *lipolysis* (fat breakdown). Only time will tell if the name change is as successful as the switch to mahi-mahi has been.

The Real Deal on Ketosis

So what is this thing called ketosis, and why should we care?

Note: I'm going to go into a little biochemistry here. I'll try to make it painless, though I understand that, for many, the term *painless biochemistry* is an oxymoron. If you want to skip the next few paragraphs, believe me, I won't be offended. If, however, you'd like to *skewer* the next person who tells you how dangerous your low-carb diet is because of ketosis, you might want to read the next few hundred words.

Your body has three main sources of fuel: carbohydrates (glucose), protein (amino acids), and fat (fatty acids). These are broken down and combined in different ways—fats and carbs to produce energy or be saved as fat, and protein to build up tissues, bones, muscles, enzymes, and the like. Remember that the whole purpose of a low-carb diet is to make your metabolism more of a fat-burning machine than a sugar-burning machine. As Lyle McDonald, one of the best known authorities on the ketogenic diet, says, "Ketosis is the end result of a shift in the insulin/glucagon ratio and indicates *an overall shift from a glucose (sugar)-based metabolism to a fat-based metabolism.*" (Emphasis mine.) In other words, the whole idea is to get your body to switch fuels from primarily carbs, its preferred immediate source of energy, to primarily fat.

Carbs, or sugar, are the first source of energy used by the body, with fats providing the best *long-term* source of energy. Yet high levels of carbohydrate produce, for many people, higher than desirable levels of the hormone insulin, and fat cannot be "burned" or "released" to any significant degree in the presence of insulin. So for someone with a weight problem, high carb intake will provide all the fuel they need for living (and probably plenty for storage as fat in addition) and will raise insulin levels enough so that fat isn't released or burned.

Normally, carbs are broken down into glucose, and then pyruvic acid, and then a substance called acetyl CoA. Fats are broken down into their component parts—fatty acids and glycerol—then *further* broken down (by a process called beta-oxidation) into two carbon fragments which *also* combine to make acetyl CoA (see illustration below).

On a "normal," high-carb diet, two things happen to the acetyl CoA. First, some of it gets broken down in the liver into ketone bodies. It's important to remember that this is a *normal* part of metabolism. You are making ketone bodies right now while you sit reading this book. The liver is *always* producing ketone bodies. As McDonald says, "Ketones should not be considered a toxic substance or a by-product of abnormal human metabolism. Rather, ketones are a normal physiological substance that

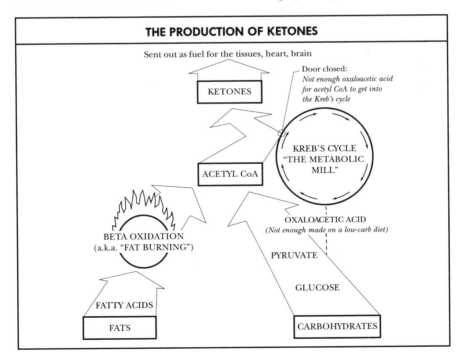

THE PRODUCTION OF KETONES

Sent out as fuel for the tissues, heart, brain

KETONES

Door closed:
Not enough oxaloacetic acid for acetyl CoA to get into the Kreb's cycle

KREB'S CYCLE "THE METABOLIC MILL"

ACETYL CoA

BETA OXIDATION (a.k.a. "FAT BURNING")

OXALOACETIC ACID
(Not enough made on a low-carb diet)

PYRUVATE

FATTY ACIDS

GLUCOSE

FATS

CARBOHYDRATES

plays many important roles in the human body." (This, of course, did not stop Jane Brody of *The New York Times*—one of the biggest apologists for the high-carbohydrate/low-fat diet in America—from calling ketones "toxic compounds that can damage the brain" and "pollute the blood.")

So the liver makes ketones—which are essentially by-products of fat metabolism (specifically the breakdown of acetyl CoA)—*all the time*.

What's the *other* thing that happens to the acetyl CoA?

Well, on a diet with plenty of carbohydrates, the acetyl CoA combines with a by-product of *carbohydrate* metabolism called oxaloacetic acid. When acetyl CoA combines with oxaloacetic acid, it enters an energy-production cycle called the Krebs Cycle. (This is what is meant by the old saying "Fat burns in a flame of carbohydrate." Without the carbohydrate necessary to produce the oxaloacetic acid, the acetyl CoA cannot gain admission to this energy cycle and be burned.)

So those are the two pathways that acetyl CoA (which you remember is produced *both* by fat breakdown and by carbohydrate breakdown) can take when there's carbohydrate in the system.

But what happens when there isn't?

What happens when you go on a very restricted carbohydrate diet and there is not enough carbohydrate (glucose) coming down the pike to produce the oxaloacetic acid necessary to take the acetyl CoA into the Krebs cycle? Well, the acetyl CoA *accumulates* in the liver. And the liver promptly breaks it down into ketones (also known as ketone bodies—if you really want to get technical, there are three of these ketone bodies, and their names are acetoacetate, beta-hydroxybutrate, and acetone; it's the release of the acetone that gives you that "fruity" breath). The major determinant of whether the liver will produce a significant or negligible amount of ketone bodies is the amount of sugar (liver glycogen) that's around. In a low-carb diet, there's not a lot. So all of the acetyl CoA has to be broken down into ketones, and these ketones—products of *fat* breakdown—are now being made in sufficient quantities that you can detect them in the urine. The "normal" level of ketones in the blood is about 0.1 mmol/dl; mild ketosis is 0.2 mmol/dl. Ketogenic diets typically produce between 5–7 mmol/dl (see chart opposite).

Please remember: these ketones are benign products of normal metabolism, and the fact that you can actually see their presence in the urine (by the use of ketone test strips) simply means that your body is breaking down fat for energy in measurable, significant amounts.

So how did ketone bodies get such a bad rap?

There are two reasons.

COMPARISON OF KETONE CONCENTRATIONS UNDER DIFFERENT CONDITIONS	
Metabolic State	**Ketone Body Concentration (mmol/dl)**
mixed (regular) diet	0.01
ketosis	0.02
fasting 2–3 days	1
after exercise	up to 2
fasting 1 week	5
ketogenic diet	5–6
fasting 3–4 weeks	6–8
ketoacidosis	8+
diabetic ketoacidosis	up to 25

Note: Ketone body concentrations are higher when fasting than during a ketogenic diet due to the slight insulin response from eating.

Reprinted from Lyle McDonald, *The Ketogenic Diet: A Complete Guide for the Diet and Practitioner* (Kearney, Neb.: Morris Publishing, 1998), by permission of the author.

After data from G.A. Mitchell et al, "Medical Aspects of Ketone Body Metabolism," *Clinical and Investigative Medicine* 18 (1995):193–216, and A.M. Robinson et al, "Physiological Roles of Ketone Bodies as Substrates and Signals in Mammalian Tissues," *Physiological Reviews* 60 (1980): 143–87.

Ketosis and Diabetic Ketoacidosis

To understand the primary reason keytones have been vilified, we have to look at the type 1 diabetic. As you may remember from earlier discussion, insulin is responsible for getting sugar *out of the bloodstream* and *into the cells*, thus keeping blood sugar (glucose) within a tightly controlled range. Insulin also keeps fat from being broken down, which is why it needs to be in balance with its sister hormone, glucagon. Glucagon is responsible for *releasing* fat into the bloodstream, where it can be broken down and used for energy. Insulin is responsible for *storing* it.

The type 1 diabetic cannot make insulin.

With no insulin, two things happen, neither of them good. One, blood sugar rises to very dangerous levels. Two, with no insulin to put the brakes on glucagon, fat is broken down and released into the bloodstream faster than it can possibly be used, and the production of ketone bodies is seriously ramped up. In addition, these ketones *cannot* be used by the body tissues like they can in normal dietary ketosis. This is because there's tons of glucose around, which is the preferred fuel, so the ketones just keep accumulating at an alarming rate. This state is called *diabetic ketoacidosis*, and it is indeed very dangerous and life-threatening to an untreated type 1 diabetic. Remember, a ketogenic diet produces, on average, 5 to 7 mmol/dl of ketones, and does it in the presence of *normal to low* blood sugar. The untreated type 1 diabetic will produce ketones in the range of 25 (350 to 600 percent higher than normal!) and will do it in the presence of *extraordinarily high and dangerous* levels of blood sugar. There is absolutely no comparison between the two states. The person *without* uncontrolled type 1 diabetes has a number of normal feedback mechanisms that will always keep the ketones in a safe range, mechanisms that *do not exist* with the untreated type 1 diabetic. Diabetic ketoacidosis *cannot happen* when there is even a small amount of insulin around, as there *always* is in those not suffering from type 1 diabetes, even when the person is on a ketogenic diet.

COMPARISON OF DIETARY KETOSIS WITH DIABETIC KETOACIDOSIS			
	Normal Diet	**Ketosis**	**Diabetic Ketoacidosis**
blood glucose (mg/dl)	80–120	~65–80	300+
insulin	moderate	low	absent
glucagon	low	high	high
ketone production (g/day)	low	115–180	400
ketone concentrations	0.1	4–10	
blood pH	7.4	7.4	<7.3

Reprinted from Lyle McDonald, *The Ketogenic Diet: A Complete Guide for the Diet and Practitioner* (Kearney, Neb.: Morris Publishing, 1998), by permission of the author.

The second reason ketosis has gotten a bad rap is a reversal of a medical fact. Ketosis is one of the metabolic adaptations to starvation. When you're starving, the body uses ketones for fuel. Starving is bad. Therefore, people who didn't think about it very clearly reversed the order and assumed that since ketosis is one of the *reactions* to something bad, ketosis *itself* must be bad. That's like assuming that umbrellas cause rain. Ketosis in starvation is very, very different from ketosis in the ketogenic (high-fat or high-protein) diet. Why? In starvation, the body is *breaking down muscle* in the absence of dietary protein. In the low-carb diet, dietary protein is plentiful and prevents the loss of muscle that occurs with true starvation. The loss of body protein is actually what causes death from starvation. When you supply sufficient protein in the diet, this simply doesn't happen.

Are Ketones Dangerous?

Hardly. They're a perfectly good source of energy. Drs. Donald and Judith Voet, authors of a popular medical biochemistry textbook, say that ketones "serve as important metabolic fuels for many peripheral tissues, particularly heart and skeletal muscle."[1] And a recent paper coauthored by a number of distinguished researchers, including one from Harvard Medical School, stated that ketones provide an efficient source of energy for the brain and that mild ketosis—the kind you achieve on a low-carb diet—could have a wide range of benefits for conditions ranging from Alzheimer's to Parkinson's.[2]

A ketogenic diet should not be used by three groups of people: (1) uncontrolled type 1 diabetics (for the reasons outlined above); (2) pregnant or nursing women (not because higher levels of ketones in the blood are dangerous, but just because we don't know for sure if they have any effect on the baby); and (3) people with existing kidney disease (see myth #3 for a full explanation of the connection between protein and kidneys).

If you are not in one of these three groups—type 1 diabetics, pregnant or nursing women, or people with existing kidney disease—*the ketogenic diet is perfectly and utterly safe.*

Let's take a look at the science.

A recent study in the *Journal of Nutrition* looked at the effects of a six-week ketogenic diet on risk factors for cardiovascular disease.[3] The study found *improvements* in triglycerides and insulin levels plus a slight *increase* in HDL cholesterol (the "good" kind). Most importantly, the *type* of LDL ("bad" cholesterol) tended to change from the kind that's dangerous (pattern B) to the kind that's not (pattern A). Other studies have shown similar results.[4]

A recent study at the University of Cincinnati and Children's Hospital Medical Center in Cincinnati specifically looked at the effects of a very low-carbohydrate diet on cardiovascular risk factors in fifty-three obese but otherwise healthy women. The women were placed on either a very low-carbohydrate diet with unrestricted calories or a low-fat diet that was calorie-restricted. The low-carb group lost significantly more weight and, more importantly, more *body fat* than the low-fat diet group. (Interestingly, after the study, both groups of women wound up maintaining their weight loss on about the same number of calories—1,300.)

This last study is particularly interesting for a couple of reasons. One, the low-carb group *was* in ketosis, but as the authors noted, the level of ketones wasn't even close to that seen in starvation or diabetic ketoacidosis and presented no problems whatsoever. Two, the subjects on the very low-carbohydrate diet experienced significantly *more* weight loss than the low-fat group *and* maintained great readings for blood chemistries and cardiovascular risk factors *while consuming more than 50 percent of their calories as fat and 20 percent as saturated fat*. Current standards for healthy eating include reducing total fat intake to less than 30 percent of total calories and decreasing saturated fat to less than 10 percent, which is supposed to both lower cholesterol and decrease the risk of obesity. These subjects accomplished the same thing while eating a heck of a lot more fat—and saturated fat—than the current standards, *plus* they lost more weight in the bargain. The authors wisely conclude that "this study provides a surprising challenge to prevailing dietary practice."[5]

Finally, ketogenic diets have been used as treatments for childhood epilepsy for more than seventy years. They are currently used at seventy-eight centers in the United States alone, including Children's Hospital in Los Angeles, John Hopkins in Baltimore, the UCLA School of Medicine, Children's Hospital in Boston, the Montefiore Medical Center and Columbia Presbyterian Medical Center in New York, and the Lucille Packard Children's Hospital at Stanford, whose website states, "No patient has had serious complications."

Do You Have to Be in Ketosis to Lose Weight on a Low-Carb Diet?

No. You don't.

Ketosis is actually only a feature of some low-carb diets, and not even that many. It is stressed in Atkins; it is likely (but not mandatory) in Protein Power; it is a feature of the Lindora program and the GO-Diet. Many other low-carb programs don't even mention it. The point is that it is *not* something to fear. Many nutrition experts—myself included—feel that you don't have to be in ketosis to get the benefits of a low-carb diet. You can "flirt" with ketosis, be on the cusp of ketosis, but unless you are very metabolically resistant, you may be able to get the benefits of low-carb eating without ever worrying about your ketone levels.

Perhaps the most sober and rational summary of the ketogenic diet is given by Lyle McDonald, who wrote the definitive book on the subject and accumulated the greatest number of scientific references on ketosis ever seen in one place. He says: "After years of experimenting with the [ketogenic] diet myself, and getting feedback from hundreds and hundreds of people, about the best anyone can say is that the ketogenic diet is a diet that works very well for many but not for all."

Amen.

> **BOTTOM LINE**
>
> *Dietary ketosis is not the same as diabetic ketoacidosis. The ketosis of a low-carb diet is not the same as ketosis in starvation. Many studies have demonstrated the safety of ketogenic diets, even for children. For references, go to What's New?/For Your Doctor on JonnyBowden.com.*

MYTH #2: Low-Carbohydrate Diets Cause Calcium Loss, Bone Loss, and/or Osteoporosis

This criticism of low-carb (or high-protein) diets is based on the fact that higher levels of protein result in higher levels of calcium in the urine, leading some people to the erroneous conclusion that protein causes bone loss. But a tremendous number of recent studies are showing something quite the opposite.

Want Strong Bones? Eat More Protein!

The Framingham Osteoporosis Study investigated protein consumption over a four-year period among 615 elderly men and women with an average age of seventy-five. The amount of protein eaten daily ranged from a low of 14 grams a day to a high of 175 grams. And guess what? The people who consumed *more* protein had *less* bone loss! Those who ate *less* protein had *more* bone loss, both at the femoral bone and at the spine. The study also found that "higher intake of animal protein *does not appear to affect the skeleton adversely.*"[6] (Emphasis mine.)

Calcium is better absorbed on a higher-protein diet, even if there is somewhat more *urinary* calcium excretion. High-protein diets in two recent studies resulted in *significantly more* calcium absorption than the low-protein diets, which were associated with *decreased* absorption.[7, 8] Interestingly, the actual "low-protein" diet that caused decreased calcium absorption in these studies had about the same amount of protein that the government recommends for adults! The authors concluded that this fact "raises new questions about the optimal amount of dietary protein required for normal calcium metabolism and bone health in young women."[9] And a recent study in *Obesity Research* looked at a high-protein versus low-protein diet to determine whether the protein content of the diet impacted bone mineral density. It did. *Bone mineral loss was greater in the low-protein group.*[10]

In other words, without enough protein, you just ain't gonna build (and preserve) strong bones, and the definition of "enough protein" may turn out to be a lot more than we previously thought.

The Verdict on Protein: Not Guilty

So how did protein get this bad reputation for causing calcium loss and osteoporosis? It partly stems from something in the body called the acid-base balance. All foods eventually digest and present themselves to the kidneys as either acid or alkaline. When there is too much acid, the body needs to buffer it, and calcium is one of the best buffering agents. Meats—along with many other foods, especially grains—are known to be acid-producing; hence the deduction that high-protein diets would cause a leeching of calcium from the bone in order to alkalize the acid content.

But here's the thing: we now know that if you take in enough alkalinizing nutrients, this doesn't happen. If you balance your high-protein foods with calcium (and potassium), you will not lose calcium from your bones! An interesting side note: you can take all the supplemental calcium you want; if you don't get enough protein, it's not going to make much difference to your bone health. The studies are very clear on this: *extra calcium is not enough to affect the skeleton when protein intake is low.*[11]

In short, it doesn't matter if there is a little more calcium in the urine as long as the body is holding on to more calcium than it's losing (i.e., is in "positive" calcium balance). And it will do that when there's plenty of protein plus calcium (and other minerals) in the diet.

BOTTOM LINE

Higher protein intakes do not cause bone loss or osteoporosis, especially in the presence of adequate mineral intakes. In fact, lower protein intakes are associated with more bone loss. For references, go to What's New?/For Your Doctor on JonnyBowden.com.

MYTH #3: High-Protein Diets Cause Damage to the Kidneys

You will often hear from ill-informed sources that a high-protein diet damages the kidneys. Not so. Consider the following: everyone knows about step classes and aerobics. They are great calorie burners, get the blood and oxygen flowing, are good conditioners of the cardiovascular system, and, with certain variations, can even be good for muscle toning. So they're a good thing, right?

Yes.

Except if you have a broken leg.

If you have a broken leg, or a sprained ankle, or shin splints, I'm going to suggest to you that you not take a step class until the injury heals. Under these special circumstances, the very weight bearing that does so much good for the normal person is going to be more stress than you need during the healing phase. I'm going to tell you to stay off the leg, let it heal, and avoid putting additional stress on it at this time.

Does the fact that step class is not good for a person with a broken leg mean that the step class *led* to the broken leg?

No. And ketogenic diets do not—I repeat, *do not*—cause kidney disease. If your doctor says they do, politely ask him or her to show you the studies. (They don't exist.) Ketogenic diets are, however, not a good thing if you have an existing kidney disease, much the way a step class is not a good thing if your leg is already broken.

High Protein Causes Kidney Disease? Not.

The oft-repeated medical legend that high-protein diets cause kidney disease came from reversing a medical fact. The medical fact is that reducing protein (up to a point) lessens the decline of renal (kidney) function in people who already have kidney disease. Because restricting protein seems to be a good strategy for those with *existing* kidney failure, some people drew the illogical conclusion that the reverse must also be true— that large amounts of protein *lead* to kidney failure.

In any case, it is not proteins per se that cause problems, even for those who already have renal disease; it is the *glycolated* proteins (see chapter 2). These sugar-sticky proteins, you may remember, are the result of excess sugar in the blood bumping into protein molecules. These sugar-coated proteins are called AGES, **a**dvanced **g**lycolated **e**nd-products. The AGES themselves then stick together, forming even bigger collections of molecules, which are too large to pass through the filtering mechanisms of the *glomerulus*, the network of blood capillaries in the kidneys that acts as a filter for waste products from the blood. This reduces GFR (glomerular filtration rate), a measure of kidney function.

I was warned that going on a low-carb, high protein diet would make me lose calcium from my bones. Yet my last two bone scan screenings showed just the opposite— at age 50 I have the bones of a 30-year-old!

—Ada K.

High-protein intake *does not* cause this to happen in normally functioning kidneys. A recent study of 1,624 women enrolled in the Nurses' Health Study concluded that "high protein intake was not associated with renal function decline in women with normal renal function."[12] Another study in the *American Journal of Kidney Disease* showed that protein intake had *no effect* on GFR in healthy male subjects.[13] And a third study in the *International Journal of Obesity* compared a high-protein with a low-protein weight loss diet and concluded that healthy kidneys adapted to protein intake and that the high protein diet caused no adverse effects.[14]

If you don't currently have kidney disease, a low-carbohydrate diet is actually an ideal way to help control the blood sugar levels that can eventually lead to kidney disease. Of course, just to be safe, you should check with your doctor to make sure you don't have any undiagnosed kidney impairment; but if you don't, you're sure not going to develop it from being on a low-carb diet.

BOTTOM LINE

Higher protein intakes do not cause any damage whatsoever to healthy kidneys. For references, go to What's New?/For Your Doctor on JonnyBowden.com.

MYTH #4: The Only Reason You Lose Weight on a Low-Carb Diet Is Because It's Low in Calories

The short response to this myth is simple: *so what?*

This accusation—that low-carb diets work only because they are low in calories—is particularly amusing because it is never made against high-carb weight loss diets that are *equally* low in calories. In fact, there is only a 121-calorie difference between the most stringent induction phase of the Atkins diet and the Dean Ornish ultra-low-fat diet. And after the first couple of weeks, when you get into the ongoing weight loss phase of Atkins, you're actually consuming 354 calories *more* than you would be on the Dean Ornish diet and 165 calories *more* than you would be on Weight Watchers![15] Yet you never hear the establishment say that the Ornish low-fat diet works only because it's low-calorie!

Look, on virtually every weight loss diet in the world, you ultimately wind up consuming fewer calories than you did while you were putting on weight. I don't care if the diet is low-fat, high-fat, low-carb, high-carb, vegetarian, Food Pyramid, raw food, you name it—ultimately, they are *all* reduced-calorie diets. One of the primary reasons most of them fail is hunger. By now we know that insulin is called the hunger hormone for a very good reason, and insulin is elevated *most* by high-carbohydrate diets. So if you have a choice of gritting your teeth and staying on a 1,200-calorie, low-fat, high-carbohydrate diet that leaves you hungry and craving sweets all the time or of going on a diet with the *same number of calories* that allows you to eat rich, satisfying, natural foods and *doesn't* leave you hungry all the time, which would *you* pick?

Exactly. That's why the short answer to this myth is "Who cares?" Even if it *were* true that low-carb diets work only because they are low-calorie, who gives a rat's tail? If two "diets" with an equal number of calories produce equal weight loss but one is easier to stay on, why in the world wouldn't you go with it?

I used to find that I'd have fewer cravings—actually be less hungry—if I forgot to eat. Now that I understand how insulin works as "the hunger hormone" it all makes sense. These days I choose my food with an eye on how it's going to affect my blood sugar and insulin levels. I'm much more in control of my appetite when I choose low-sugar, unprocessed foods
—Jeremy N.

More Food on a Low-Carb Diet?

Because a low-carbohydrate diet is able to reduce insulin levels and is far more likely to induce hormonally balanced states than conventional high-carb diets, it is possible—though we're not 100 percent sure—that you may be able to consume somewhat more calories on a low-carb diet than you would on a high-carb diet and still lose weight. One dramatic study compared a low-fat diet to an Atkins-type diet in two groups of overweight adolescent boys. After three months, the low-carb group lost almost twice as much weight as the low-fat group (19 pounds for the low-carb group and 8.5 pounds for the low-fat group); the low-fat group averaged 1,100 calories a day, while the Atkins group averaged 1,803![16]

Recently, a number of studies have come out showing that weight loss is actually greater on a low-carb diet than on a conventional low-fat diet that has the same number of calories.[17, 18] To be fair, there are plenty of studies showing that both diets produce identical weight loss. (Interestingly, there are virtually *no* studies that show that low-carb diets produce *less* weight loss!) But even in the studies that show identical weight loss, triglycerides and HDL levels almost always improve on the higher-protein diets. For example, Alain Golay, a respected researcher who is no particular advocate of low-carb diets, recently tested a low-carb (25 percent) diet against a typical higher-carb (45 percent) diet for weight loss and found that, while there was not much difference in weight loss, the low-carb group had significantly greater improvements in fasting insulin and triglycerides.[19] In another study, he pitted a low-carb (15 percent) diet against a higher-carb (45 percent) diet and again found similar weight loss but marked improvements in glucose, insulin, cholesterol, and triglycerides on the low-carb diet *only*; no such benefits were seen on the high-carb diet.[20] If two "diets"—high-protein/low-carb and high-carb/low-fat—are equal in calories and produce equal weight loss but the first produces significantly improved blood chemistry and lowers the risk for heart disease and diabetes, why in the world wouldn't you choose that one?

Many studies have been done comparing all kinds of different diets for weight loss, but the truth is that very few studies have lasted more than a year, leading many experts to conclude that while you can basically lose weight on any diet, we really have no idea whether any particular regimen is easier to stay on over the long haul. The action is clearly in *maintaining* weight loss, and since the lower-carb diets seem to be much more satiating, we can speculate that they may turn out to be a lot easier to maintain as a lifestyle than a diet that simply reduces fat, which is turning out to be a lot less

I had no idea that by raising my triglycerides my high-carb, low-fat diet could actually be putting me at risk for heart disease.

—Adrienne W.

important than previously thought. In fact, Dr. Walter Willett, chairman of the department of nutrition at Harvard University's School of Public Health and one of the most respected researchers in the field, recently declared in two articles—one in *Obesity Review*[21] and one in the *American Journal of Medicine*[22]—that dietary fat is *not* a major determinant of body fat and plays virtually no role in obesity.

What About Calories?

Since most low-carb diet authors do not advocate counting calories (at least at first) and because most low-carb diets are based on the premise that it is critical to control the hormonal responses to food, many people have gotten the idea that low-carb theorists think calories don't matter at all. This is simply not so. As I wrote in a previous book, calories are still on the marquee, but they are not starring players anymore. Of *course* calories still count—there isn't a responsible low-carb diet writer out there who would argue the point. But controlling hormones counts *at least as much*, if not more. If I take in 1,500 calories a day from sugar and insulin-raising carbohydrates, I will find it notoriously difficult to lose any weight, since the high levels of insulin I produce are going to effectively block fat from being released from my fat cells. Yet if I take in the same 1,500 calories— or even a few more!—from a diet with less carbs and more protein and fat, the resulting balance between insulin and glucagon is going to be much more favorable to fat release. And I'm likely to lose a lot more weight for the same caloric price.

On the other hand, to play devil's advocate, if I take in 15,000 calories, all from fat with a little protein, producing the absolute minimum amount of insulin, I'm *still* going to gain weight. Why? Because even though the "doors" to the fat cells are now open for business, there is simply no reason for my body to *release* any of the fat inside them for fuel, because I'm already consuming way more fuel than I could possibly need.

Now, can you lose weight on a low-calorie diet that is not low-carb? Of course you can. People do it all the time. But consider the following: most weight loss diets—of any kind—wind up being lower in carbohydrates *even if they are not "low-carb" diets*. The average overweight American man is easily able to consume 3,500 calories daily, and let's hypothetically say 65 percent of it is from carbs. That's a total of 2,275 calories from carbs, or 569 grams of carbohydrates a day. The National Weight Control Registry, which follows people who have successfully lost at least 30 pounds and kept it off for more than a year, has found that the average man on a successful weight maintenance diet consumes 1,724 calories, of which 56 percent come from carbohydrates.[23] So our typical National Weight Control Registry man is consuming 237 grams of carbs a day, *a 59 percent reduction in carbohydrates from what he was eating when he put the weight on!*

The average successful *woman* on the registry maintains her weight at 1,297 calories, 55 percent from carbohydrates.[24] We can postulate that if she was 50 pounds overweight to begin with, she was eating *at least* 2,000 calories a day minimum (probably more), and even if only 60 percent of that came from carbs, that's 300 grams of carbs a day. At her present maintenance level, she's consuming 178 grams, a 41 percent reduction in carb intake, certainly enough to make a major impact on insulin levels.

Yes, calories count. But so do hormones, and way more than the dietary establishment believes.

BOTTOM LINE

Calories count, but so do hormones. Many studies show more weight lost on low-carb diets than on high-carb diets with the same number of calories, and more of that weight comes from fat. Even those studies that show equal weight loss invariably show better blood chemistry on the low-carb diets. Lowering fat in the diet is not the answer to obesity. For references, go to What's New?/For Your Doctor on JonnyBowden.com.

MYTH #5: Low-Carb Diets Increase the Risk for Heart Disease

In Denmark, the number of storks is positively correlated with the number of babies born.

This interesting fact was taught to me in graduate school by a wonderful psychology professor named Dr. Scott Fraser, who used it to teach a lesson about scientific studies that has allowed me to understand a great many things about research. I will pass it on to you, and you may never look at research studies in quite the same way.

So let's repeat: in Denmark, the more storks, the more babies. This positive correlation holds up year in and year out.

Okay, class, what shall we conclude from this?

A LITTLE INTERNET HUMOR

1. The Japanese eat very little fat and suffer fewer heart attacks than the British or Americans.

2. The Mexicans eat a lot of fat and suffer fewer heart attacks than the British or Americans.

3. The Japanese drink very little red wine and suffer fewer heart attacks than the British or Americans.

4. The Italians drink excessive amounts of red wine and suffer fewer heart attacks than the British or Americans.

5. The Germans drink a lot of beers and eat lots of sausages and fats and suffer fewer heart attacks than the British or Americans.

Conclusion: Eat and drink what you like. Speaking English is apparently what kills you.

I hope you see what I'm getting at.

Here's what *actually* happens. In the particular part of Denmark where the study was done, single people live mainly in the cities. When they get married and decide to raise a family, they move to the suburbs. The architectural design of the suburbs in Denmark favors angled roofs made of tar. Storks nest in angled roofs made of tar. Both storks and young married couples wanting to have children gravitate to the same area, albeit for somewhat different reasons.

But they are *found together,* consistently, year after year. They are *positively correlated.*

The lesson: *correlation* does not equal *cause.* When two variables are found together, it does not mean that one caused the other. Diabetes went way up during the Clinton presidency, so an increase in diabetes is positively correlated with the Clintons. Statistical studies have also noted that the number of new radio and television sets purchased correlates with an increased number of deaths from coronary disease.[25] In Stockholm, Sweden, there was a correlation between the municipal tax rate and coronary mortality, leading to the interesting proposition that if tax rates were lowered, there would be less heart disease![26]

One scholar described this as the "yellow finger" phenomenon. Men with yellow fingertips are more likely to die of lung cancer. The reason: they are *smokers*. That's why they *have* yellow fingers. The yellowed tips of their fingers are the result of holding twenty cigarettes a day for twenty years. Washing off the yellow will not reduce their risk for lung cancer.

This brings us to cholesterol, heart disease, and the low-carb diet.

The Birth of the Diet-Heart Hypothesis and the Demonization of Saturated Fat

When the diet-heart hypothesis—the idea that saturated fat causes heart disease—was first proposed in the 1950s by Ancel Keys (see chapter 1), very little was known about either fat or cholesterol. Cholesterol, which is actually not a fat at all but a waxy molecule classified as a sterol, is the parent molecule for all the sex hormones in the body. Without it, you would not have testosterone, the estrogens, progesterone, or DHEA, not to mention cortisol and aldosterone. Most of the cholesterol in your body is *produced* by your body. *Dietary* cholesterol has virtually *no effect* on the amount of cholesterol in your blood. Two major long-term studies, Framingham and Tecumseh, confirm this (see tables below)[27]; they show that those who ate the most cholesterol had exactly the same level of cholesterol in their blood as those who ate the least. Even Keys, the author of the diet-heart hypothesis, knew this and said in 1991 *"There's no connection whatsoever between cholesterol in food and cholesterol in blood and we've known that all along. Cholesterol in the diet doesn't matter at all unless you happen to be a chicken or a rabbit."*[28]

CHOLESTEROL INTAKE—THE FRAMINGHAM HEART STUDY			
	Average Cholesterol From Food	Below Average Cholesterol From Food	Above Average Cholesterol From Food
		Blood Cholesterol	
	mg/day	mmol/L	mmol/L
Men	704 ± 220.9	6.16	6.16
Women	492 ± 170.0	6.37	6.26

CHOLESTEROL INTAKE AND BLOOD LIPIDS—THE TECUMSEH STUDY			
Blood Cholesterol in Thirds	Lower	Middle	Upper
Daily Intake of Cholesterol (mg)	554	566	533

What we do know is that dietary fat has an effect on serum cholesterol. What is a lot less clear is whether it matters much. (The Eadeses call "Cholesterol Madness" the most important chapter in their book "not because we believe cholesterol is such an important problem but because *everybody else does*.") Fully 50 percent of heart attacks happen to people with completely normal cholesterol numbers.[29] The Tokelauan Islanders get 63 percent of their diet from the healthy saturated fat in coconuts, and though their cholesterol levels are a bit high, they have virtually no heart disease.[30]

Fats: The Good, the Bad, and the Ugly

We know a lot more about fat than we did back in the '50s and even in the '80s, when the message was "All fat is bad." Most people are now aware that there are "good" fats and "bad" fats, and most people believe that the bad fats are saturated. Not so fast. It's turning out to be even more complicated than that. We now know that there is a type of fat far more dangerous and insidious than saturated fat—*trans-fat*—and virtually all of the data we have "linking" saturated fat with heart disease did not distinguish between *saturated fats* and *trans-fats*. Therefore, it is almost impossible to know whether or not saturated fats got the blame for something that was really being done by trans-fats.[31] Saturates, for example, *lower* lipoprotein(a), a risk factor for heart disease, and *raise* protective HDL cholesterol; trans-fats not only do the exact opposite but also raise LDL cholesterol![32] Many of us now believe that saturated fats have gotten the blame for damage that is actually caused by trans-fats. Virtually every low-carbohydrate diet, by definition, contains incredibly low amounts of trans-fats.

Furthermore, we also know that "saturated fat" is not a homogenous entity. It consists of many different types of fatty acids, and some of them are downright beneficial for health. For example, lauric acid has antimicrobial and antiviral properties and is able to fight bacteria. Caprylic acid is used to fight yeast. Short- and medium-chain saturated fatty acids like those found in coconuts are actually much more likely to be burned for fuel than stored as fat, and can be a great adjunct to a weight loss program.[33] And others, like stearic acid, have no effect whatsoever on cholesterol, except to possibly *raise* protective HDL.

Consider this, as the brilliant investigative reporter and three-time National Association of Science Writers' Science in Society Award winner Gary Taubes did in a recent article in *Science*. A porterhouse steak cooks down to about half fat and half protein. Of that fat, 51 percent is monoun-saturated, mostly all from oleic acid, the same monounsaturated fat found in heart-healthy olive oil. Forty-five percent is saturated, but a third of that is stearic acid, which at worst is harmless and at best raises HDL choles-terol. The remaining 4 percent is polyunsaturated. Thus, a porterhouse steak may actually be better for your heart—especially if eaten with a generous helping of vegetables—than a no-fat meal of high-glycemic, triglyceride-raising pasta.[34]

There's More to Cholesterol Than Just "Good" and "Bad"

Most people are aware that cholesterol comes in two "flavors," good (HDL) and bad (LDL). But most people do not know that both HDL and LDL have different subclasses, and these subclasses behave quite differently in the body. For example, LDL cholesterol has at least two types—pattern A, which are large, fluffy, cotton ball–like molecules, and pattern B, which are small, dense molecules that look like BB gun pellets. It is these small, dense LDL molecules that cause plaque and contribute to heart disease; the fluffy LDL is fairly harmless. In recent years, studies have begun to look at the factors that affect these particle sizes.[35] We are finding out that while the traditional high-carb, low-fat diet may in fact lower *overall* LDL, it *raises* the dangerous pattern B molecules and *lowers* protective HDL cholesterol. So while your overall cholesterol number may go *down*, your overall risk may go *up*. Not only that, high-carbohydrate diets significantly raise triglycerides—this is inarguable and has been shown in virtually every major study comparing high-carb to low-carb diets. The combination of high triglycerides and low HDL is far more predictive of heart disease (and far more dangerous) than an overall elevated cholesterol number.[36]

In the following story, you can see cholesterol madness in action: I have a dear friend who is in great shape and exercises every day. He came to me because he and his doctor were very concerned that his cho-lesterol was too high. I looked at his blood tests. He had normal lipopro-tein(a), a fasting glucose under 100, a fasting insulin of 5, triglycerides under 100, an HDL of 60 (giving him a triglyceride/HDL ratio of less than 2!), a cholesterol ratio itself of 3, normal C-reactive protein (a measure of inflammation), and a homocysteine (a huge risk factor for heart disease) under 7—but his overall cholesterol was 240. I wish I had those numbers! This man had a better chance of winning the lottery than he did of ever getting heart disease. He will never have a heart attack. Yet his doctor was ready to put him on a lifetime of expensive medication with potentially damaging side effects to bring down a number that *did not matter*!

You might reasonably ask at this point: if cholesterol is not as important an issue as we thought, how is it that the statin drugs (which reduce cholesterol) save lives?

Good question.

The statin drugs probably do save some lives (though at what cost remains to be seen). However, whether they do so by reducing cholesterol is an open question. What the statins do *in addition* to lowering cholesterol is reduce *inflammation*, which *is* a cause of heart disease. What they do to cholesterol, in my opinion, is the least important thing that they do in the body. You can reduce inflammation by consuming omega-3 fatty acids and reducing consumption of grains without the possible statin drug side effects of liver toxicity, and mitochondrial damage, and without the increased risk for death from other causes that is associated with cholesterol numbers that are too low.

Do Low-Fat Diets Prevent Heart Disease?

So, then, what about that famous Dean Ornish study that showed that low-fat diets reverse heart disease?

Actually, it showed no such thing. The Ornish study took forty-eight middle-aged white men with existing moderate to severe coronary heart disease. The researchers then did five—count 'em, *five*—simultaneous interventions with these men. They put them on a stress-reduction program. They got them to stop smoking. They gave them group therapy and support. They had them do daily aerobic exercise. *And* they put them on a very high-fiber diet, which also happened to be low in fat. Why anyone would conclude that it was the low-fat part of this multiple intervention that caused their improvement is a mystery. If we put those same men on a program of exercise, stress reduction, smoking cessation, group support, and meditation and included a pack of M&M's in their diet every day, would we conclude that M&M's reduce heart disease? I would argue that Ornish would have gotten the identical results—perhaps even *better* ones—using all those good interventions plus a diet loaded with fiber, absent of trans-fats, absent of sugar, containing very low amounts of vegetable fats, *and* containing plenty of good-quality protein from grass-fed animals plus saturated, monounsaturated, and omega-3 fats. We'll never know, because when five factors are involved, it is impossible to say which of them—or what combination of them—is responsible for the results.[37]

On a personal note: in researching this book, I read through literally hundreds of studies on cholesterol, fat, and heart disease. I could have rented a cot in the National Library of Medicine. I read the papers that appeared in the medical journals, I read the reanalysis of the data by scholars who questioned the cholesterol/saturated fat hypothesis of heart disease, I studied their arguments, I read the rebuttals to their arguments, and I read the rebuttals to the *rebuttals*.

I have, I confess, come to believe—along with a growing number of health professionals—that saturated fat and cholesterol are, for the most part, innocent bystanders. They were in the wrong place at the wrong time, Your Honor, and they hung out with the wrong crowd. As I mentioned earlier, virtually every epidemiological study that linked saturated-fat consumption with increased risk of cardiovascular diseases failed to separate saturated fat from its extremely dangerous cohort, trans-fatty acids.[38] Nor did the studies implicating saturated fat distinguish the *source* of the saturated fat consumed: saturated fat from natural foods like butter, eggs, and grain-fed cattle is *not* the same as saturated fat from fries and burgers; most people in industrial nations consume their saturated fat from hot dogs, fast-food hamburgers, and processed deli meats like salami and bologna. The people consuming the most saturated fat in those studies ate few fruits and vegetables and little fiber. But they ate something like 150 pounds of sugar per year (the latest figures from the USDA from 1997, projected to soon rise to 170 pounds). And for the most part, they did not exercise. Although it is extremely convenient to blame a single factor (like saturated fat) for heart disease, the fact is that a matrix of lifestyle and dietary characteristics such as the ones just mentioned are found *together*. In my opinion, saturated fat and cholesterol are not the bad guys here.

New research is beginning to support this. When a recent study in the *British Medical Journal* factored in fiber intake, the usual association between saturated fat and coronary disease risk practically vanished. The study concluded that the adverse effects of saturated fat and cholesterol are "at least in part explained by their low-fiber content and their associations with other risk factors." The researchers further stated that "benefits of reducing intakes of saturated fat and cholesterol are likely to be modest *unless accompanied by an increased consumption of foods rich in fiber.*" The study also commented on how the inclusion of omega-3 fats in the diet had a protective effect on heart disease.[39]

However . . .

I realize that this is a radical position and a hard sell to a population that has been raised on the premise that saturated fat and cholesterol are basically the children of Satan. So let me put you at ease: you do *not* have to accept the position that cholesterol and saturated fat are relatively harmless to do a low-carb diet. In fact, many of the low-carb authors don't accept that position either, so you will be in good company (notable exceptions—with whom I agree—are the Eadeses, Schwarzbein, and Atkins). You can do the GO-Diet, in which almost all of the fat comes from monounsaturated sources. You can do the Zone, which limits saturated fat and stresses omega-3s. You can do the Paleo Diet, which is about as anti–saturated fat as you can get. Or you can do Protein Power or Atkins and just make sure you're getting a ton of omega-3s.

On virtually all low-carb diets, blood lipid chemistries improve. That's what is important, and that is the take-home point here. Even those studies that showed identical weight loss with low-carb versus high-carb diets demonstrated this: low-carb diets beat the pants off high-carb diets every time when it comes to lowering triglycerides and raising HDL, even in those few cases where weight loss was identical.[40]

And here's the pièce de résistance. If you and/or your doctor are still concerned about the amount of fat in low-carb diets, consider the following (see table below): if you are a male who is 40 to 50 pounds overweight, you have probably been consuming a diet of *at least* 3,500 calories a day (probably more: one fast-food order of fries alone is 700). Let's say you've been adhering to the dietary guidelines of no more than 30 per-

MALE, 40 TO 50 POUNDS OVERWEIGHT: FAT INTAKE ON CURRENT DIET COMPARED WITH LOW-CARB DIET					
	Calories	% Total Fat	Fat Calories	% Saturated Fat	Saturated-Fat Calories
Current diet (follows dietary guidelines for fat)	3,500–4,000	30%	1,050–1,200	10%	350–400
Low-carb, high-fat diet	1,700	50%	850	20%	340

cent of your calories from fat, with no more than 10 percent of the total diet from saturated fat. That means you have been consuming about 1,050 calories a day from fat, of which 350 are from saturated fat.

Now look at what happens if you go on a typical low-carb weight reduction diet. You would consume in the ballpark of 1,700 satisfying, filling calories. Let's give the worst-case scenario, from your doctor's point of view, and say that a full 50 percent of those 1,700 calories come from fat—that's 850 fat calories, definitely a high-fat diet in anyone's book. Say that 20 percent (twice the dietary guidelines) of your total calories comes from saturated fat (340). Even with these numbers, you would actually consume 20 percent *less* overall fat on a low-carb diet than you were before, when you were following the dietary guidelines. This should put both you and your doctor at ease.

BOTTOM LINE

Low-carbohydrate diets do not increase the risk for heart disease. If anything, they improve blood lipid profiles. For references, go to What's New?/For Your Doctor on JonnyBowden.com.

CHAPTER 6

Frequently Asked Questions

In this chapter, I've posed and then answered the questions that I see most often on my "Ask Jonny Bowden" bulletin board on iVillage.com, as well as those I'm asked most frequently in seminars and workshops around the country. I've also incorporated the questions that I've seen come up time and time again on Internet sites dealing with low-carbohydrate diets. The questions are organized into categories, such as Losing Weight on Low-Carb, Food and Drink, and Exercise. If you have a question that's not answered here, you're always welcome to post it to me directly through my website, JonnyBowden.com.

Losing Weight on Low-Carb

How Long Will It Take Me to Lose 10 (or 100) Pounds?

There is absolutely no way to know the answer to this question. A lot depends on how much you have to lose and how you respond to your program. Everyone is fundamentally different on a metabolic, genetic, and biochemical level, and each body responds differently. Even people on identical programs are likely to experience different amounts of weight loss on different timetables. Rule of thumb: in the first week or so of a low-carb diet, you may lose a bunch of weight—maybe even 7 to 10 pounds if you are considerably overweight—but eventually you should settle in to an *average* of 2 pounds of weight loss per week, more or less. Don't be discouraged if your weight loss is less—many other things could be going on. And even at the rate of 1 pound a week, you'll still lose 50 pounds a year.

Is a Low-Carb Diet for Everyone?

Memorize this and tattoo it behind your eyelids: no single diet is for everyone. The Bantu of South Africa thrived on a diet of 80 percent carbs, and some groups of Eskimos thrived on a diet of nearly zero carbs. However, here in America and in most of the industrialized nations, it's fairly safe to say that nearly everyone would benefit from a *lower*-carb diet than is currently the norm. And *everyone* would benefit from changing their carbs from the highly processed, sugar-laden, fiberless fare of convenience, fast, and packaged foods to what we might call "real" carbohydrates—things you could pluck, gather, or grow.

How low in carbohydrates you personally need to go must be determined by trial and error. If you are a basically healthy person looking to stay that way and weight loss is not a real issue for you, the best template to start with is the one advocated by Barry Sears, which is approximately 40 percent of your food as carbohydrates, 30 percent as protein, and 30 percent as fat. Interestingly, this is very close to what many of the plans discussed in this book—among them the Atkins diet, Protein Power, and the Fat Flush Plan—recommend for maintenance after your weight target has been achieved. Sugar Busters! recommends this proportion from the beginning, although the authors don't credit it to Dr. Sears. And no less a luminary than the renowned Harvard epidemiologist Dr. Walter Willett has said, without actually mentioning the Zone diet, that a diet containing 40 percent carbs, 30 percent protein, and 30 percent fat may well be the healthiest alternative to the moribund USDA Food Pyramid's recommendations.

Once I Reach My Goal Weight, Can I Add Carbs Without Gaining Weight?

Posts on Internet bulletin boards respond to this type of question with the acronym YMMV, which means "your mileage may vary." Translation: everyone responds differently, so try it out. All of the classic programs basically suggest adding carbs back in a controlled and measured way until you discover for yourself the "magic" amount that allows *you* to maintain your goal weight.

Should I Weigh Myself Regularly?

Yes. The scale is a great way for you to check in with reality, as long as you know how to use it right. You need to learn *not* to beat yourself up about the number. You need to understand that water retention can mask fat loss. You need to understand that body composition can change with weight training exercise, and that you could be losing fat while gaining muscle (which would not necessarily show up right away on the scale). And you need to understand that everyone loses at a different rate. You may go for a period of time with no change whatsoever and then all of a sudden have a "whoosh" of weight loss. That said, the scale *will* keep you honest. *Eventually*, the scale will reflect fat loss. It will tell you—in combination with other cues, like how you're feeling and what your measurements are—whether what you're doing is working or not. If you want to figure out your critical carb level, you'll have to use the scale at some point to find out whether additional carbs are slowing you down. Many people have been delighted to find out that they actually could have a few more carbohydrates than they previously thought, and that it didn't slow down their weight loss appreciably or, if they were already at their goal weight, it didn't cause them to gain. But you'll never know any of that if you don't watch the numbers.

What Are Net Carbs? What's the Difference Between Net Carbs and Effective Carbs?

There is none. Net carbs and effective carbs are the same thing. The idea is that fiber, even though it's "counted" as a carbohydrate on food labels, isn't absorbed, so it shouldn't really be counted. To get the net, or effective, carbohydrate content of a food, simply go to the label and subtract the number of grams of *fiber* from the number of grams of *carbohydrate*. For example, 1 cup of raspberries has 14 grams of carbohydrate, but 8 of those are from fiber. Subtract the 8 grams of fiber from the 14 grams of *total* carbohydrate, and you get the number of net carbohydrate grams per cup: 6.

What Is the Minimum Daily Requirement for Carbohydrates?

Zero. There is no biological requirement for dietary carbohydrate in human beings. You would die without protein and you would die without fat, but you can live just fine without carbohydrate. I'm not suggesting that you should—just that you can.

Low-Carbing and the Body

Why Am I Getting Headaches During the Induction Phase of My Diet?

Headaches are a frequent side effect of switching abruptly from a high-carb to a low-carb diet. One of the reasons for this is that your body and your brain need to adapt to using fat and ketones as a primary fuel source after being accustomed to using sugar. Your brain can certainly use ketones, but it takes a few days to make the adjustment, during which you may get a headache. It usually goes away by itself, but one thing you can definitely do is drink more water. In fact, if you don't drink enough water, you may get a "ketone headache" even *after* your body has adapted to the diet. The other thing you can do is up your carbs by 5 to 10 grams a day until you're feeling better, then lower them gradually. Preventing some of the side effects is one reason for doing a three-day transition from your previous way of eating into this new low-carb lifestyle.

I'm Getting Leg Cramps, Especially at Night. Why?

This is almost always due to a mineral deficiency, particularly potassium, calcium, and magnesium. Remember that insulin tells the body to hold on to salt and water. When your insulin levels fall, especially during the first week on your low-carb diet, the kidneys will release that excess sodium— and you will begin to lose a lot of water. This will usually result in a loss of potassium as well, and one of the symptoms of potassium loss is muscle cramping (as well as fatigue). Dr. Alan Schwartz, medical director of the Holistic Resource Center in Agoura Hills, California, recommends taking one to two potassium supplements (99 milligrams) with each meal, especially in the first week of your low-carb diet. Magnesium supplementation is also a good idea.

Note: nuts help prevent potassium and magnesium imbalances. While you have to watch your intake of nuts during the weight loss phase of your program, they nonetheless are chock-full of these valuable minerals.

Does a Low-Carb Diet Cause Kidney Problems?

No. This is one of the great myths about low-carbing, but it is exactly that—a myth based on an incomplete understanding of the facts. It is true that people with preexisting kidney or liver problems should not go on very high-protein diets, but it is *not* true that either high-protein diets or low-carbohydrate diets in general *cause* kidney problems. If your doctor tells you otherwise, ask him or her to show you the research that confirms that finding. Your doc will not be able to, because there is none. There is not even a problem with protein in the diet of diabetics, who are frequently given to kidney problems. "There is no evidence that in an otherwise healthy person with diabetes eating protein causes kidney disease," says Frank Vinicor, director of diabetes research at the Centers for Disease Control and Prevention.[1] (For a more detailed explanation, see chapter 5; for studies showing that protein does not harm the kidneys of healthy people, click on What's New/For Your Doctor on JonnyBowden.com).

Is Low-Carbing Good for Diabetes?

It is not only good; it is *essential*. "Diabetes is a disease of carbohydrate intolerance," says physician and diabetes specialist Lois Jovanovic, chief scientific officer of the Sansum Medical Research Institute in Santa Barbara, California. "Meal plans should minimize carbohydrates because *people with diabetes do not tolerate [them]*."[2] (Emphasis mine.) Dr. Richard Bernstein, author of *The Diabetes Solution* and a diabetic himself, has been fighting the medical establishment over this since the 1970s. "What is still considered sensible nutritional advice for diabetics can over the long run be fatal," Bernstein writes.[3]

The American Diabetes Association's high-starch diet is so behind the curve that it's ludicrous. Jovanovic sums up the conventional high-carb advice for diabetics in one word: "Malpractice!"

Can Stress Stall Weight Loss?

You bet. Not only can stress stall weight loss, it can *reverse* it. Stress—which can come from lack of sleep, extremely low-calorie dieting, and, of course, from life itself—causes the release of hormones such as cortisol and adrenaline. These stress hormones send messages to the body to break down muscle for fuel, resulting in a lower metabolic rate. They send compelling messages to the brain to eat (i.e., the well-known "stress eating" phenomenon). Cortisol also tells the body to store fat around the middle. Because cortisol basically breaks down biochemicals in the body, chronic elevated levels of cortisol can trigger a protective reaction from the body in the form of insulin secretion (since insulin builds up structures in the body, including, of course, the fat cells). This makes chronically high levels of cortisol one possible cause of insulin resistance.

Another way stress can screw up weight loss is by its effect on serotonin. Stress *eats up* serotonin. Less serotonin is produced because stress interferes with the good, deep, restful sleep needed by the body to replenish its serotonin stock.[4] The demand for serotonin becomes greater, while the production of it is lower. Serotonin depletion is never, *ever* conducive to weight loss, as it works against you in very powerful ways.

What Is Leptin?

Leptin is a hormone involved in appetite control. Early research at Rockefeller University showed that obese mice were very low in leptin, leading to a lot of excitement about the possibility that giving leptin to obese people would somehow result in weight loss. No such luck. It turned out that obese people have plenty of leptin. What seems to be happening is that they have what might be called leptin resistance—their cells don't respond to it, in a scenario not unlike that of insulin resistance.

Leptin is produced by fat cells—when the fat cells are full, they release leptin, which sends a signal to the brain to stop eating—but this mechanism doesn't seem to work in obese people. *Less* leptin means *more* appetite; as body fat is lost, leptin levels drop,[5] which in turn sends a message to the brain telling you to eat more. This mechanism may be one of the many that makes regaining weight after a diet so easy; it's as if this feedback mechanism is hard at work to preserve you at a set weight. Drugs to treat this "leptin resistance" are in development and, if they prove promising, may one day help to fight obesity.

This Is My First Week on a Low-Carb Diet. Why Do I Feel Lightheaded?

Loss of minerals could be the culprit. Remember that when you lower your insulin levels, you lose salt and water (but, in the process, lose potassium as well). This, plus the tons of water I hope you're drinking, could conceivably result in enough electrolyte loss to lower blood pressure to the point where you might feel lightheaded or even faint. Replace some of the lost salt with either salty foods or with some table salt. Try ¼ teaspoon of potassium chloride (Morton Lite Salt) and ¼ teaspoon of table salt to start, and see if that helps. Don't forget to take potassium supplements.

How Do I Know If I'm Insulin-Resistant?

The best way is with a fasting insulin test. This test tells you what your baseline level of insulin is when no food is around to spike it. If you're not insulin-resistant, you shouldn't have a lot in your bloodstream when you haven't eaten. Lab ranges will vary; you should not be above seventeen, and the optimal level is below ten. A blood sugar test won't tell you if you're insulin-resistant. You could have blood sugar in the normal range, but it could be taking an enormous amount of insulin to keep it there.

Without a fasting insulin test, the best "low-tech" way is to look at your body's "insulin meter"—your waistline. If you're storing a bunch of fat around your middle, chances are you're somewhat insulin-resistant. And though the argument about which comes first—obesity or insulin resistance—continues to rage, the fact is that they are so often found together that for all intents and purposes, if you're extremely overweight, you can assume you are also insulin-resistant. (There are exceptions; some heavy people are insulin-sensitive, and some thin people—who usually exercise a ton and never overeat—are insulin-resistant. These are not the typical cases.)

Does a High-Protein Diet Cause Bone Loss or Osteoporosis?

No. If anything, a diet high in protein does the opposite, particularly in the presence of adequate calcium intake and plenty of alkalinizing vegetables. There are a tremendous number of studies now showing that protein is essential for healthy bones and that, indeed, low protein intake can be an obstacle to bone building. (For a list of representative studies showing the positive effect of protein on bone health, see For Your Doctor on JonnyBowden.com; for a more in-depth discussion of calcium, high protein, and bone loss, see chapter 5.) It's also worth remembering that the total amount of protein consumed on the typical low-carbohydrate diet of 2,000 calories (or less) is in no way excessive, even if it is a higher percentage of your diet than it had been before you revised your eating habits.

Can a Low-Carb Diet Cause Gallbladder Problems?

No, but if you have been overweight and have been on a very low-fat diet for a long time, a high-fat diet can make your gallbladder problems—like gallstones—apparent. Here's why. The gallbladder basically responds to fat in the diet with contractions that release the bile necessary to digest fat properly. When you've been on a very low-fat diet, there's not much for the gallbladder to do, so it gets lazy, and sometimes deposits accumulate and form stones, kind of like sediment forming in stagnant waters. When you suddenly go on a high-fat diet, the gallbladder now has work to do—it contracts in response to the fat, and it *may* pass these stones. The high-fat (low-carb) diet didn't *cause* the stones; they were already there and developed most likely in response to your very low-fat diet! But switching to a high-fat diet could trigger an attack. The solution: a moderate-fat version of the low-carb diet will trigger gallbladder contractions that are strong enough to release bile, but not vigorous enough to dislodge any stones.

What Can I Do About Constipation?

The two main causes of constipation on low-carb diets are not drinking enough water and not eating enough fiber, both of which you should be doing even if you're *not* constipated. Drink more water (see "How Much Water Should I Be Drinking?" on page 243), and make sure the vegetables and fruits you consume are high in fiber—spinach, broccoli, and raspberries are all good choices. Consider a fiber supplement (even sugar-free Metamucil, though I prefer Meta-Fibre by Metagenics; see Resources). Exercise almost always helps. And drinking hot water with a squeeze of fresh lemon juice first thing in the morning can help get things going as well.

A terrific "cure" for constipation is magnesium. Get the magnesium citrate form, start with 400 milligrams a day for a few days, and then, if needed, increase to 800. That almost always does it.

Cravings

Why Do I Get Cravings?

Cravings have many causes. Some are caused by nutrient deficiencies (see chapter 4 for information on supplements). In this case, what you crave is a clue to what's missing; for example, craving fatty foods could indicate that you're not getting enough essential fatty acids. Try adding omega-3 fats like fish oil; women can also try flaxseed oil. Many cravings are caused by blood sugar imbalances. The common craving for carbohydrates in the evening can be caused by not having eaten enough protein and/or fat earlier in the day. Frequent small meals that contain protein and fat will help control the blood sugar roller coaster that is often responsible for cravings. If a carb craving is absolutely irresistible, as a transition technique you should satisfy it with fruit (though you can blunt the insulin effect by adding some peanut butter or turkey).

A lot of cravings are caused by low serotonin states. Eating high-carbohydrate foods in this scenario is a kind of self-medication. The problem is that it creates a vicious cycle that results in weight gain and more cravings. Some supplements can help boost serotonin naturally (see chapter 4), and there are a number of lifestyle ways to boost it as well, such as having a pet, being out in the sun, and making love! You also need to understand that some cravings are simply conditioned responses to stress and are more emotionally driven than anything else. That's why "comfort foods" are so named—we have been conditioned to eat them when things aren't going well and we need a little TLC. The more you work on developing alternative behavioral responses to these situations—like taking warm baths or going for a walk—the better off you'll be.

What Can I Do to Combat Sugar Cravings?

There are two supplements that are phenomenal for sugar cravings. One is glutamine—I recommend that you take a spoonful or two of the powder in water (available in health food stores or through Internet sources). A spoonful of glutamine mixed with the sweetener xylitol and dissolved in a few tablespoons of half-and-half or heavy cream will knock the socks off even the worst sugar craving.

> *I don't care how much the experts say it's harmless, I know how sugar makes me feel: crazy. I start craving it like an addict, and once I start eating it I can't stop.*
>
> —Jean N.

You might also investigate a new product called Crave Arrest, a blend of ingredients such as tyrosine (a precursor to dopamine), 5-HTP (a precursor to serotonin), and B_6, which is necessary for the conversion of tryptophan to serotonin. (Crave Arrest is made by Designs for Health and can be purchased through a link on my website, JonnyBowden.com.)

Here are the top five techniques for busting cravings.

1. Control blood sugar by eating protein and fat every few hours, at every meal and snack.
2. Avoid *any* junk carbohydrates made of white stuff (rice, bread, pasta) as well as those that contain highly concentrated sweeteners, even if their carbohydrate content is permissible on your program.
3. Never let yourself become famished. Carry protein-based snacks like nuts, cheese, and hard-boiled eggs with you at all times.
4. Get enough sleep. Lack of sleep increases appetite and stimulates stress eating.
5. Learn to recognize the emotional triggers for cravings, such as fear, tension, shame, anger, anxiety, depression, loneliness, resentment, or any unmet needs. Don't pretend they're not there—recognize them, accept them, embrace them, and own them. Then explore behavioral ways of dealing with them besides eating.

Supplements

Do I Need to Take Supplements?

The technology exists to give you health-protective and therapeutic amounts of vitamins, minerals, phytochemicals, antioxidants, and other compounds, many of which are simply not available from our food supply or, if they are, not in the amounts needed to make a difference to your health and well-being. You don't *need* to take vitamins, but then you don't need electricity either. The question is, why would you do without either of them if you didn't have to? (See chapter 4 for complete recommendations on supplements.)

Doesn't Taking Vitamins Just Result in Expensive Urine?

If it does, then why bother to drink water? You just urinate it out at the end, right? Do you see how ridiculous this concept is? The expensive urine comment, which is perpetuated by doctors who don't really understand nutrition and vitamins, implies that just because something eventually winds up in the urine, it didn't accomplish anything in the body. Why does a drug addict take drugs or an athlete take steroids? Drugs, both recreational and prescription, are detected in the urine, right? Does the fact that they're detectable in the urine mean that they didn't *work*? If that were the case, there's an awful lot of people wasting an awful lot of money on drugs and medications! It's funny how the same doctors who cry "expensive urine" in response to vitamin therapy never make the same remark about their prescription drugs that are just as detectable in the urine as vitamins are!

> I definitely noticed a difference in my skin when I began to supplement with fatty acids like fish oil. My hair and scalp weren't as dry and even my fingernails got stronger.
> —Bernice D.

The fact that drugs—or vitamin residues—are detectable in the urine means absolutely nothing except that those substances went through the body and did their job. They didn't pass through and accomplish nothing, or else steroids wouldn't be banned by athletic organizations! The body takes what it needs, uses it, and excretes the rest. In addition, there's no way to know exactly how much of a given vitamin a specific individual actually needs. It's a lot better to take too much (with a few exceptions that might be toxic in very large amounts over an extended period of time, such as very high-dose vitamin A or selenium) and let the tissues decide how much they need and how much is excess. As nutritionist Robert Crayhon says in answer to this question, "Hey, I *want* expensive urine! In fact, I want the most expensive urine money can buy!"

What About Ephedra?

A recent post on an Internet diet board asked the following question: "Do people die from taking ephedra?" The question produced the single best response I've ever seen: "No, people die because they are *morons.*"

When ephedra has been used in supervised weight loss research studies, it's been used in the dosage of 60 milligrams per day in three divided dosages (20 milligrams each) combined with 200 milligrams of caffeine per dose. In every supervised study using this dose, it has not shown itself to be dangerous, and the side effect of "jitters" was usually pretty well tolerated. It is *not*—I repeat, *not*—for people with high blood pressure; for people who are sensitive to ephedrine or caffeine; for people who have any kind of heart, kidney, or liver problems; or for people who are on *any* medication, including over-the-counter meds (unless cleared by a doctor). Ephedra works by stimulating brown fat metabolism, thereby increasing the bodily production of heat (upping your metabolism *slightly*) and by suppressing your appetite. The possible side effects are very annoying and include nervousness, insomnia, and possibly dizziness. The benefits in the way of fat loss are very mild but probably do exist.

But here's the thing. While I'm no great fan of ephedra, it has also been blamed for an awful lot of things it doesn't deserve. When a college athlete dies on the football field while practicing in one-hundred-degree heat in full uniform, dehydrated, with a few hundred milligrams of ephedra plus who knows what else in his system, it's not exactly fair to blame ephedra. A recent field trip to my local vitamin shop uncovered ephedra pills with 250 milligrams *per pill*—more than ten times the recommended dose—and believe me, there are people who are taking several of these pills at a time. Let's also keep in mind that there are a couple of thousand deaths directly related to aspirin per year. Ephedra in small amounts, under controlled conditions, is not dangerous.

I'm more concerned about the adrenal burnout factor with ongoing ephedra use. This drug *is* a metabolic stimulant, and like any stimulant, it taxes the adrenal glands, which over the very long haul can not only hamper your weight loss efforts but damage your health.

This discussion is probably moot, however. "Its time is over," says Dr. C. Leigh Broadhurst, who has herself used ephedra without incident. There's just too much bad publicity and public outcry about it, and it will almost certainly be taken off the market soon. The new "ephedra-free" diet pills have simply replaced ephedra with citrus aurantium (bitter orange), which has many of the same fat-burning/appetite-suppressing effects but doesn't yet have the bad rap. (See next question.) If you *do* use ephedra, make sure you do not fit in any of the categories mentioned above, and never take more than the recommended dosage.

What About Over-the-Counter "Ephedra-Free" Diet Pills?

The new "ephedra-free" diet pills have simply replaced ephedra with bitter orange (citrus aurantium), an herb that contains the active ingredient synephrine. Synephrine is chemically very similar to ephedrine and pseu-doephedrine and has similar effects in terms of providing an energy boost, suppressing the appetite, and increasing metabolic rate and caloric expenditure. By stimulating specific adrenergic receptors, it is theorized that synephrine stimulates fat metabolism without the negative cardiovascular side effects experienced by some people with ephedra (also called ma huang).

Bitter orange usually contains between 1 and 6 percent synephrine, but some manufacturers boost the content to as much as 30 percent.[6] It *does* have a thermogenic (fat-burning) effect.[7] In animal studies, synephrine caused weight loss, but it also increased cardiovascular problems.[8]

Bitter orange can also increase the side effects of many medications, including (but not limited to) Xanax, Zocor, Sudafed, Buspar, Celexa, Zoloft, Allegra, prednisone, Meridia, Viagra, and a number of blood pressure medications.[9] Do *not* take bitter orange if you have high blood pressure or are pregnant.

The bottom line is this: it *is* a stimulant, and the same cautions about other stimulants (like ephedra) apply. Just because the pill is "ephedra-free" does not mean that you should use unlimited amounts of it.

What's in Those "Fat-Burning" Formulas I See Everywhere, and Do They Help with Weight Loss?

A recent field trip to my local vitamin store to inspect a dozen of these formulas—labeled everything from "metabolism boosters" to "fat burners" to "lipotropics"—revealed a pretty standard revolving door of ingredients. Most used some combination of:

- **bitter orange** (citrus aurantium), a stimulant that increases metabolism (thermogenesis) slightly and is discussed above (see "What About Over-the-Counter 'Ephedra-Free' Diet Pills?")
- **guarana**, which is herbal caffeine
- **white willow bark**, which is basically aspirin and really doesn't add anything to the mix
- **green tea extract, a.k.a. EGCG** (epigallocatechin gallate), which *does* have thermogenic properties (see chapter 4)

Combinations of these ingredients can definitely suppress appetite, give you the jitters, and maybe, just maybe, burn a few extra calories.

Some "fat burners" include a mix of carnitine and chromium (both of which are discussed in chapter 4). They almost never contain the best form of carnitine (tartrate) and rarely contain more than 500 milligrams (most nutritionists think the minimum amount necessary to impact fat burning in an overweight person is 1,500 milligrams). As far as chromium is concerned, while I *have* seen formulas with 200 micrograms (the absolute minimum needed), I saw one that loudly proclaimed "contains chromium" and actually had a ridiculously low 13 micrograms. Understand that the amount most often given to people with blood sugar problems is in the neighborhood of 600 to 1,000 micrograms; 13 micrograms would do absolutely nothing and is only there so that the manufacturer can say "contains chromium"—a complete rip-off.

Other ingredients that show up in the formulas, especially the ones labeled "lipotropics," are inositol, an essential nutrient and relative of the B family, and choline, another relative of the B family that mobilizes fat. Both choline and inositol (plus methionine) are involved in the liver's ability to process fats, so there's reason to think that these nutrients might help the liver move fat through it. If a sluggish liver is part of the reason you're holding on to fat, these nutrients could be helpful. As lipotropics go, I like the Fat Flush Weight Loss Formula from unikeyhealth.com, which contains reasonable amounts of choline, inositol, and methionine, plus the good form of carnitine, 400 micrograms of chromium, and an herbal mix that's good for the liver.

The other pair of ingredients often found in these formulas are tyrosine, an amino acid helpful for improving mood, and phenylalanine, an essential amino acid that can be converted into tyrosine. Both of these are precursors to dopamine, a neurotransmitter that makes you feel peppy and bright. Tyrosine is needed for the making of thyroid hormone, but it is highly unlikely that tyrosine will boost low thyroid, even though some supplement makers claim it does.

The important thing is to read the ingredients on the labels of the products you are considering. These formulas vary widely in their effects, depending on the amounts and quality of the ingredients included. At worst, they do nothing. At best, they'll give you a bit of a speedy feeling and maybe increase metabolic rate by a very small amount.

Ketosis

What Is Ketosis?

Ketosis is a term used to describe what happens when the body switches to fat as its main source of fuel, which is exactly what you want to happen when you're using a low-carbohydrate diet to lose weight. When fat is the main source of fuel, there is an increase in the number of ketone bodies made as a by-product of fat metabolism: ketones can be measured in the urine by means of ketone test strips.

> *It was absolutely amazing to me when I really studied ketosis and found out that almost everything I had heard about how dangerous it was was utter hogwash.*
>
> —Dana McG.

Is Ketosis Dangerous?

Absolutely not. Ketones are a natural part of human metabolism —your body is always producing ketones. When you are in benign dietary ketosis, you are just making *more* of them, because fat, rather than sugar, has become the main source of fuel for your body. A strict ketogenic diet has been very successful in treating epilepsy in children and has been used for years at the Children's Hospital of New York-Presbyterian.[10] Children have been kept on it for years at a time. If there were dangers associated with ketosis, we would have heard about it by now. (For a full discussion, see chapter 5.)

Do I Need to Be in Ketosis in Order to Lose Weight?

No. First of all, ketosis doesn't *cause* weight loss. You can easily be in ketosis eating 10,000 calories of fat a day, but you'll never lose any weight that way. Ketosis is simply a by-product of fat burning. There have been many people who've lost weight on low-carb diets without being in ketosis, and there are many who have been in ketosis and not lost weight. Ketone loss, in the urine and the breath, accounts for only about 100 calories a day.[11] That said, there are some extremely metabolically resistant people who truly seem to do much better on Atkins-like induction plans in which they *are* in ketosis, carbohydrates are kept to very low levels (20 to 30 grams or so a day), and calories are moderately low.

You may want to go into ketosis just to get started, but the vast majority of people can lose weight over time on a low-carb diet by hovering around the border of ketosis. And as we saw in chapter 3, many of the programs don't emphasize ketosis at all—some programs deliberately keep you at a slightly higher carb level (50 to 90 grams a day) to prevent it. The point is this: if you keep your carbs low enough (and your calories reasonable), you will be lowering your insulin levels and breaking down fat. Exactly how low they have to be for you to continue to lose weight is something you will have to experiment with.

Why Don't My Ketone Test Strips Show a Positive Reading?

There are a number of reasons you may not get a positive reading, and you probably don't need to be too concerned about it. There are three ketone bodies—beta-hydroxybutyric acid, acetoacetic acid, and acetone—and the strips detect only the latter two, which are less than one-fifth of the total ketones produced. Beta-hydroxybutyric acid goes completely undetected. So it's entirely possible that you might not test positive on the ketone strips, yet if you performed a more sophisticated urinalysis, you'd find plenty of ketones floating around!

Other things can influence whether the strips change color, such as how much water you're drinking. If you're drinking a lot, which you should be, that'll very likely keep the strips from turning a deep color.

Of course, the possibility exists that they're not turning color because you're not in ketosis, probably because you are eating more carbs than you think or there are hidden carbs in your food choices. (See Resources for a hidden carb counter.)

Food and Water

How Many Calories a Day Should I Be Eating?

For weight loss, a good rule of thumb is to take your goal weight and multiply by 10. If you've got more than about 25 pounds to lose, multiply your *current* weight by 10 and then deduct 500 calories from that number. This formula doesn't work as well if you are at a relatively low weight—say 125 pounds—and are trying to drop only a few pounds. You should never, ever let your calories fall below 1,000 per day.

If you'd prefer not to do any calculations, you can remember it this way: the average weight loss diet for men is about 1,500 calories and the average for women is about 1,200.

Remember that these formulas are only approximations. Every person's situation is going to be different based on one's own metabolic and historical factors, genetics, age, hormonal profiles, muscle mass, activity levels, and so on. The calorie calculators found on diet Internet sites woefully overestimate how many calories you "need," especially for weight loss. Ignore them. And remember that calories are important, but they're not the whole picture; the kinds of food you eat determine what messages are sent by your hormones, and the hormones are what control the whole shebang.

I'm a Vegetarian. Can I Low-Carb?

Yes, depending on the type of vegetarian diet you are following. If you're a vegan, it's going to be next to impossible, but if you can eat eggs and whey protein, it's definitely doable. If you can also eat fish, it's a snap. Check out *The Schwarzbein Principle Vegetarian Cookbook* (see "The Schwarzbein Principle," page 142) as well as the cookbooks in the Resources section.

A note on vegetarianism: if you're not eating animals for spiritual, ethical, or moral reasons, I am in great sympathy with you. I myself am a believer in animal rights, am a card-carrying member of PETA, and understand your feelings profoundly. But if you're doing it for health reasons, I urge you to rethink your position. Most people do better with some animal foods, and some people do a *lot* better on a *lot* of animal foods. Maybe one way to reconcile this for yourself is to patronize only those who sell meat from animals that have *not* been factory-farmed, have been *organically* raised, and have had a good and happy life. Just something to think about.

Why Is Water So Important for Fat Loss?

Drinking plenty of water is absolutely necessary for fat loss. When you're not drinking enough water, the kidneys can't work properly, so they start dumping part of their load onto the liver. The liver is the main fat-processing plant in the body, but if it has to take over some of the kidneys' work, it can't work at full operating capacity. It metabolizes less fat, so more fat remains in the body, and weight loss stalls.[12] Water is also necessary to get rid of the toxic wastes released from fat stores.

Water is also the absolute best treatment for water retention. The less water you drink, the more the body perceives this as a threat and sends signals that result in holding on to as much of that scarce water as possible. Sometimes this shows up as swollen hands, feet, and legs. When you're drinking enough water, this doesn't happen. There's no more "emergency," and the body releases stored water instead of retaining it.

How Much Water Should I Be Drinking?

More than you think. "Larger people have larger metabolic loads," says Dr. Donald Robertson. "Since we know that water is the key to fat metabolism, it follows that the overweight person needs more water." Robertson recommends 3 quarts a day. Many personal trainers recommend a gallon. I think the absolute minimum is 64 ounces plus an additional 8 ounces for every 25 pounds of excess weight you are carrying.

How Can I Get More Fiber in My Low-Carb Diet?

If your program permits it, include a serving of All-Bran or Fiber One cereal, which are the only commercial cereals that have a significant amount of fiber. Get some wheat or oat bran (not the cereals, the actual *bran*; you'll find it in the section of the health food grocery that sells dry bulk items). You can mix the brans together in different proportions and cook it to make your own hot cereal mix, or you can use it as a breading or a filling. I also recommend adding fiber supplements (like psyllium husks or flaxseeds) to your program, but don't take them at the same time as other medications or supplements, because the fiber can inhibit absorption.

What Are Sugar Alcohols? Do They Count as Sugar?

Sugar alcohols—also called polyols—are sugar-free sweeteners that are carbohydrates but are not sugar. Common ones include maltitol, mannitol, sorbitol, and xylitol. They have fewer calories per gram than sugar: sugar has 3 calories per gram, while sorbitol has 2.6, xylitol has 2.4, and mannitol has 1.6. They don't cause sudden increases in blood sugar; instead, they are slowly and incompletely absorbed from the small intestine into the blood, and the portion that *is* absorbed requires little or no insulin. Since they aren't technically sugar, manufacturers are able to say "sugar-free" when they use sugar alcohols as sweeteners, but they're required to include these sweeteners in the carb count on the nutrition label (though not everybody does).

Scientists call them sugar alcohols because part of their structure chemically resembles sugar and part chemically resembles alcohol. They're certainly a lot better for you than pure sugar. Xylitol actually has health benefits. But some of them can cause slight gastric upset for some people, like a little gas or a mild laxative effect. And you have to be careful with portion sizes—even though the food may be technically sugar-free, the calories and grams of sugar alcohol can add up. And some folks—particularly carb addicts—say that products sweetened with sugar alcohols can trigger cravings just like products sweetened with sugar.

What Are the Best Oils?

There's a new star on the horizon: coconut oil. It can be used for anything and has amazing health benefits (see also next question).

For cooking, I recommend extra-virgin olive oil, virgin coconut oil, grapeseed oil, or butter (I know it's not an oil, but it is fine for cooking and sautéing). Peanut oil is stable and can be used occasionally for stir-fries, but it is very high in omega-6, so don't overdo. You can use sesame oil, which is very good for frying, but remember that it contains a larger proportion of omega-6s, so don't use it exclusively. Almond oil is good for baking.

Flaxseed oil is terrific, of course, but *never* use it for cooking. It is a great source of alpha linolenic acid (an omega-3 fat), but for that reason it can't be heated (though it can be poured or drizzled on hot foods such as vegetables). Omega-3 fats are very unstable and become extremely damaged when heated. Another terrific new oil that is a great source of the same omega-3 fat is perilla oil (a plant extract), but it should not be used for cooking.

For salads, try coconut oil, extra-virgin olive oil, any of the nut oils (macadamia, hazelnut, almond, walnut), avocado oil, or sesame oil. You can also use flaxseed oil or perilla oil. I don't recommend canola oil. To be used commercially, it has to be partially hydrogenated, refined, and deodorized, and in the process its omega-3s become a potent source of trans-fatty acids.[13] If you do use it, make sure to get organic, cold-pressed, or expeller-pressed canola oil (such as Spectrum), and only use it cold.

Oils you can say good-bye to permanently include safflower, sunflower, corn, soybean, and cottonseed. Buh-bye.

What's the Story with Coconut Oil? I Heard This Is a "Bad" Fat!

You heard wrong. Virgin coconut oil is a good, stable, healthy fat that actually has a number of healing properties, not the least of which is that it is anti-inflammatory.[14] The original bad rap for coconut oil came four decades ago, when researchers fed animals *hydrogenated* coconut oil that was purposely altered to render it devoid of essential fatty acids. The animals that were fed the hydrogenated coconut oil (as the only fat source) naturally became deficient in essential fatty acids, and their serum cholesterol increased.[15] Early commercial coconut oil was often hydrogenated (loaded with trans-fats), and all the good, healing stuff had been removed. That coconut oil *wasn't* very good for you. But *real* coconut oil is a health bonanza. The Pukapukans and the Tokelauans of Polynesia, for whom coconut is the chief source of energy, have virtually no heart disease, and research on these populations concluded that there was no evidence that their high saturated-fat intake (from coconut) had any harmful effects.[16] The saturated fat in coconut oil comes mainly from MCTs (medium-chain triglycerides), which are preferentially burned as energy and less likely to be stored as fat, making them a good choice for a weight loss program.[17] Coconut oil also contains a high proportion of the antiviral and antimicrobial lauric acid, as well as the antimicrobial capric acid and the potent "yeast fighter" caprylic acid.[18] Be sure to purchase the virgin or cold-pressed kind.

What Are the Good Fats?

Good fats include all the oils mentioned above as "good" *plus* natural, undamaged fats like butter, coconut, avocado, nuts, and the fat in fish.

The dietary establishment has long fostered the myth that fats are "good" or "bad" depending on whether or not they are saturated: saturated fats = bad, unsaturated fats = good. Not so. A much better way to categorize fats is by whether they are damaged or undamaged. You can damage fats in a number of ways. One way is by overheating any vegetable oil by frying at high temperatures—this creates toxic substances known as lipid peroxides. Another is through an industrial process known as partial hydrogenation, which creates something called trans-fats, by far the most dangerous of all fats. Trans-fats are found in almost all fast foods (french fries, for example, are doused in them), most margarines, virtually all commercially baked goods (including children's cookies), and movie popcorn, and in any products containing partially hydrogenated vegetable oils (look for these in the ingredients list on the package). Trans-fats are the true demons of the fat world, and the ones we want to avoid completely, as they are associated with all of the degenerative diseases common in the modern world.

Unfortunately, until recently, there has been no separation in the research between saturated fats and trans-fats, so saturated fats have been blamed for a great deal of the damage to the body that is actually the fault of trans-fats.[19] This may soon change, as identifying trans-fats in the Nutrition Facts on food packaging will be required of manufacturers as of January 2006, and researchers are starting to make a distinction between the two very different classes of fats. Many labels already carry this information, so be sure to check the products you buy.

There probably *are* prudent reasons to keep saturated-fat intake at a reasonable level; for one thing, in *some* people, it can increase insulin resistance. For another, the nonorganic and fast-food meats that are our biggest sources of saturated fat are loaded with bovine growth hormone, steroids, and antibiotics, not to mention toxins from the grains that factory-farmed cattle consume. The danger is probably not so much from saturated fat itself, but from what's *in* the kinds of saturated fat we typically consume. Also, the lack of balance in our diet between omega-6s and omega-3s is a big health concern that has many ramifications. Fats that are too high in omega-6s, such as vegetable oils (corn, safflower, sunflower, soybean), just add to the tremendous imbalance between omega-6s and omega-3s (found in fish) and should be avoided for that reason alone.

> *Every time I drink [alcohol] my diet goes out the window and I eat way more than I ever intended to. Cutting out alcohol—at least for now—has been the best thing I ever did for my waistline.*
> —Kelley F.

What About Alcohol?

Here's the deal with alcohol: the body has no way to store the energy in it (7 calories per gram), so all "fat burning" is put on hold while the body burns off the alcohol. Alcohol can also produce cravings, both for itself and for carbohydrates—Kathleen Des Maisons, Ph.D., an expert in addictive nutrition, considers alcohol dependence simply an extension of sugar sensitivity.[20] She also believes that although hard liquor is not technically a sugar, the beta-endorphin effect is a powerful trigger for cravings.[21]

That said, a lot of low-carb plans permit some alcohol, particularly red wine (in 4-ounce servings), which contains about 3 grams of net carbohydrate. Do the math and see if it works for you.

What Is the Glycemic Index?

The glycemic index is a numerical way of describing how carbohydrates in foods affect blood sugar levels (an even more accurate measure is the glycemic *load*; see next question).[22] The index measures how quickly a 50-gram serving of a particular food converts to sugar. Foods with a high glycemic index cause a dramatic rise in blood sugar (and subsequent demand on insulin levels). That's why all low-carb diets suggest that you eat *low-glycemic* carbohydrates; these carbs (green vegetables, for example) have a much lower impact on your blood sugar and insulin.

What's the Difference Between the Glycemic Index and the Glycemic Load?

The glycemic load is a more accurate predictor of what's going on with blood sugar and insulin than the glycemic index. Here's why. Suppose I put an empty bucket under a faucet and I want to know how much water is going to wind up in the bucket. You can see immediately that there are two variables I need to know: the water pressure (how high I turn on the faucet) and how *long* I'm going to leave it on. In the same way, if I want to know the impact of a particular food on blood sugar and insulin, I need to know two things: the glycemic index *and* how *much* of that food I'm going to eat!

The glycemic *index* tells you the impact that a 50-gram serving of a particular food will have on your blood sugar. The glycemic *load*, on the other hand, also takes into account the amount of carbs actually in the food. Remember that all the low-carb plans consider the number of net, or effective, carbohydrates in a serving because we need to know that in order to determine the total impact the food is going to have on your blood sugar. Some foods have only a few grams of available carbs, so even if their glycemic index is high, their overall impact will be reduced because there are so few of them. The glycemic load is a measure of that *overall* impact. To find the glycemic load, multiply the glycemic *index* by the number of *net carbohydrates in a standard serving* (find the glycemic index for various foods at glycemicindex.com).

Consider the difference between carrots and pasta. Carrots have a glycemic index of 47, higher than that of whole-wheat spaghetti, which is only 32. If this was the only information you based your decision on, you'd think carrots were much worse from a blood sugar point of view. But while there are only 6 net (or effective) grams of carbs in a carrot, there are a whopping 48 grams of net carbs in the pasta! Let's calculate the glycemic load (index times net carbs): carrots would be 47 times 6, which is 282. But the calculations for the spaghetti would be 32 times 48, which is 1,536—more than 500 percent higher than carrots!

What's the Best Type of Protein Drink to Use?

Whey. It seems to be the best all-around source of protein, followed by soy that has been enriched with methionine (an amino acid not found in soy). Whey is absorbed the best and is the most available; it also increases levels of glutathione, perhaps the most powerful antioxidant in the body. There are a lot of people on the antisoy bandwagon right now, but I think soy protein *in moderation* is fine. Whey, however, is better.

What's the Difference Between a Protein Drink and a Meal Replacement Shake?

Protein powders are 100 percent (or almost 100 percent) pure protein. You can drink them by themselves or make a "meal replacement" drink with them by adding a controlled amount of carbohydrates (berries are a good choice) and maybe some fat like nuts or nut butter (women can add flaxseed oil if they don't mind the taste). Designs for Health makes an excellent protein powder called PaleoMeal that is enriched with omega-3s and a number of other terrific ingredients (see Resources). You can also get Designer Protein, which, though not quite as good as PaleoMeal, is widely available and fairly inexpensive.

Meal replacement shakes have carbs, protein, and fat in different proportions depending on the philosophy of the company making them. Many are very high in carbs.

What's Wrong with Grains? Aren't They Supposed to Be Healthy?

Grains, grain products, starches, and sugars all share some common links: they turn into glucose (sugar) in your body very quickly, they promote addictive eating habits in a large percentage of people, and they trigger insulin release. All of these things result in weight gain and other health problems.[23] Grains also contain compounds called phytates and pyridoxine glucosides that block absorption of B vitamins, iron, zinc copper, and calcium and lead to possible mineral deficiencies that can slow metabolism. (For a full discussion of grains, see "The Problem with Grains" in "The Paleo Diet" on page 126.) In addition, both gluten and certain protein fractions of gluten are a big problem for many people. It used to be thought that celiac disease—a sensitivity to gluten—was rare. We now know that it probably affects one in thirty-three people. That's a lot. There are an amazing number of toxins used in the processing of wheat and grains, and it is entirely possible that some of the problems that people have with wheat are actually caused by these toxins. (Other problems are certainly caused by the wheat itself.)[24] Clinically, an awful lot of problems seem to just magically "clear up" when you take grains, especially wheat, out of the diet. While whole grains are in theory better than refined grains, they're not nearly as common as you might think. The making of flour is itself a refining process. And the "wheat breads" in your grocery are no better than white bread. Couple this with the fact that grains usually have a very high glycemic load, and you can see the potential problem. Obviously, not everyone will have a problem with grains, but cutting them out during the initial stages of a low-carb weight loss program is definitely a good idea.

Is Coffee Okay?

Probably. Those who argue against coffee are concerned with its possible effects on insulin and on the adrenal glands. Atkins didn't like it because he felt it caused unstable blood sugar. There *is* some research that suggests that caffeine increases insulin resistance[25, 26] and that it raises insulin levels.[27] How much this matters as a practical consideration is debatable— the insulin insensitivity it produces in studies may be an insignificant amount as a practical matter and may be only temporary. There is also research showing that coffee actually *improves* insulin sensitivity[28] and con- tributes to *reducing* insulin,[29] as well as some research that says it has no effect on insulin at all.[30] And in one study, coffee was actually associated with a much *lower* risk of type 2 diabetes.[31]

While coffee is obviously a stimulant, drinking it is also a very pleasant experience for a lot of people, and that has to be factored into the mix. Those who are very concerned about adrenal health (Dr. Diana Schwarzbein) recommend dumping it, but others say it's fine. From a weight loss perspec- tive, it's probably not going to hurt at all, but if you're looking to go the last mile for ultimate health, you'd be better off without it.

Important note: it's not just the caffeine that's a problem—there's caffeine in green tea too, and that doesn't seem to hurt anyone—it's the enormous amount of toxins in the coffee plant. You can go a long way toward reducing any negative health impact of coffee by purchasing organically grown beans.

Are Diet Sodas Acceptable on My Low-Carb Diet?

You'd be *much* better off without them. If you can't give them up right away, put it on your goal list and at least start cutting back. Most of them use aspartame, which should definitely be eliminated (see next question); in addition, diet soda can stall weight loss in some people (up to 40 to 50 percent, by some estimations), possibly due to the citric acid they contain.

Many people do drink soda addictively (I had one client who routinely consumed sixteen cans a day), and the amounts consumed by people like this have never been tested for safety in long-term studies. Through a classical conditioning mechanism, like the one used to teach Pavlov's dogs to salivate at the sound of a bell, drinking diet soda may well trigger insulin production (as may the consumption of other artificial sweeteners). And the chemicals, food colorings, flavorings, and other stuff in diet soda make it no picnic for the liver, either.

What About Aspartame?

Aspartame, the most common of the artificial sweeteners and the one used in most diet sodas, is a real problem. Even though it has been declared "safe," the FDA has received numerous reports of seizures and other problems that have been linked to it.[32] There's also good reason to believe that aspartame may be neurotoxic.[33] In a report to the Senate Labor and Human Resources Committee, Dr. Richard Wurtman, professor of neuroendocrine regulation at the Massachusetts Institute of Technology, stated that the most common side effects linked to aspartame include dizziness, visual impairment, disorientation, ear buzzing, a high level of SGOT (a liver enzyme), loss of equilibrium, severe muscle aches, episodes of high blood pressure, and other not-so-lovely stuff.[34] Other reports claim that in susceptible people, aspartame can produce symptoms ranging from sleep disturbances to headaches to fuzzy thinking to mood disturbances, and one recent article in the *Townsend Newsletter for Doctors and Patients* suggested that in susceptible people (called aspartame responders), the substance could be somewhat addictive. Kathleen Des Maisons, Ph.D., an expert in addictive nutrition, believes that the taste of any sweetener, for sugar-sensitive people, evokes a beta-endorphin response in the body which will create cravings.[35]

No integrative or holistic practitioner I interviewed had anything good to say about aspartame. The consensus of advice: stay away.

What About Artificial Sweeteners in General?

You basically have six choices.

- **Aspartame** (Equal), is probably the most commonly used artificial sweetener these days, but it's also one that I *cannot* recommend (see previous question).
- **Saccharin** (Sweet'n Low) has been around for about a hundred years, and at one time it had a reputation as a cancer-causing agent because of studies in which rats got bladder tumors when they were fed incredibly high amounts (equivalent to what a human would get drinking eight hundred cans of diet soda a day). Recently, saccharine was declared safe, and probably is in reasonable amounts. Next to sucralose and stevia, it's probably the best choice.
- **Cyclamate** (Sugar Twin, Sucaryl) also continues to have a cloud of smoke around it concerning cancer in rats, but it too has been added to food and beverages since the 1950s and is probably safe in small amounts.
- **Acesulfame-K** (Sunette) is in the same family as saccharin but isn't widely available in the States.
- **Sucralose** (Splenda) is the most promising of all. It is basically a slightly chemically altered version of sucrose (sugar) and is six hundred times sweeter. The chemical alteration prevents the digestive system from "recognizing" it and absorbing it, so it doesn't cause the rise in blood sugar and insulin associated with sucrose, unless of course it turns out to cause an insulin rise through a conditioned response mechanism. The only possible problem with Splenda—and it is only theoretical—is that the chemical "alteration" involves adding chlorine molecules. Is that a good thing? Only time will tell. For now, it's the sweetener most recommended by people in the field.
- **Stevia** is an herb sold as a food additive, which has basically no downside except a somewhat weird aftertaste that some people don't mind at all. You can get it at any health food store.

Note that the only ones you can cook with are Sweet'n Low, Sugar Twin, Sunette, and Splenda.

Is Fructose Okay?

No. Fructose doesn't raise blood sugar a lot, so it used to be thought of as the perfect sweetener for diabetics. Bad idea. Even though it doesn't raise blood sugar very fast, it induces insulin resistance in both animals[36] and humans.[37] Fructose is turned to fat in the liver, so it raises your triglycerides. High-fructose corn syrup is the worst offender of all. When you consume fructose, make sure it comes in its natural container—fruit—surrounded by fiber. Never use it as a sweetener, and don't make a habit of eating foods that are sweetened with it.

What About Protein Bars?

The problem is that many of these products are deceptively labeled. A lot of them will tell you they have only 2 or 3 grams of "usable" carbs, but don't be too quick to buy it. They are sweetened with sugar alcohols, which the manufacturers often decide not to count when telling you how many carbs the bar contains. The argument is that sugar alcohols don't have the same effect on blood sugar, which is true. But they're still carbs. Nutrition labeling regulations don't require manufacturers to put the number of grams of sugar alcohols per serving *unless* they are making a claim related to sugar content, in which case it's mandatory. Since most of the low-carb bars don't claim to be sugar-free, they can get around this mandatory clause. Even Atkins does not count the glycerin (glycerol) that sweetens his Atkins Nutritional Bars as part of the carb gram count. The problem is that like all sugar alcohols, glycerin *is* a carbohydrate. The FDA's Office of Food Labeling states: "FDA nutrition labeling regulations require that when glycerin is used as a food ingredient, it must be included in the grams of total carbohydrate per serving declaration." So although sugar alcohols do behave differently in the body than sugar, you should still be aware of their presence.

The other concern about low-carb bars is calories. Just because they are low in carbs doesn't mean they're low in calories, so factor that in. In sugar-sensitive people, they can *easily* trigger cravings; these bars are, after all, very sweet, which is why they taste so good. And while most of them are better than candy bars, none is as good as real food.

So use them occasionally, but beware. Some low-carbers have found that these bars can stall weight loss, so if you're eating them a lot and you're stuck, they might be a good thing to let go of.

Can I Eat Dairy Products?

For many people, dairy—especially milk and cheese—will slow or stall weight loss. Many holistic practitioners recommend eliminating wheat, dairy, and sugar as the three biggest triggers of food reactions, subclinical allergies, and the like.

I don't believe homogenized, pasteurized milk is a good food. In addition to the pus cells (the FDA allows 1.5 million per cc of milk as "safe"), factory-farmed cows are treated with antibiotics, bovine growth hormone, and other drugs to fatten them and keep their milk production elevated to unnatural levels. The grain they eat, which is not their natural food, is irritating to their stomachs (one reason for the antibiotics) and contains a whole different set of toxins. (Raw organic milk, which may be available from local farmers, is a whole different story, but note that some states prohibit the sale of raw milk. For more information, see realmilk.com.) If you're not ready to eliminate milk, or if you want to consume it in small amounts, at the very least buy the organic kind. Excellent substitutes are the nut milks, like almond milk, or try goat's milk, which does not present the same problems for most people, for reasons that are not fully understood. Many people who have a problem with milk are still able to tolerate fermented dairy foods like kefir and yogurt.

Cheese has stalled many a low-carber's weight loss. Although some plans allow it, if your weight loss isn't progressing, this might be one food to cut back on.

I'm Getting Bored with the Usual Low-Carb Fare. What Else Can I Eat?

Here are some terrific suggestions from low-carb chef and Internet guru Karen Barnaby.

- Thinly sliced raddichio, endive, and fennel with a fresh basil dressing, sprinkled with crisp bacon and goat cheese. Eat with roasted chicken.
- Raw, sautéed, or grilled mushrooms on romaine with blue cheese dressing. Eat with a steak.
- Fried peppers, mushrooms, and garlic. Serve on arugula, sprinkled with feta cheese, and eat with good Italian sausage.
- Thinly sliced cucumbers, radishes, and celery. Toss with lemon mayonnaise and serve on butter lettuce, along with a piece of salmon. Sprinkle with fresh dill.

- Cooked asparagus and Swiss chard. Serve a piece of halibut, cod, or sole on top and drown it in Hollandaise sauce.
- Sautéed spinach or julienned daikon seasoned with soy sauce and a few drops of sesame oil. Serve with grilled tuna on top and mayonnaise mixed with wasabi as a sauce.
- Marinated cubes of feta, Brie, or Camembert in basil, garlic, and lots of olive oil. Eat with sliced cucumbers as a snack or sprinkle on a salad. Have it alongside a hamburger. Use as an omelet filling with one-fourth of a tomato, chopped.
- Make a cabbage slaw and jazz it up with mint, cilantro, green onions, and a bit of lime juice. Put canned tuna or salmon and hard-boiled eggs on top.

Here are some other ideas.

- Make omelets with fillings like bacon and Swiss cheese, mushroom and avocado, goat cheese and mushrooms, spinach and feta, or bacon and avocado.
- Add chopped nuts or sunflower seeds to cottage cheese.
- Make a "wrap" out of sliced turkey with cream cheese inside.
- Make a "wrap" out of sliced roast beef with cheddar, scallions, and a drop of sour cream (if dairy is on your program).
- Try deviled eggs.
- Use low-carb tortillas and make your own breakfast burritos.
- Keep varying the toppings on your salads. Try warm meats or shrimp, crab, or lobster. Try different cheeses, if that's on your program. Mix and match.
- Make a low-carb burger by putting a hamburger patty between two lettuce leaves (or red cabbage leaves). Add mayo and mustard if you like.
- Pan-fry some chicken and add feta cheese and olives.
- Eat a hot dog minus the bun and use mayo and mustard as dipping sauces.
- Steam some veggies and add butter, lemon, a handful of nuts, and maybe some soy sauce.
- Fill celery sticks with peanut butter, cream cheese, or tuna salad.
- Try beef jerky, turkey jerky, or veggie jerky.
- Mix sugar-free, all-natural peanut butter with whey protein powder and roll in cocoa powder.
- Combine whey protein powder with sour cream and Splenda—kneading this mixture renders a pretty interesting taffy. You must eat it within a couple of days, but it is great.

And here's one of my favorite ideas courtesy of the diet website 3fatchicks.com: "muffins" made with eggs and your choice of sausage, hamburger, shredded zucchini, mushrooms, onions, broccoli, cheeses, etc. Just pour the mixture into muffin tins, bake, and freeze for easy breakfasts on the go!

Plateaus

What Could Be Causing My Plateau?

The underlying premise of this book, and my philosophy of weight loss in general, is that *everybody's different* (the theory of biochemical individuality). So you will not be surprised to find that I wholeheartedly believe there are *at least* a dozen or more reasons for the dreaded plateaus that you will inevitably reach in your weight loss efforts. The Drs. Eades have called plateaus "the purgatory of dieting" for good reason. They drive everyone crazy (plateaus, not the Eadeses, who are very lovely people). Nevertheless, you need to learn to *expect* them and to deal with them. There is virtually no one who has successfully lost weight who has not experienced them. And the very first (and maybe most important) rule of dealing with them is this: don't panic, and don't give up.

Here are the top twelve reasons plateaus occur.

1. **You are losing fat but building muscle.** If you are exercising, especially for the first time, you may be putting on muscle while you are losing fat. This change for the better will not show up on the scale, though it would definitely show up in a body composition analysis. You will likely notice a small but definite change in your shape or the measurement of your waist, even though the scale isn't really moving. Don't worry—eventually, the scale will reflect the loss of body fat.
2. **Water retention masks fat loss.** You may be losing fat while holding on to water. This happens more often than you might imagine. Make sure you are drinking plenty of water (see page 243). Not drinking enough water is one of the top reasons for plateaus and stalls.
3. **You are experiencing a period of adjustment.** Remember that when it comes to weight, your body operates something like the feedback loop of a thermostat. Your body needs periods of adjustment to catch up with the different amount and type of fuel it's getting, just like the thermostat needs to "catch up" with changes in

the temperature of the air in your apartment. If you're resetting your "set point," it happens not all at once, but in stages. Being stuck at a certain weight for a few weeks may just be your body's way of reprogramming itself. Eventually, the scale will move again.

4. **Your carbohydrate level is too high.** The plans discussed in this book are contingent on careful monitoring of carbohydrates. Your carbohydrate intake may simply be too high for what *your* body needs to lose weight. You could easily be taking in more carbs than you're aware of, as many foods and drinks have what are known as "hidden carbs." There is a great hidden carb counter listed in the Resources. If you suspect this may be the problem, check it out.

5. **Your carbohydrate level is too low!** This is one of the great paradoxes of low-carb dieting because it is completely counterintuitive. Nonetheless, I've seen it in action many times. More than one person wrote to me of weight loss stalled at a carb intake of 20 grams per day, which they were able to get going again by simply moving their carb intake *up* to about 40 or 50 grams. One possible explanation for this comes from the work of Dr. Diana Schwarzbein, who would argue that too low an intake of carbs creates higher levels of adrenaline and cortisol (which ultimately work against weight loss). While this scenario may not be true for everyone, upping your carbs is certainly worth a try.

6. **You are undereating.** Remember that the body responds to too few calories by simply becoming more efficient at extracting every single ounce of energy from its limited food supply. Too few calories literally slow down the metabolic rate.

7. **You are overeating.** At some point, every low-carber has to look at calories. Low-carb diets don't usually stress calorie counting, because you're much less likely to overeat on healthy proteins and good fats than you are on junk carbohydrates. Nonetheless, calories still count to some degree. You may be eating too many of them.

8. **You aren't eating enough protein.** If you don't eat enough protein, you're more likely to break down your body's own protein for fuel. That means muscle loss, which in turn means a lowering of your metabolic rate. Make sure you're eating at least the minimum recommended amount of protein for your plan.

9. **You are not exercising.** Though weight loss is 80 percent diet, exercise definitely helps things along. The many things it does for both your health *and* your weight loss (and weight maintenance!) efforts are too lengthy to go into here. Just trust me. Do it.

10. **Medications are preventing optimum weight loss.** Many medications can interfere with weight loss. Steroid medications like prednisone are among the worst offenders, but there are plenty of others. Check this out with your doctor.

11. **You are experiencing food intolerances.** The usual suspects are foods that are generally reduced or eliminated on low-carb programs, but if you're consuming them, try your own version of a modified elimination diet: remove the suspect food for a week or two and see what happens. The "sensitive seven" are wheat, milk, sugar, peanuts, soy, eggs, and corn.[38] You may want to expand the wheat category to include all grains and the milk category to include cheese. Other well-known stallers that you might want to cut out for a while include artificial sweeteners, especially aspartame (Equal); citric acid, found in diet sodas; glycerin, found in many low-carb meal replacement bars, including those by Atkins; and alcohol.

12. **You have nutritional deficiencies.** A deficiency in some nutrient or nutrients may very well be interfering with how smoothly the energy-making cycles in your body run. This could easily account for you not burning fat at an optimal level. (See the section on supplements in chapter 4.) At the very least, take a high-potency multivitamin and mineral, although this is only the first line of defense—you probably need a lot more. Just as an example, in a paper in *Medical Hypotheses*, Dr. L.H. Leung noted that for reasons not completely understood, he had had a lot of success with weight loss patients by simply adding pantothenic acid to their program.[39] (Nutritionist Barbara Marquette, M.S., who teaches nutritional therapeutics in the University of Bridgeport's master's program in nutrition, has seen the identical effect.) This could be because of pantothenic acid's direct effect on the adrenal glands. However, this is only one example; there are easily a dozen other vitamin or mineral deficiencies that could prevent optimal fat loss.

How Do I Break a Plateau?

You can try a lot of things. You could up your carbs if the amount you've been eating is very low, or you could try lowering them (see the list of reasons for plateaus in previous question). Try cutting out treats and going back exclusively to unprocessed meat and dark green vegetables for a few days. Cut out the low-carb bars. Drink a lot more water. Or try one of the following techniques, which have been known to knock people off plateaus.

Try a vegetable and fruit fast. Eat nothing but vegetables and some fruit for about three days. This is very alkalinizing, in addition to being low in calories and very high in nutrients. Eat all you want, and feel free to add some good fat like flaxseed oil (for women), olive oil, or butter.

Try a vegetable juice fast. This is a favorite of Dr. Allan Spreen, the "Nutrition Physician," and it's one of my favorites as well. Go a day or two on nothing but freshly squeezed vegetable juices. I'm not talking V8 here; I'm talking the kind you make at home with a juicer. You can also drink hot water with lemon juice and, of course, all the fresh water you like.

Try raw foods for a few days. Be aware that not all people can tolerate this, and if your digestion isn't great, this may not be the best intervention for you.

Add digestive enzymes. Dr. John Hernandez, medical director of the Center for Health and Integrative Medicine in San Antonio, Texas, has found this to be one of the most useful weapons he has in his weight loss arsenal (see also chapter 4).

Try the all-meat diet for a few days (no more than three). Eat nothing but meat and drink plenty of water. (The Lindora program uses a variation on this technique once a week, only with more choices for protein.) Another variation on this technique is to use the Stillman diet, which I consider to be absolutely ridiculous as an eating program but perhaps useful for a couple of days to get things going again. On the Stillman version of the meat fast, you eat only lean meats, chicken, turkey, all lean fish, eggs, and cottage, farmer, or pot cheese made with skim milk. No extra fat, zero carbohydrates, and nothing but water to drink.

Do the Fat Fast. This is an Atkins technique, but it should be reserved for *only* the most metabolically resistant people who have been absolutely unable to move the scale any other way. It's based on the Kekwick and Pawan study in which researchers placed patients on a 1,000-calorie diet that was 90 percent fat and got better fat loss than on any other plan.[40] In the Atkins version, you eat only 1,000 calories, with 75 to 90 percent of it coming from fat. Atkins recommends five small meals of about 200 calories each. Sample 200-calorie choices include 1 ounce of macadamia nuts, 2 ounces of cream cheese or Brie, or two deviled eggs with 2 teaspoons of mayo. (For more choices and a full explanation, see *Dr. Atkins' New Diet Revolution*, pages 272–74.) Atkins emphasizes that this is actually *dangerous* for anyone who is not metabolically resistant—the rate of weight loss is too rapid to be safe. Atkins used it only with people who could not lose weight any other way, to encourage them and to show them that weight loss was possible—but even then, he used it for only four or five days.

Exercise

What About Exercise?

Exercise is probably the most important predictor of whether or not you will keep weight off. Unfortunately, it doesn't really account for a great deal of the weight you will lose (maybe a few pounds a month), but if you don't do it, the odds of keeping the weight off tumble. Some lucky people are able to lose weight just by adding a lot of exercise to their daily routine without changing their diets much, but these are very rare people who usually don't have an awful lot of weight to lose.

That being said, there are many, many excellent reasons to begin an exercise program if you are not exercising already. The health benefits alone are legion, and exercise is one of the things that helps change your biochemistry to that of a leaner person. Exercise has an insulinlike effect on lowering blood sugar, it increases serotonin, and—except when very high-intensity—it decreases stress hormones.

Low-carb exercise gurus Graeme and Kate Street recommend full-body circuit training for beginners (plus cardio interval training for all levels) as the ideal programs for low-carbers. I agree. These programs will maintain or even build a little muscle yet are not so overwhelmingly intense that you won't have the energy for them. You can supplement with cardio as you see fit, probably the more, the better. And don't worry about the fat-burning zone (see the following question). Just go as long and as hard as you can without exhausting yourself, or mix short, intense workouts with longer, slower ones.

Whatever you do, do *not* neglect weight training. Walking by itself is just not going to cut it as an exercise program for weight loss. Without using and challenging your muscles, you will lose them, slowly but surely, and that will slow down your metabolism. Weight training is the best way to boost a sluggish metabolism. The more muscle you have, the more calories you burn.

Do I Need to Exercise in the Fat-Burning Zone?

The need to exercise in the so-called fat-burning zone is a complete myth. You should exercise for as hard and as long as you safely and reasonably can, and go for the maximum amount of calories you can burn. It makes no real difference whether those calories come from fat or from sugar any more than it matters if you pay for something with a check or with cash.

The average person uses about 70 percent fat and 30 percent sugar as "fuel" while they're sitting, sleeping, or relaxing. As they become more active, the percentages shift—the harder they exercise, the lower the proportion of fuel from fat and the higher the proportion of fuel from sugar. This is where the misunderstanding comes from. While the *percentages* of fuel do indeed change, so does the amount of calories burned. So, sure, at low levels of exercise, I'm burning about 70 percent of my calories from fat, but I'm burning only a couple of calories a minute! When I exercise harder, I may be burning only 40 percent fat, but I'm burning a lot more calories. Would you rather have 90 percent of all of my money or 10 percent of Donald Trump's?

I Have No Stamina for Exercise When I'm on a Low-Carb Diet. What Gives?

Lyle McDonald, one of the foremost experts on the ketogenic diet and author of a textbook in the field, works with many athletes, particularly bodybuilders. He believes that with very high-intensity exercise, the ketogenic diet can present a problem as far as energy goes. He therefore recommends that on exercise days you consume more carbohydrates than usual, then go back to your usual amount at the next meal. It's important to realize that he's talking only about super-high-intensity exercise. For more "regular" folks, a ketogenic—or any reduced-carb—diet will supply more than enough energy for circuit training, conventional weight training, and/or moderate aerobics. If it doesn't, it may be that you're not eating enough fat.

> *I've recently started both low-impact circuit training and a low-carb diet, and I haven't had any problems. As long as I don't overdo my workout, I have more energy than ever before.*
> —Janice K.

If, however, you still find that getting through your workouts is nearly impossible, try eating a small amount (5 to 25 grams) of carbohydrate about thirty minutes before your workout and see if that helps. If it does, you'll know that you are one of those people who need more carbs to work out effectively.

I'm a Runner and I Like to Run Races at My Local Runner's Club. I Thought "Carb Loading" Was a Must for Athletes. Can a Low-Carb Diet Work for Me?

Remember that the fuel you most want to use during endurance exercise is fat, not sugar. "Carb loading" simply ensures that your glycogen stores are full, which translates into using sugar for fuel. The better you are at fat-burning, the longer you'll be able to go. For what it's worth, Stu Mittleman, an exercise physiologist, nutritionist, ultramarathoner, and one of the greatest endurance athletes of all time, generally eats a diet of about 40 percent carbs, 30 percent protein, and 30 percent fat, but when he is in training for an event, he ups the *fat* to about 50 percent—not the carbs.

CHAPTER 7

Tricks of the Trade: The Top 50+ Tips for Making Low-Carb Work for You

I've put together more than fifty of the most useful tips for making low-carb eating a part of your life. The tips are organized into three categories—food and drink, motivation, and general. Occasionally, a tip in the general category may seem like it has nothing to do with low-carb eating, but believe me, if it's there, it has everything to do with making low-carb weight loss a success. Remember that no program that results in changing your body *and* your life can be based *just* around what foods to eat or not eat. We also need to know how to deal with the kinds of issues—boredom, anxiety, disappointment, failure, perseverance, and so on—that inevitably come up when we're talking about changing lifelong habits. By the way, before we get started, let me tell you the first and most important tip of all. . . .

Don't Try to Do All the Tips

In low-carb dieting, as with many other things in life, you can easily and quickly get intellectually fatigued from information overload, a pitfall that causes many people to just throw up their hands and give up. Don't do this. Use the tips that make sense to you and that you can incorporate easily into your life. Don't worry about the rest. You can always go back and revisit them.

Now, let's get started!

Food and Drink

Drink Water

No kidding. This tip has been all over this book in various forms, including in the FAQ chapter, but it's so important that I'm going to stick it everywhere you might possibly see it. *Water can—and does—affect fat loss*. If you're on a ketogenic diet (Atkins induction phase, Protein Power phase one, etc.), it's essential to flush out the ketones and waste products from the fat you're losing. Even if you're not on a ketogenic diet, it's essential to prevent constipation and to optimize kidney and liver function (remember that the liver is the main fat-processing factory in the body, and if it's not working properly, neither is fat metabolism). Eight glasses a day is the *minimum* and is not enough for most overweight people. For more specific recommendations on how much water to drink, see page 243.

P.S.: If you need more motivation, water is number one in the anti-aging arsenal of Dr. Nicholas Perricone, formerly of Yale University and the chairman of the International Conference on Aging and Aging Skin. Perricone says, "If I could teach my patients and students three things that would keep them forever young, they would be: one, drink water; two, drink water; and three, drink more water."

Watch Out for Protein Bars

You gotta be careful with these. I definitely don't recommend them during the first two weeks, when you're adjusting to this new way of eating. For one thing, the market has been saturated with this new class of candy—I mean snack food—and predictably, the bars vary in quality from complete junk to not so bad. Some of the best are PaleoBar, available only through Designs for Health, Sears Labs' Omega-3 Zone (don't confuse them with the Zone bars found in every grocery store)—see Resources for where to purchase—and the Atkins bars, available everywhere.

All protein bars are not created equal, and the term *energy bar* is a complete marketing scam. "Energy," in the parlance of nutrition, simply means "calories," but manufacturers want you to think that eating one of their bars will make you feel like running a marathon. Not so. In fact, most "energy" bars are loaded with carbs. Almost all have hydrogenated fats (trans-fats). Protein bars specifically have more protein and often less carbs, but you still have to read labels. Some are as high as 330 calories, not exactly snack food. In addition, they have sweeteners like sorbitol or mannitol, which are sugar alcohols that still need to be counted if you're counting carbs. Mannitol, especially, may give you gas. And even dear Dr. Atkins doesn't count the glycerine (also known as glycerol) when he tells you there's only 2 or 3 grams of effective carbs in his bars. That's controversial: glycerol—an odorless, colorless, sweet-tasting liquid—is used as a sweetener and is classified as a carbohydrate, but Atkins claims that because it does not impact blood sugar in the same way sugar does, it shouldn't be counted as part of the net (effective) carb content in his bars. Maybe; maybe not. Many low-carbers do find that it slows down their weight loss; others don't. In any case, stick with real food and hold off on the bars for a few weeks until you get your bearings in this new way of eating.

Consider Salmon for Breakfast . . . or Lunch or Dinner

I told you that not all tips would be applicable to all readers, but if you can make this one work, you'll reap a lot of results. Unfortunately, farmed salmon— which is what you'll get most often in restaurants—has all the problems other farm animals have. The fish are raised in pens, fed grain, and given antibiotics. As a result of the grain diet and the lack of exercise, their omega-3 fat content is not nearly as good as that of their wild brethren. However, with wild fish there is always the slight risk of mercury. So what to do? There are such huge benefits to eating salmon that I recommend it anyway. If you can get Alaskan wild salmon, that's great. Consider, however, some amazingly healthy varieties of canned salmon, which also taste delicious. The red sockeye kind is the best. You can get my *absolute* favorite, the hard-to-find gourmet Vital Choice salmon (which is also the choice of many other well-known nutrition and health gurus), through a specially arranged link on my website: JonnyBowden.com.

Eat Breakfast Every Day

When you skip breakfast, among the many other negative things that happen is that insulin release is greater at the next meal than it would otherwise have been. Blood sugar is destabilized. You're more likely to be subject to cravings. In all likelihood, you're running on empty and masking it with coffee. If you're one of those people who has no appetite in the morning, it's probably because you've just conditioned yourself to this unnatural way of eating. A good place to start with the rehabilitation of your appetite is with a protein shake. Even people who are not hungry in the morning can get one of these babies down, especially if it's delicious and made with good extras like berries or a tablespoon of peanut butter. Eventually, you should transition to a real-food breakfast (at least for most days), and make sure it contains protein and some good fats.

If you need some additional motivation: at least seven studies have found a correlation between being overweight and skipping breakfast.[1-3]

Memorize This: Water Retention Can Mask Fat Loss!

This is one of those paradoxical situations that doesn't make sense on the surface of it—the less water you drink, the more water you retain. Why? Because when not enough water is coming into the body, a hormone called vasopressin acts upon the kidneys to tell them to reabsorb the existing water in the body rather than urinating it; another hormone, aldosterone, tells the body to conserve sodium, leading to more water retention. Other factors—such as medications, hormones, menstrual cycles, and birth control pills—can also affect water retention. So sometimes your body is actually dropping fat, but because you're holding on to water, you might not notice it on the scale. Once again, the best advice is to keep drinking water.

Shop for Color

I read the women's magazines all the time to stay up-to-date on the kind of nutrition information being disseminated (I read the men's magazines too, but only, of course, for the articles.) One of the very best tips I ever read was this one: shop for color. If you don't want to memorize a whole bunch of antioxidants and proanthocyanidins and phytochemicals, the easiest way to ensure you're getting the best nutritional bang for your money is to look at what the contents of your cart look like on the checkout counter. Does it resemble one of those great postcard pictures of a European outdoor market? It should be overflowing in greens, reds, oranges, and even blues. All those colorings in fruits and vegetables are there because they are natural antioxidants that will serve a similar purpose in your body. If everything you buy is the color of cardboard, you're doing something wrong.

Shop the Outside Aisles

Want to magically reduce the number of calories you're eating from sugar, processed foods, and junk carbohydrates? Here's a simple trick: step away from the inner aisles of the supermarket. All the good stuff is on the outside. Spend your time in the periphery of the supermarket. (It also seems to be the secret to a good singles pickup; after all, no one ever turned to a stranger to ask, "How do you tell if this cereal box is fresh?")

Carry Protein-Rich Snack Food with You

Forget the vending machines, the airport kiosks, and the 7-Eleven stores. Start thinking of snack food in terms of *real* food, and start thinking of real food in terms of *protein* (and fat)—just what your hunting and gathering ancestors would most likely have been munching on while taking a break from stalking wild game. Think nuts, cheese (string cheese is a great choice), hard-boiled eggs, jerky, or some leftover chicken in a plastic bag. You can occasionally add a piece of fruit to the mix if your particular plan permits it, but what you *can't* do is grab a bag of chips or pretzels or a chocolate chip cookie—not if you want to get or stay slim!

Buy Some Cookbooks

If I had a mere nickel for every client who asked me "What can I eat?" or who complained of being bored with the same old choices, I would be one very rich nutritionist! The answer to the question became abundantly clear to me while researching this book. There are dozens—I mean *dozens*—of amazing cookbooks and recipes out there for virtually every level of ability and interest in cooking, from complete novice (me) to gourmet chef. (Look at some of the marvelous suggestions for meats and snacks from Internet chef superstar Karen Barnaby on page 253, or visit lowcarb.ca, and those are only the beginning!) The best of the cookbooks are listed in Resources, and there are more coming out every month. In addition, the websites (see Resources) that I list nearly all have recipe sections, some of them incredibly diverse and interesting. There's a *lot* more to low-carb eating than just chicken and vegetables.

Don't Do Anything Else While You're Eating

You're trying to bring mindfulness and consciousness to the table when it comes to eating so that you can reduce some of the automatic eating that takes place when you're thinking about other things. A good way to do that is to make eating time *eating time*, not reading the paper time or watching television time. The more you can do this, the better, and the less likely you are to consume food while you barely notice you're consuming it!

Eat Slowly and Savor Every Bite

Here's another tip you can file under "Grandmother knew best." The fact is that chewing your food slowly and thoroughly, putting your fork down between bites, and actually *enjoying* what you're eating can help you lose weight. Here's why. The brain doesn't really get the message "Hey, he's full!" from the stomach until about twenty minutes after you've eaten enough. That's how long it takes for the hormone CCK to do its job and signal "Enough!" to the brain. So fast eaters frequently overeat before their brain gets the signal that they're not really hungry anymore. You can go a long way toward enhancing natural appetite control by taking advantage of your body's excellent communication network, but you need to give it enough time to work! Also, eating slowly and actually *experiencing* your food works against the kind of unconscious, mindless eating that caused you to put on weight in the first place.

Eat the Bulk of Your Food Earlier in the Day

Adelle Davis used to say, "Eat breakfast like a king, lunch like a prince, and dinner like a pauper." She was right. One important study showed that when people were fed a 2,000-calorie meal for breakfast (and nothing else during the day), they lost weight, but when they were fed the exact same meal at night, they gained.[4] Spread your food out during the day to control your blood sugar and insulin levels, but try not to eat too much in the evening.

Add Yogurt or Kefir to Your Daily Program

Cultured milk products restore healthful bacteria to your body and are usually well tolerated even by people who have problems with dairy. You need to eat the *plain yogurt* with the *real live cultures* (not the junk food with the tons of fruit on the bottom). Even better, use kefir. Here's the deal with the carb content: it's not as high as the package says. In fact, for ½ cup of yogurt, kefir, or buttermilk, you need to count only 2 grams of effective carbohydrate!

How can this be? It's because of the way the government measures carbs. They measure everything in the food—water, ash, protein, fat—and then assume that what's left is carbohydrate. This works fine for everything, including milk, but it doesn't work for *fermented* milk products. As Dr. Jack Goldberg of GO-Diet fame points out, when you ferment milk, you inoculate it with lactic acid bacteria, which then "eats up" almost all of the milk sugar (lactose) and converts it into lactic acid, the stuff that curds the milk and gives the product its unique taste. So the milk *sugar* that the government thinks is left in the product is really just about gone—it's been "converted" in the fermenting process by the lactic acid bacteria. The "real" amount of carbohydrate left in ½ cup of plain yogurt or kefir is only 2 grams—this has been measured by Goldberg in his own lab. I recommend that you get the full-fat variety of kefir or yogurt and enjoy it on an almost daily basis.

Repeat After Me: Fruit Juice Is Not—and Never Was—a Health Food

One of the many triumphs of marketing by the giant food conglomerates was convincing America that fruit juice is good for you. There are ads that proclaim proudly that some stupid sugar-laden soft drink is actually 10 percent real fruit juice. Fruit juice is *not* fruit (and for carb addicts, even fruit itself has to be watched, at least in the beginning). Fruit juice is plain and simple junk food. It's loaded with sugar, it has none of the fiber of real fruit, it has a high glycemic load, and it contributes absolutely nothing of value to your diet except for a few measly vitamins that you can easily get elsewhere.

Eat Protein at Every Meal

Every single meal should have protein in it. Ideally, so should every snack (but see "Choose Your Battles" on page 288). Protein has less of an effect on insulin than carbs do, is more satisfying,[5] and requires more energy (calories) to break down and assimilate. The body recognizes protein (and fat) as something that you have a need for; therefore, the appetite-control mechanisms that send messages from your gut to your brain signaling that you've had enough food work well with protein (something they do not do with carbohydrates, as we saw in chapter 2). A greater ratio of protein to carbohydrate at a meal stabilizes blood sugar and reduces insulin response.[6] And new research suggests that leucine, an amino acid found in protein, specifically helps you to maintain muscle mass while losing body fat during weight loss.[7]

"All-Natural" Doesn't Mean All-Good

Another triumph of the marketers was convincing us that "natural" on a food label actually *means* something. The term *all-natural* is a wholly unregulated, utterly meaningless term. Anyone can use it on anything. What's all-natural about frozen dinners, "energy" bars, or even cut-up chicken parts in the meat section of your supermarket? You mean they were "naturally" fed a diet they normally wouldn't eat, fed "natural" antibiotics, and then all by themselves just "naturally" morphed into chicken parts in little yellow "all-natural" Styrofoam containers? Forget the term *natural*. Toxic mushrooms are all-natural, and so is crude oil, but we don't eat those. Look for *real food*, preferably without a bar code. Think about what you could have hunted, fished for, gathered, plucked, or grown if you were with your original ancestors on the savanna. *That's* natural food. Eat it.

Replace Grains with Greens

There are lots of reasons why grains may not be the healthiest food in the world for most people. According to Dr. Joseph Mercola, grains contain little vitamin C and no vitamin A, and two of the major B-vitamin deficiency diseases are almost exclusively associated with excessive grain consumption.[8] Fiber—with very few exceptions—is present in paltry amounts in most processed grain products like cereals and breads and, in any case, can be gotten from vegetables and other sources. Though some people do okay with grains, if you've got a weight problem, you are probably not one of them. Get your carbohydrates from vegetables, at least most of the time. C. Leigh Broadhurst, Ph.D., author of *Diabetes: Prevention and Cure*, once told me that if she could have her overweight and diabetic clients make only a single change, the one that would have the most impact on their lives would be to remove wheat from their diets. Think about it.

Bring Your Own (Food, That Is)

One problem for a lot of my clients is that they don't know how to stay on their eating plan once they're out and about, running around, or stuck at the office. That's probably because the whole world is set up for quick and easy junk food, and chicken breasts don't fit in a vending machine. Don't be a victim of circumstance. Take control of your own life. Start thinking about packing your own lunches, or at the very least your own snacks. Bodybuilders have been doing it for decades. You can, too.

Use Green Drinks

Green drinks is the general category name for juices from barley, wheatgrass, or any combination of whole green foods. Green drinks pack an incredible nutritional wallop and usually have amazing phytonutrient and vitamin profiles. They are very alkalizing (and are thus a terrific balance to a higher-meat diet), they're usually made from organic sources, they're very low in calories, and most have no more than 3 to 4 grams of (low-glycemic) carbohydrate, an insignificant amount unless you are on the strictest of induction-stage diets (and even then you can work them in). You can find them in most health food and whole food supermarkets, and you should definitely consider making them part of your program. One of my favorites is Barley Power, a completely organic product. I'm also a fan of Green Magma by Green Foods, Greens First by Doctors for Nutrition, Perfect Food by Garden of Life, and my personal favorites, Pro-Greens by Nutricology and Paleogreens by Designs for Health.

Consider Eggs Rocky Style

That's right. Raw eggs. I put two in a glass just about every day and drink 'em down. When I tell my clients this "tip," most look at me like I just stepped off a spaceship, but here's the deal: *there is no more perfect food on earth, and there is no more healthy way to eat it.* Dr. Joe Mercola says, "Raw whole eggs are a phenomenally inexpensive and incredible source of high-quality nutrients that many of us are deficient in, especially high-quality protein and fat." He also believes that the reason eggs are often allergenic is that they are cooked: heating the egg protein changes its chemical shape, which can lead to allergies. When consumed raw, the incidence of egg allergy virtually disappears. One great way to consume them—if you don't want to drink them straight—is in a protein shake. It'll add a creamy, delicious texture to the drink and beef up the protein and nutrient count.

  What about salmonella? Well, first of all, understand this: the risk of getting an egg contaminated with salmonella is one in thirty thousand.[9]

Second, nearly all of those contaminated eggs come from sick hens; if you get organic, free-range (and preferably omega-3-enriched) eggs, the risk virtually disappears. Third, even if you get it—and you probably won't—salmonella is a relatively benign, self-limiting illness in healthy people.[10] Ninety-four percent of those who get it don't even see a doctor.[11] And before you dismiss the idea of a raw egg or two as just too weird, remember how an egg cream was made at virtually every soda fountain in the world back in the "old days": chocolate syrup, seltzer, milk, and a raw egg!

Use Cabbage Leaves for "Bread"

You could use lettuce leaves, but red cabbage is stronger. You can make a "sandwich" (or a grain-free "wrap") of virtually any meat you like—deli turkey, real turkey, chicken, even a hamburger—by wrapping it in a big, hard leaf of cabbage or an outer leaf of lettuce. Try chicken with a few avocado slices or beef with tomato. Consider using this tip in conjunction with "Bring Your Own"!

Get a Coffee Grinder and Use It for Flaxseeds

This is just an all-around great health tip in general, but it can be especially useful to low-carbers for the following reason: flaxseeds (as opposed to flaxseed oil) are a significant source of fiber, which is not only protective against diseases like colon cancer but is also demonstrably related to weight loss. Fiber blunts blood sugar response and adds to a feeling of fullness. At least a dozen clinical studies demonstrate the effect of fiber on weight loss (see chapter 4). In addition, flaxseeds are one of the best sources of the omega-3 fat ALA (alpha linolenic acid), which has documented heart-protective effects as well as being anti-inflammatory. Inflammatory chemicals (cytokines) are produced, among other places, in the fat cells, so if you're very heavy, you're also likely to have a problem with inflammation. All in all, freshly ground flaxseeds are a terrific addition to your program.

Sardines: The Health Food in a Can

You simply cannot beat sardines as a quick, easy, inexpensive source of first-class protein and omega-3 fats. I learned the usefulness of sardines as a fast and easy pick-me-up when I was traveling in Florida with the famous New York nutritionist Oz Garcia and giving seminars. We had a brutal schedule and almost no time between events to grab anything to eat. Whenever Oz felt his blood sugar dropping or his energy flagging, he would stop and run into the nearest convenience store or bodega and grab . . . *a can of sardines*! I learned firsthand how energizing and satisfying this food can be, right out of the can! If your particular low-carb program permits it, eat sardines with some low-carb, low-sugar crackers like Wasa bread. If you're in somewhat more relaxed circumstances than we were, sardines over any kind of green salad makes the perfect low-carb meal. The best kind (if you can find them) are packed in sardine oil. Do not buy the kind in soybean or cottonseed oils, as these are way too high in omega-6s.

When Eating Out, Send Back the Bread

Don't even let the waiter put it down. If it sits there, two things can happen to it—you can eat it, or you can *not* eat it. If you send it back, you eliminate the first possibility.

Eat Almonds—but Portion Them Out

Nuts are a great addition to the low-carb lifestyle—but they can also slow weight loss because they are so easy to overeat and are so high in calories. If you're going to eat them during the weight loss phase of your program, divide them into appropriate portions. Fifteen almonds is a portion. If you buy those big convenience bags, don't take the whole bag with you to "snack" on—portion out your serving, put it in a little bag, and put the rest away.

Craving Sugar? Try Sautéed Almonds

Here's a neat treat that'll satisfy a craving for dessert: sauté some raw almonds in butter, or bake them and melt a little butter on top. Use a bit of sea salt if you like. Remember to watch the portion size (see previous tip).

Try This Super Craving Buster

Mix together 1 tablespoon each of sesame tahini and organic soy miso, and use the mixture as a spread on celery, lettuce, or even low-carb crackers like Wasa. It'll satisfy cravings and help reduce mineral deficiencies.

Crave-Bust with This Amino Acid

A tablespoon of powdered glutamine (an amino acid) sweetened with xylitol and dissolved in a tablespoon or two of heavy cream or half-and-half will disarm even the most demanding sugar craving.

Do Damage Control with Pasta

You don't have to give up pasta forever, especially once you're at your goal weight. But lower the glycemic load significantly by cooking it al dente. The less time you boil it, the more the long chains of starch molecules in the pasta remain closely packed, making it difficult for enzymes to break them down and thus lowering the impact the pasta has on your blood sugar. Better yet, get one of the new lower-carb, higher-fiber pastas and cook *that* al dente.

Here's a Way to Become a Vegetable Lover Instantly

Even the most ardent antivegetable person is won over by a plate of roasted vegetables. Take a bunch of veggies—all kinds of peppers and root vegetables like carrots, parsnips, beets, and onions respond well to this method—cut them up, and arrange them in a roasting pan. Drizzle with olive oil and put 'em in the oven for thirty or forty minutes. The roasting brings out sweetness and flavor you never knew existed.

Read Labels and Be a Sugar Detective

Manufacturers are required to list ingredients in order of amount; the first ingredient makes up the largest proportion of the product, and the last ingredient is present in the lowest proportion. Most manufacturers don't like saying that sugar is the main ingredient, even though it's true. So they label their products with small amounts of a ton of different forms of sugar—sucrose, glucose, corn syrup, corn sweetener, dextrose, fructose, lactose, maltodextrin, invert sugar, concentrated fruit juice, sorbitol, xylitol, mannitol, barley malt, malt extract, and the

> *Giving up sugar was almost as hard as quitting smoking, but after about three months I found I didn't crave it anymore, and I felt 100 percent better.*
> —Patricia M.

absolute worst of all, high-fructose corn syrup. By putting in small amounts of a mix of these, they can legally disguise the fact that the main ingredient in the packaged food you are holding is . . . sugar! If you want to know how many teaspoons of added sugar is in a food you are eating, just divide the number of grams of sugar on the label by 4. You'll be amazed to find that some cereals have 7 teaspoons of sugar per serving, and those serving sizes are tiny!

Watch Those "Legal" Desserts

Just because something is low-carb does not mean it is no-calorie and definitely does not mean you can eat unlimited amounts of it. Don't make the same mistake the low-fat dieters did when they consumed massive amounts of junk food, thinking it was perfectly okay because it was low-fat. There are plenty of delicious low-carb desserts, and it's nice to be able to have them once in a while, but if they trigger eating binges, then step away from the dessert! It's also not a good thing if they start to replace real food on a regular basis (same problem with low-carb bars).

If You Need Dessert, Ask for Cheese and Berries or Berries and Cream

Dr. Jack Goldberg of the GO-Diet recommends this one, and adds that you can sweeten with the no-calorie sweetener on the table if you like. If it fits into your carb allowance and you're doing the berries and cream at home *and* you must have sweetener, try xylitol (see Resources).

Motivation

Keep a Journal

Virtually all of the successful low-carbers I interviewed for this book routinely kept food diaries, and journaling is one of four key behaviors consistently cited as a winning strategy by people who were successful in losing weight (at least 30 pounds kept off for at least one year) in the National Weight Control Registry. It's also probably the one technique that every specialist, no matter where they stand on the "dieting" spectrum, recommends.

In my own "Shape Up" program, run successfully on iVillage.com for more than five years, the journal is essential. Here's why. You can't change something unless you know what it is you're changing—keeping records of what you're eating allows you to see what's working and what's not; it allows you to track changes in your eating behavior against changes in your weight (and energy, mood, and sleep); and it causes you to be aware of what you're eating, which keeps you rigorously honest.

In addition, for those who are so inclined, the journal can also be a terrific tool for self-discovery and has been for many great artists throughout time. You can add recollections of the day's events as well as notations about your feelings, your moods, your resentments, your anxieties, and your joys. But don't feel you *have* to—all you really need to do to make this work from a weight loss perspective is to keep a record of what you eat and drink—every single day. You don't have to do it forever, but the more you do it, the more successful you are likely to be.

Visit a Support Community Online

One of the best things about the Internet—besides instant messaging—is the way it has allowed people with similar interests to form long-distance communities of support and information sharing. I've spent literally hundreds of hours on the Internet exploring the various online communities for low-carbing, and I've distilled the best (and steered you from the worst) in the Resources. Take a look. You'll find bulletin boards with posts from people just like you (no matter what level you're at, your particular interest or concern, how much weight you have to lose, your age, or how sophisticated or unsophisticated you are about this stuff). If you don't like the first one you go to, just pick another; eventually, you'll find one where you feel at home. Many of the low-carb sites also have links to the diet journals, called diet blogs, of people just like you who have been successful at losing weight. And many of the sites listed in the Resources are personal sites and journals of individuals whose lives have been transformed by low-carb living. If one day you happen to feel unmotivated, look at some of their pictures!

Expect Stalls and Plateaus

There is no one on the planet who has lost weight who hasn't experienced these. They're a natural part of weight loss. Think of them as your body's way of "catching up" with the changes you're introducing to your lifestyle, kind of like a "reset" of the thermostat. They can occur for a million different reasons (see "Plateaus," page 255), but the important point is that they *do* and *will* occur, and you will be better off if you're prepared so that you don't get thrown when they happen.

Find a Diet Buddy

This works for both exercise and dieting. It may even be the secret behind the success of personal training. If you have a commitment that involves another person, you are far more likely to actually *do* it. A diet buddy is like your committed listener. By stating your goals—saying out loud to another person what you're going to eat, do, or accomplish today (or this week, or whenever)—you are giving your word a much greater reality than it might have if all you did was make a vague promise to yourself. And with the omnipresence of the Internet, there is no longer any reason not to take advantage of this secret dieting weapon. You can find a diet buddy anywhere, and you can set up the ground rules to include "check-ins" as frequently as you both need. As a frequent contributor to the iVillage.com online community, I've seen this tip work time and time again.

Don't Let Yourself Get Too Tired, Angry, Hungry, Lonely, or Bored

Emotional eating is a huge factor in weight gain, as virtually everyone reading this book knows. In many ways, it is virtually impossible to separate the emotional component from the physiological components. All of these states of being—anger, sleep deprivation, hunger, loneliness, and boredom, not to mention anxiety, fear, nervousness, and stress—have been known to trigger overeating, nervous eating, comfort eating, or binge eating. The best cure in this case is a healthy dose of prevention.

Give Yourself a Nonfood Treat

Remember that changing your lifestyle is about breaking some old habits and replacing them with more empowering ones. One of the mental habits most in need of overhaul is telling yourself that food is your only reward and comfort. That doesn't mean there won't be a place in your life for comfort food or recreational eating, but you need to increase your repertoire of things that make you feel good.

Start looking for things that make you feel good besides food, and start finding time to do them! Give them to yourself as a reward, either for reaching a weight loss goal or just for the hell of it. (I had one client who cut out a picture of the Armani suit he was going to buy when his waist got down to a 34 and put it on his refrigerator.) It might be a trip to a day spa, a manicure, some time on the golf course, reading a beach novel, or going to a museum. Better yet, take a tip from Julia Cameron's *The Artist's Way* and make a "play date" with yourself: just you, doing whatever you want, no agenda, no greater purpose than to have fun. It doesn't have to be an all-day deal. It would be really great if you could come up with a number of *little* things you could do that don't take a lot of time and that can be incorporated into your daily life—take a bath or spend some time meditating or even listening to one absolutely great song from the disco era ("To Be Real" brightens almost every day). When you feel the need to compulsively dig into the cookie jar, start to train yourself to substitute one of these nonfood treats. You'll be conditioning a new repertoire of behaviors that has nothing to do with food.

Focus on the Weight You Have Lost and Kept Off—and Remember "the Bowden Equation"

Focusing on the weight you have lost is a gem of a tip from Internet guru and low-carb chef Karen Barnaby. I can't tell you the number of times I have seen a weight loss effort bite the dust because the person continued to focus on how far she had to go rather than how far she'd come. Many studies have shown that weight loss expectations tend to be greatly out of sync with what can realistically be attained. For example, most obesity programs consider the loss of 10 percent of original body weight a success, but when clients who are entering the program are asked what *they* think would be a successful outcome, they typically say that anything less than 25 percent would be a failure. This does not mean you should set your sights low—not at all. Go to some of the "real people" sites listed in Resources and look at some of those pictures. They are amazing! You can do this, too. But if you're expecting to lose 7 pounds a week consistently, you are going to be very, very disappointed, and if you are disappointed, you are going to feel like you failed, and if you feel like you're failing, you're much more likely to give up.

Remember my famous "Bowden Equation": *disappointment* equals the difference between *expectation* and *reality*. If you focus on the weight you have lost so far—even if it's a pound or two—you will be way better off in the long run and much more likely to keep going. Even better, focus on nonscale-related benefits, such as how you feel, lack of bloat, increased energy and well-being, lack of headaches, no more brain fog, or, best of all, lost inches and a changing shape. Remember that you lose weight exactly the same way you put it on—one pound at a time.

If You Get Stuck, Do Something Different

While stalls and plateaus are to be expected, they can be very frustrating. You may need to do something counterintuitive to start weight loss back up again. Some people have found that, strangely enough, adding *more* carbs gets things going again. Or try the Fat Fast outlined in Atkins or an "all-meat" day. Alternatively, go the other route and try a fruit and vegetable fast for a few days. None of these techniques will hurt—the fruit and vegetable one will probably do a lot of good—and any one of them may push you off a stall.

Take the Word "Cheating" Out of Your Vocabulary

Cheating implies lying or dishonesty. It's much more empowering to think about the low-carb lifestyle in terms of being "strict" or "not so strict." You may have some days when you are "not so strict." More than one very successful low-carber told me he would occasionally have days when he just had to have pizza, so he did. Then he'd get back on the "strict" track at the next meal. Usually, he didn't lose much momentum, and over time, the occasional lapse became meaningless. These people still lost a ton of weight over time by being strict more often than they were not so strict.

Look in the Mirror and Talk to Yourself

Here's another one from Dr. Jack Goldberg, who is clearly of the tough-love school of weight loss. He says that you shouldn't be angry with yourself if you lapse from your diet. Just look at yourself in the mirror and say the following to your image, in a loud voice so you can really hear yourself: *"Are you serious about losing weight? Then I don't want this to happen again. You are not a child. Grow up and take responsibility for yourself. There was no reason to eat that unhealthy junk."*

General Tips

Read a Book

Actually, that's good advice for life in general, but it's essential for low-carbing. I've had dozens of people tell me they were "on Atkins," yet they had absolutely no idea what Atkins really said and had heard only diluted information thirdhand from their hairdresser. Obviously you're not averse to the act of reading or you wouldn't have bought this book, so in a sense I'm preaching to the choir. But let *this* book whet your appetite for more info. Although you can clearly do the basic low-carb approach outlined in chapter 8 and get great results, one (or more) of the structured programs discussed in this book may have spoken to you in some way or piqued your interest. Consider my discussions of the diet programs in chapter 3 like Cliffs Notes. Find a plan that appeals to you and invest in the book itself— it will give you far more detail, you'll know how to do the program correctly, and you'll probably learn a lot in the bargain. Even if you don't wind up sticking with that exact program, it'll give you a great jumping-off point.

Take Your Measurements

You want to know where you're starting from so that you can monitor your progress. Keeping your head in the sand accomplishes nothing. Many people lose inches before they lose pounds (or they lose both, which is even better). If you measure your waist, at the very least you'll be able to track changes that may be happening independently of the scale, and that can be a big motivator during those times when your actual weight doesn't move (and there *will* be those times—see "Plateaus," page 255). Measuring your chest, waist, hip, upper thigh(s), and upper arm(s) is best. Don't look for a significant change in measurement every week, but check in every now and again to see how far you've come. You won't be able to do that if you don't measure first!

Use the Scale

Yup. This suggestion meets with a lot of protest, so let's first deal with the objections. Many people, especially those who have suffered eating disorders in the past, have experienced the tyranny of the scale and have been obsessive about using it, driving themselves crazy in the bargain. For these people, throwing the scale out—and relying on how they feel and how they look—has been nothing short of a psychic liberation. I get that.

But here's the thing: there's a way to use the scale as an ally, as a means to an end, as a tool for empowerment. First of all, you have to get that the readout is just a number and not make it "mean" anything other than what it is. That number is not a statement about your self-worth, who you are, or anything else—*it's just the number of pounds you weigh at the moment.*

Second, you have to realize that, imperfect as it may be, the scale is your reality check. I've seen clients assume that they *must* have lost weight because they jogged that day or, conversely, that they gained all kinds of tonnage because they overate at the family barbecue. Don't kid yourself. Check in with the scale. Sure, you may gain some muscle while you're losing fat, and that won't be reflected on the scale, but eventually fat loss *will* be reflected in that digital readout! Using the scale also keeps you accountable and honest: if you see your weight go up the morning after you did some midnight pigging out, it's a good lesson in associating cause and effect. And don't think for a minute that you won't feel great when you finally see the scale move toward your goal, even if it is a pound at a time.

Speaking of the Scale, Use It the Right Way

Don't compare your weight on different scales at different times of day (like how much you weighed at the doctor's office versus how much you weighed at the gym). Scales are like clocks: no two agree perfectly, but if you keep checking the same one, it will accurately tell you how much time is passing. I recommend daily weigh-ins. There are two rules to using the scale correctly. One, always do it in the morning, wearing no clothes, before eating. Let that number be your reference. Two, average the results of the week. There are simply too many variables that can be responsible for a half-pound to pound variation, day to day, and it can make you crazy to see these minor variations (especially when they're in the wrong direction). Use the totals for the week to compute where you're going. (With all that said, some people may find daily weigh-ins emotionally just too tough. If that's you, at the very least do a weekly weigh-in, which will help you stay on track and prevent you from obsessing too much about the numbers.) Incidentally, I have seen clients of mine completely transform their weight loss results simply by making everyday weigh-ins a part of their program.

Eat Before You Shop for Food

Ever go shopping when you're hungry? Then you know why people buy things like chocolate-covered artichokes. *Anything* sounds good when you're starving. When you're hungry is *not* the time to hit the supermarket. You won't make any kind of rational decision about food. Much better: go after you've eaten, when your choices won't be dictated by a growling stomach and a craving brain.

Get a Calorie/Carb Counter

This is just part of the overall mandate for conscious eating. *You need to know what's going into your body.* It will keep you honest. If you're counting carbs, a carb counter is a must. It's nice to know the calorie, protein, and fat content as well. My own *Living the Low Carb Life Pocket Carb Counter* gives you net carbs, calories, protein, fat, fiber, glycemic load rating (where applicable), and my assessment of how a particular food fits into the low-carb lifestyle. Both Atkins and Protein Power also have very good pocket carb guides.

Get Enough Sleep

There is no way to overstate the effect sleep can have on your weight loss efforts. Sleep, and lack of it, affects the body in several ways. One, lack of sleep is a stressor; stress raises cortisol, which in turn sends a message to the body to store fat around the middle. (Chronically high levels of cortisol also produce a counterresponse from the body in the form of insulin release.) Two, the absence of deep, restful, restorative sleep prevents the body from building up a reserve of serotonin. Low serotonin states are associated with cravings and overeating (not to mention good old garden-variety depression). Three, without deep, restful sleep, your pituitary will not produce any significant amount of growth hormone, which assists in the building of muscle and the loss of fat. Fourth, lack of sleep causes people to be hungry and to overeat during the day.

Some experts feel so strongly about the role of a full night of uninterrupted sleep in successful weight loss that they will even prescribe medications (typically trazadone, brand name Desyrel) to regulate sleep patterns. They feel that you are much better off taking a fairly innocuous medication than you would be with not getting enough sleep.

Volunteer

Nothing contributes to your own life more than contributing to the lives of others. Too many of us have made weight our sole focus for too long. Try putting the focus on others. Choose an activity in which your weight is of no significance, like putting in some volunteer time in a hospital or an animal shelter, moderating an Internet group, mentoring a kid, or even helping out a friend or family member with a yard sale. Get out of the house and get out of your head. It'll help keep things in perspective.

Buy or Rent an Exercise Video (Then Use It!)

One great thing about living in a city is that there's always at least one video rental place, and virtually all of them carry exercise videos. There's a million of them, for every possible taste and style, from *Dancing to the Oldies* to the latest, hippest body-shaping video by the Firm. You'll find everything from hard-core boot-camp stuff to the gentlest stretching. Try them on for size. If you're a beginner, just do one for a few minutes and watch yourself progress until you can do the whole thing. The best part of videos is that you don't have to be intimidated by anyone else in the class. And if you're not intimidated—and why in the world should you be anyway?—there's always an exercise class at the local gym, YMCA/YWCA, or studio. Try one.

Clean Out Your Kitchen Cabinets and/or Your Refrigerator

Man, I can't tell you how many clients I've had who have lost weight just by doing this one thing! I call it *bulletproofing your environment*. In fact, whenever I go up a few pounds and need to lose it, this trick has been my salvation. For many people, the attitude about food—at least in the beginning, before they've really adopted this new Way of Life—is this: *if it's there, I'm gonna eat it.* Since a lot of our sabotage happens at night, when defenses are down (with television snacking or even midnight refrigerator raids), the best defense is a good offense. If it ain't there, you can't eat it. So get it out of there. That's not to say you couldn't get dressed, get in the car, go to the twenty-four-hour convenience store, and buy some junk, but most of us won't go that far, even for a carb or sugar fix. We *will*, however, go as far as the freezer. So dump the junk from your house and give yourself an advantage. If you live with other people and this isn't really practical, try sectioning off parts of the fridge for your stuff and theirs, then think of the sections as truly separate. Pretend you're living with roommates who will get mad if you eat their food.

Stop Watching Television (Okay, Okay, Then Cut Back)

I know it seems like heresy to suggest this, but study after study has linked increased television watching with expanding waistlines,[12] not to mention the development of childhood obesity.[13] No one is quite sure exactly why, but it's true nonetheless. Speculation has ranged from the obvious—more TV watching means less activity and more snacking—to the slightly more subtle (the number of overt cues to eat that come with the commercials). Even the esoteric has been postulated, like the idea that certain brain states induced by staring aimlessly at the tube might be linked to a general slow-down of the metabolism.[14] Whatever. The bottom line is: you watch more TV, you tend to be fatter. Try picking a few absolute favorites and then sticking with them. Watch them, enjoy them, then shut the TV off. And try turning it off when no one is watching it.

"Listening to Your Body": Not Always a Good Idea

Face it: our bodies lie. They're especially deceitful if we've been on the standard American diet for a long time. If we were back in the caveman days, eating only the food that was available to us by hunting, fishing, or gathering, our bodies would tell us exactly what we needed. Our sweet tooth, for example, was originally a great survival mechanism. It caused us to seek out sweet-tasting plants, which were generally safe to eat, and fruits, which we needed because we humans do not make our own vitamin C. Now it causes us to roam the aisles of the twenty-four-hour supermarket looking for cookies and ice cream. Our foolproof appetite regulators—such as cholecystokinin, the hormone that is released in the small intestine when our stomachs are full and we've had enough food—responds to protein and fat. It doesn't recognize carbohydrate, which is why it is so easy to overeat carbs. So "listening to your body" may not always be such a great idea, as you can't count on it to tell the truth, especially when you begin this new way of eating. Our bodies often tell us what we *want*, which is a conditioned response, and confuse us by making us believe that it's what we *need*. They're not necessarily the same thing. We need to reeducate our bodies to tell us the truth, and we do that the same way we teach our kids to be honest—by training them. Once our bodies have been reconditioned to respond to real food, we can begin trusting them to give us reliable signals.

Finally . . .

If You Fall Off the Wagon

Don't let it be a big deal. Acknowledge that it happened, and just get back on, beginning with the very next meal.

CHAPTER 8

Controlled-Carbohydrate Eating: Putting Together Your Program

So let's talk about putting together the perfect low-carb diet.

The first step is to memorize the following: there *is* no perfect diet.

There's also no perfect dress size—the one that's perfect is the one that fits. If there's one nugget of truth that we can hang our collective philosophical hats on, it's the wisdom of the Romans: *De gustibus non disputandum est*, which means "Of taste, there is no disputing." Translated to the area of weight loss and diet, it means quite simply this: *everybody's different*. Each individual has his or her own emotional, psychological, and physical blueprint, as unique and special as fingerprints. No two people respond exactly the same way to anything—not to life, not to medicine, not to food, not to diet.

In interviewing dozens of people who have been low-carbing successfully for years, I was struck by the number of people who have done their own versions of programs discussed in this book or who have come up with their own solutions, spins, and variations to make low-carbing work for them. Rick, for example, lost 50 pounds in five months by using the basic Atkins program, but deviated from Atkins orthodoxy by never bothering to check for ketosis and drinking one glass of red wine per day right from the beginning. Laurie lost 144 pounds and went from a size 26 to a size 8 not by following any specific plan but by eating "only low-carb food, exercising every day, and, for the last 25 pounds, lowering the fat in my diet." Ari, who lost 50 pounds, did the Protein Power plan but monitored calories with an online diet tracker, making sure "not to go over 2,500 a day." Leigh—40 pounds, 10 inches down and still counting—is a strict lacto-ovo vegetarian and lost her weight on a pretty unusual low-carb diet without meat. She attributes her success to completely cutting out sugar in all forms. Carl, an award-winning amateur figure skater from Alaska, has dropped 116 pounds by lowering his carbs to 50–80 grams a day—higher on days he has to train hard—and carefully monitoring calories, which he keeps to about 1,500 to 1,800 a day. And Annie, a low-carber from England, lost 50 pounds on the Atkins program but found that she had to *increase* her carbs to continue losing weight. When she reached her goal weight, she switched to the Schwarzbein Principle.

Many people begin with a strict version of one of the programs discussed in this book and then "graduate" to a more customized variation of their own making. That is a terrific way to go for many people. The original structure serves a purpose, like training wheels on a bike. For some others, a program "off the rack" is going to fit them just fine and they can follow the recommendations of the plan precisely and get great results. Some of us are lucky enough to be able to buy clothes off the rack with no alterations. For most, custom tailoring will be necessary.

One-size-fits-all diets are finished. In the not-so-distant future, we will probably be able to determine, through a kind of functional genetics, which patients are most likely to respond to which medicines and nutrients and, possibly through a metabolic typing, who does better on what kinds of foods. But for now, we have only the low-tech way, a kind of informed version of trial and error: if it works, great. If not, move on to something else.

Low-Carb Is Not a Religion

Don't treat a low-carb lifestyle as a religion; it's much better to think of it as a *strategy*. Like any strategy, you use it to achieve a goal, and you use it until it stops working. Your goal may be to lose 10 pounds or 100, and to maintain that goal weight forever. Or your goal may be to live a healthier, richer life free of many of the risks from heart disease and diabetes that come with the standard American diet. In either case, or in *both* cases, you might find that you do much better on a more restricted plan, at least in the beginning. If that's the strategy that works for you, great. If you have less weight to lose and are less metabolically resistant, you may find that you get great results with a plan that is a little less restricted from the beginning, more like the second, ongoing weight loss phase of some of the three-phase plans (like Atkins, Protein Power, or Fat Flush). These plans allow anywhere between 40 and 90 grams of carbs per day. If you are already near your goal weight, don't have any serious problems with sugar metabolism, and simply want to improve your health and maintain your weight, the Zone, or the third phase of one of the three-phase plans, might be the perfect place for you. Find what works for you and do it. If it stops working, reassess.

Reassessment 101

Most people will lose weight on a low-carb program, whether it be on the restricted induction phase, the more lenient ongoing weight loss phase, or a more general 50-gram-a-day starting plan. If you aren't losing any weight or if your weight loss has stalled for more than a few weeks, it's time to go back to the drawing board.

You may be stalled because you need to reduce carbs further (say, to 20 to 30 grams). In some cases, it may even be because your carbs are a bit too *low*—remember that everybody's different! Equally likely is the possibility that your calories are too high, in which case you will need to begin measuring portions and keeping an eye on the amount of food you're taking in. You may have some nutrient or mineral deficiencies that could be slowing metabolic processes; consider at the very least supplementing with a high-quality multivitamin, essential fatty acids, and magnesium, and go back and read chapter 4.

You may have sensitivities to some of the foods you are eating—a good game plan would then be to cut out all the usual suspects (especially wheat, dairy, and sugar) and see if the scale begins to move. Maybe you're sensitive to some of the sugar alcohols found in those low-carb protein bars—they've been known to stall weight loss in some people. So has the citric acid in diet sodas. The point is to be willing to experiment, fine-tune, and tweak your program. And in the words of Winston Churchill, *"Never give up!"*

Choose Your Battles

When you first begin low-carbing, don't allow yourself to be overwhelmed by too much information. It's especially easy to get caught up in the small battles among low-carb diet theorists about things like coffee, artificial sweeteners, diet sodas, sugar alcohols, protein bars, cheese, wine, and other minor areas of disagreement. Don't get sucked in. I've had clients who simply can't imagine giving up coffee; I tell them not to give it up. Same with diet sodas, wine, or even raspberry mocha–flavored coffee creamers! The important thing to remember is that you are trying to make changes on a *continuum*. The name of the game is *direction*, not *perfection*. If all that's standing between you and a healthier low-carb diet is a couple of diet colas, keep the colas for now—maybe you'll give them up later (or maybe you won't). Learn to choose your battles. You don't have to do everything all at once.

Invest Time in the Kitchen

In 1970, we spent $6 billion on fast food. In the year 2000, we spent *$110 billion*—virtually 150 percent of the entire California budget deficit. Fully 90 percent of the money spent on food in this country is spent on *processed* food. The typical American eats three fast-food burgers and four orders of fries *per week*. "We are," says Dr. Joe Mercola, "exchanging our health for convenience."

It's time to stop. Spend a little time in the kitchen. Prepare your own food. Make your own snacks. Cook your own breakfast. Begin to look at food as a *prescription drug*. As one Zone dieter on the Internet said, "Treating food in this new way is definitely a challenge and a learning experience—but it certainly beats my old way of eating that left me fat, tired, and depressed."

Junk Is Junk, High-Carb or Low-Carb

Americans' taste for simple solutions and a food industry more than willing to accommodate them could easily result in the following scenario: a vast, overweight population of "low-carbers" with swelling waistlines and skyrocketing health problems. A typical specimen of this committed "low-carber" strolls through Disneyland, one hand grasping a vat-size cup of sugar-free soda, the other holding any of a zillion "carbohydrate-free" snack foods yet to be invented—hot dogs on low-carb buns, low-carb *cotton candy,* low-carb candy bars, low carb-*popcorn.* You get the picture. And it's not pretty.

Cutting carbs is not enough. We have to cut the *junk.* We have to learn, unfortunately, that in most cases the food industry is not our friend. If carb-free becomes just another slogan like low-fat did and we become a nation addicted to carb-free, high-calorie, chemically enhanced junk food, we will have traded one idiotic notion for another and our health will be in the same bad shape it was before.

This brings us to the question on the table: how *should* we proceed? What general principles can we extract from the collective wisdom of the diet authors discussed in this book and from the principles of controlled-carbohydrate eating that all subscribe to in one fashion or another? How can you put together a program that works for *your* life, that will allow *you* to lose weight, and that will promote and optimize *your* health for years to come?

Glad you asked.

Ten Simple Principles for a Successful Low-Carb Life

Principle #1: Begin with a Two-Week "Boot Camp" Period

Many of the diets discussed in this book make use of an initial restricted eating period of at least two weeks—what Atkins called the *induction phase.* This idea is common to many of the plans, and I recommend it highly and use it with my own clients all the time. During this time you:

- Eat as much meat, poultry, and fish as you like.
- Eat unlimited vegetables.
- Eat as much of the healthy fats—butter, avocados, olive oil, coconut oil, fish oil—as you like.
- Eliminate all *potatoes, rice, pasta, breads, cereals, and other starches.*
- Eliminate grains.
- Eliminate sugar.
- Eliminate dairy.
- Eliminate alcohol.

Optional: the strictest version of this two-week program also temporarily eliminates fruit. (On an "induction-lite" program, I allow my clients one or two small daily portions of berries.)

You can have one or two cups of coffee, preferably organic, and if you like, you can sweeten your coffee with Splenda or xylitol and lighten it with 2 tablespoons of cream. You need to drink *at least* eight glasses of water a day, plus an additional 8 ounces for every 25 pounds of extra weight you are carrying. Hot water with lemon juice is fine, as are teas (green, black, and oolong). I personally do not object to caffeinated teas, though you are welcome to use herbals.

> I always wondered why I felt tired after eating pasta and wide awake after eating meat. Now I know.
> —Bill W.

If you prefer more specific guidelines for amounts, keep your protein portions to 3 to 4 ounces per meal and oils and butter to 4 tablespoons a day. Vegetables are essentially unlimited. You can eat two eggs a day with no problem, and you should use the whole egg, preferably from free-range chickens.

Principle #2: In the Beginning, Don't Be Concerned with Calories

First you want to make sure you're eating the right foods. There's plenty of time later to start fiddling with portion sizes. At this point in the game, I'm not concerned with calories; centering the diet around protein, fat, and fiber will generally cause you to be full before you've overeaten. For some lucky people, that's all that's necessary—calories will self-regulate. For most people it will be necessary to deal with calories *if* weight doesn't come off (see principle #8).

Principle #3: Find Your Own Personal Level of Carb Restriction

Though to the nutritional establishment low-carb is low-carb, the truth is that low-carbing exists on a *continuum*. As you have seen, that can mean anything from the restrictive induction phase of Atkins (20 grams or less of carbs a day) to the much more lenient Zone (in the neighborhood of 150 grams a day for a man on a reduced-calorie program). That's a big range. Where you will fall on this continuum at any given time depends on a number of things:

- how metabolically resistant you are
- how much weight you have to lose
- how you feel, physically and mentally, at various levels of carb restriction
- whether your current strategy is working for you

I suggest you *begin* at about 50 grams of carbohydrate a day for the first week; use that as a baseline from which to determine whether the amount needs to be lower (or if you can tolerate more). If you're not into counting grams, simply eliminate all of the "forbidden foods" on the induction list (pastas, grains, starches, dairy, sugars, and fruits), and you will easily be where you should be to get good results without counting carbs.

The whole concept of mindful eating— not doing twenty things while I was stuffing things into my face unconsciously—was really helpful to me. It just meant learning to put some time aside to actually enjoy and experience my food.
—Melissa McN.

Principle #4: After the First Two Weeks, Begin Adding Carbs Back Little by Little

After the initial "whoosh" of loss during the two-week induction phase, your weight loss should stabilize, and you will probably wind up losing around 2 pounds a week. Some people find that they need to stay on an induction-phase eating plan to accomplish this, but most others can begin adding back *small* portions of foods on the "forbidden" list at this time. Virtually all of the plans agree on this principle and differ only on which foods should be added back and in what amounts. This is the place where you customize and individualize. I suggest that you constantly monitor how you feel, how you look, and what you weigh and, based on these factors, determine what can go back in your diet, as well as how much and how soon.

Principle #5: Add Back Foods According to the "Ladder of Desirability"

My suggestion is that you begin with low-glycemic fruits like berries. Some people will be able to add small amounts of cheese. Many will be able to add small amounts of nuts. (Remember that nuts and cheese, while perfectly

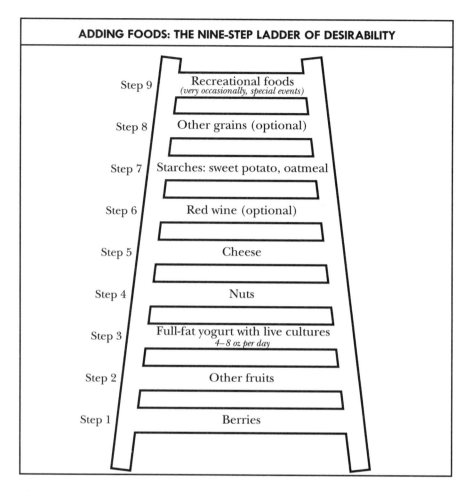

ADDING FOODS: THE NINE-STEP LADDER OF DESIRABILITY

Step 9 — Recreational foods *(very occasionally, special events)*

Step 8 — Other grains (optional)

Step 7 — Starches: sweet potato, oatmeal

Step 6 — Red wine (optional)

Step 5 — Cheese

Step 4 — Nuts

Step 3 — Full-fat yogurt with live cultures *4–8 oz per day*

Step 2 — Other fruits

Step 1 — Berries

okay for low-carb eating plans, are very dense in calories and very easy to overeat. When you get "stuck" at a plateau, it is often these foods that need to go first.) Grains should be the *last* on your "regular" diet to be added back in, if at all, and then only *truly* whole grains. The sprouted variety is best. Processed grains you can say good-bye to forever. Recreational foods include the ones we all know are not great for us but without which life would be just too boring—I include pizza, ice cream, and cheesecake on my list; you may have your own favorites. Obviously, they should be eaten infrequently!

Find the level of carbohydrate intake that suits you and allows you to keep losing consistently at a moderate rate (1 to 2 pounds a week, 3 at the most if you're very overweight), and stay at that level. Remember to expect plateaus and stalls (see page 255).

Principle #6: When You Add Back Foods, Add Them One at a Time and Watch for Reactions

One of the delightful unexpected "side effects" experienced by many low-carb dieters is that symptoms they've had for years and which are unrelated to weight begin to clear up—notably headaches, allergic symptoms, inflammation, and assorted aches and pains. This is often because the low-carb diet, by its nature, eliminates many of the foods that are triggers for unrecognized food sensitivities as well as those that contribute to inflammation and pain (namely grains and many of the omega-6 refined vegetable oils). When you begin to add back your carbs, don't do it haphazardly. Watch what you're adding, do it one food group at a time, and monitor yourself for any reactions. If you start to feel worse, the food you added back is not right for you. Dump it.

Principle #7: The Hard Work Begins with Maintenance

Difficult as it may seem, getting to a goal weight is not the really hard part. *Staying* there is. And believe it or not, developing a strategy for maintenance can actually begin while you are still in the losing phase.

When I work with someone on a weight loss program, she inevitably asks me if she will have to "eat this way forever." The dieter who asks this question is invariably gritting her teeth and simply toughing it out, waiting to get to the goal so that she can relax and eat what she wants. This is almost always a prescription for a disastrous result. You need to look at the weight loss period as a kind of driver's ed for weight maintenance. The strategy you adopt for *losing* is like the strategy of an athlete training for an event; it's tougher and more rigorous than the "off-season" (maintenance). But every athlete also knows that getting to the top is only the first part of the journey; *staying there* is where the real action is.

So the answer to the question "Will I have to eat this way *forever*?" is "No."

But you *will* have to eat differently. To think that you can go back to eating the way you did when you got fat and get a completely different result is one definition of insanity. You will probably not have to be as restrictive and structured and disciplined as you have to be during the weight loss phase, but you *will* have to be forever vigilant about preventing regain, which leads to principle #8.

Principle #8: Use the 4-Pound Rule

There will be times in life when recreational eating has an irresistible pull—weddings, birthdays, holidays, and just the plain old urge to get a couple of pizzas and beers once in a while. These situations do not have to be the end of the world; in fact, to never allow yourself these little pleasures would be a big mistake. The trick is to not allow these occasional "planned lapses" to generate a slide into chaos that culminates in a complete departure from the eating plan that allows you to keep your weight where you want it and maintain optimal health. So check in with the scale frequently. Choose a set number of pounds—let's use 4 as an example. If and when you see your weight climb 4 pounds above goal, immediately go back to your two-week induction phase, and use that restrictive plan until you get back down to goal or even a couple of pounds under. Then you can go back to maintenance eating.

Principle #9: Don't Ignore Calories

Because some of the best-known low-carb plans do not make a big deal about calories (Atkins, Protein Power, Schwarzbein, Zone, Fat Flush), many people wrongly interpret this to mean that calories are irrelevant. No responsible low-carb author has ever said this. The lack of emphasis on calories per se has been because most of us believe that the regulation of hormones (namely insulin and glucagon) takes precedence over calorie counting, which is an inefficient and unproductive (not to mention old-fashioned) way to lose weight.

The prejudice against fat people in this country is unbelievable. People always assume I have no self-control and they look at me like I'm somehow morally bankrupt.

—Emma T.

This does *not* mean that calories don't count at all—they do. But the way calories behave in the human body is far more complicated than originally thought and way more individual than any formula could convey. (An interesting side note: When Dr. Jack Goldberg and Dr. Karen O'Mara first did a clinical test of the GO-Diet in a Chicago hospital, the person who lost the most weight on the diet consumed 1,200 calories a day—but the runner-up consumed 2,600!)

Just as your level of carbohydrate restriction has to be determined by trial and error, so does your calorie intake.

Many low-carbers have been stalled because, although they are eating all the right foods, they are just eating too darn many of them! This is where monitoring calories can come in handy. Though the point cannot be made strongly enough that each individual has to determine the appropriate number for his or her body, *in general*, women will lose on 1,200 to 1,300 calories per day and men on 1,500 to 1,600.

There will probably come a point at which it will be productive for you to know how many calories you are actually consuming so that you can make adjustments if necessary.

Principle #10: Low-Carb Doesn't Mean No-Carb

There is not a single low-carb diet writer who ever recommended a *no-carb* diet. You wouldn't know it from all the people who chatter on about their "all-protein" diet, but such a diet does not exist anywhere in the responsible literature. Low-carb diets restrict carbohydrates, sometimes to very low amounts (especially in induction phases), but *never* to zero, and even the induction phases are not meant to last indefinitely. You can always have vegetables. You *should*

> It was almost like a religious experience for me when I finally gave up all the "white stuff"—potatoes, rice, pasta, bread. For the first time in 20 years I didn't feel bloated all the time.
>
> —Brian C.

always have vegetables. And even at the strictest induction levels, you can eat a fair amount of them for your 20 to 30 grams of effective carb content (much, much more when you move up to ongoing weight loss and finally to maintenance phases).

Make Low-Carb Part of a System of Self-Care

If you think of low-carbing as nothing more than a way to get skinny, you are missing out on one of the great benefits of this lifestyle. Low-carbing does not have to be merely a weight loss strategy. It can, and should, be the cornerstone of an entire system of self-care that enhances your health and your life in dozens of ways. Keeping carbs low is only the first step, and not even the most important. You can use the tools in this book to change your entire relationship to food and, by extension, to the whole notion of how you care for yourself. Some of the terrific benefits noted by low-carbers have to do with other changes in their diet and lifestyle that have accompanied their switch to low-carbohydrate foods.

Here are ten important ways in which you can make low-carbing work for you forever.

1. **Eliminate trans-fats.** Because trans-fats are found in most of the foods that are eliminated on low-carb diets, low-carbers automatically reduce their intake of this dangerous, health-robbing fat, which is found in baked goods, cookies, cakes, snack foods, and especially foods deep-fried in vegetable oils. Avoid anything that includes *partially hydrogenated oil* on the label. Fats are vitally important for the integrity of the cells and as precursors to important hormones in the body, but if the good stuff isn't around, the body will make those structures out of the reject materials. Don't feed your body damaged goods. Give it the good stuff. Dump the trans-fats.

2. **Consume more omega-3s and way less omega-6s.** Omega-3s are found in fish and flax. Omega-6s are found mainly in highly processed vegetable oils on your grocer's shelf. Many nutritionists believe that one of the greatest health problems of our time is the imbalance between these two classes of fats in the diet. Our Paleo ancestors consumed omega-6s and omega-3s in a very healthy 1:1 ratio. We currently consume something like a 20:1 ratio in favor of the omega-6s. Those polyunsaturated, highly processed vegetable oils contribute to a wide range of health problems. By reducing your consumption of vegetable oils and increasing your consumption of fish and flax (with food, supplements, or both), you help to restore the ideal ratio of fatty acids and go a long way toward improving your overall health.

3. **Eliminate sugar.** The destructive effects of sugar on human health have been addressed by nearly every one of the low-carb diet authors and have been discussed in some depth in chapter 2. For those who want to delve deeper into the subject, there are several excellent books about sugar (see Resources). There is absolutely no—I repeat, *no*—need for refined sugar in the human diet. You

may not be able to completely eliminate sugar from your diet, but you can sure try. The greater your success, the greater the benefit to your overall health and well-being.

4. **Eliminate processed foods.** In the ideal diet—low-carb or otherwise—you would eat only what you could hunt, fish, gather, pluck, grow, or possibly milk. While that may not be practical or possible in today's world, it's the bull's-eye to aim for. The more you can make foods with bar codes a smaller part of your diet, the better off you'll be. With food processing, the rule should be *none is best and less is better.* The closer a food is to the way nature created it, the better it is for your health. Eliminating processed foods also goes a long way toward eliminating a big source of exogenous toxins like chemicals, preservatives, deodorizers, colorings, flavorings, and especially trans-fatty acids.

5. **Build your meals around protein, fat, and vegetables.** As you can see from the Jonny Bowden Healthy Low-Carb Life Pyramid on page 298, these three food groups should form the basis of your diet. The exact proportions of the three will vary from person to person. There have been hunter-gatherer societies that existed on almost all protein and fat (like the Inuit) and others that existed primarily on plant foods, but there have been no hunter-gatherer societies that thrived on TV dinners. Your individual metabolism and preferences will determine how much of a contribution each of these three categories—protein, fat, and vegetables—makes to your overall diet, but whatever the mix, these should be the three major sources for most of your calories.

6. **Drink plenty of water.** Water has been discussed in many places in this book, but drinking it still earns a place on the top ten list of health habits to cultivate in order to make low-carb living synonymous with great health. Get in the daily habit of washing out metabolic waste products as well as the toxins in the fat cells you'll be emptying. Refresh, replenish, and restore your body's fluids on a constant basis with water. Just do it.

7. **Get plenty of sleep.** All together now, one more time: *stress makes you fat.* And one of life's biggest stressors is lack of sleep. Important hormones (like human growth hormone) and neurotransmitters (like serotonin) simply don't get made in sufficient quantities if you're not sleeping soundly and deeply for at least seven to eight hours a night. Sleep is a weight loss drug. It has no bad side effects. And it's free!

8. **Exercise every day.** Not only will this increase your metabolic rate and burn calories, but doing it on a regular basis—at least five days a week—is the single best predictor of whether or not you will be successful in keeping weight off. Exercise will change your mood, keep you lean, and very likely extend your life. Do you really need a better reason to get out and move?

9. **Get 25 to 50 grams of fiber every single day.** Getting the right amount of fiber will help you lose weight, help stabilize your blood sugar, lower the glycemic load of food, keep hunger at bay, and in all likelihood help protect against certain cancers. You get fiber in vegetables, nuts, and fiber supplements (see chapter 4), which are highly recommended. Don't forget the possibility of cooking up a daily "cereal" made from pure wheat, oat, or corn bran.

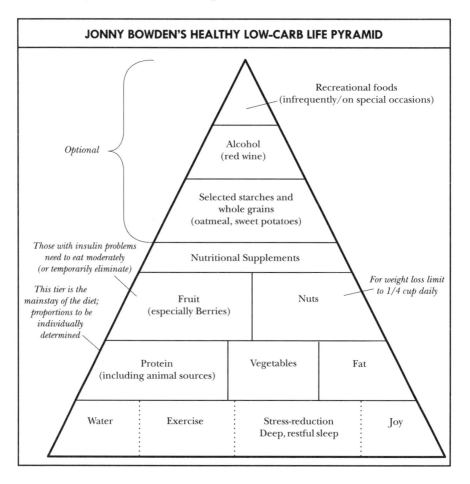

JONNY BOWDEN'S HEALTHY LOW-CARB LIFE PYRAMID

Recreational foods
(infrequently/on special occasions)

Optional

Alcohol
(red wine)

Selected starches and
whole grains
(oatmeal, sweet potatoes)

*Those with insulin problems
need to eat moderately
(or temporarily eliminate)*

Nutritional Supplements

*This tier is the
mainstay of the diet;
proportions to be
individually
determined*

*For weight loss limit
to 1/4 cup daily*

Fruit
(especially Berries)

Nuts

Protein
(including animal sources)

Vegetables

Fat

Water

Exercise

Stress-reduction
Deep, restful sleep

Joy

10. **Expand joy in your life.** In the words of Robert Crayhon, "Pleasure is a nutrient." Never forget that sadness is not a Prozac deficiency. Some natural serotonin boosters are playing with kids, petting a dog, making love, being in the sunshine, and doing for others. Find the things in your life that raise your spirits, lift your soul, and make you happy—then *do* them. Often!

You Can Lose Weight: Believing Is Seeing

Until 1954, it was generally believed that human beings could not run a mile in less than four minutes. The world agreed that there was an innate physiological limitation that prevented anyone from breaking this barrier. But the world forgot to tell Roger Bannister, a neurologist who, on May 6, 1954, ran a mile in 3 minutes 59.4 seconds, the first sub-four-minute mile.

But that's not the interesting part of the story.

The interesting part of the story is that the *next* guy after Bannister to break the four-minute-mile barrier—John Landy—did it forty-six days later. For decades it had never been done, and then it was done *twice* in less than two months. By the end of 1957, sixteen runners had surpassed the record. The number who've done it as of the writing of this book is in the hundreds.

> I was eating like a bird and still not losing a pound. I knew it had to be about more than calories.
> —Jim R.

What happened? Certainly, the aerobic capacity of human beings didn't suddenly expand in 1954. What happened was that the shared belief that it was not possible to run that fast evaporated. As soon as people *saw* that it was possible, they *believed* it could be done. Those sixteen runners who broke the sub-four-minute barrier were never stopped by a physiological barrier—they were stopped by their *belief* in a physiological barrier. When they saw that it could be done, they believed it was possible.

And then they did it.

This book has been about giving you the best information available today about weight loss and diet. But in the long run, successful weight loss has never been just about information. Information is the first step. Information puts you on a level playing field. But the real action is what you *do* with that information—how you let it empower you, how you apply it to your life.

Weight loss is about taking control of your life.

If you can *see* it for yourself, as Bannister did, you can *believe* in it. And if you can *believe* in it, you can *do* it. Weight loss is just the medium in which you can practice mastery—of your environment, your mind, and your body.

Master these things and you master your life. The only limits that are there for you are those you believe in.

Enjoy the journey.

Resources and Support for a Low-Carb Lifestyle

*T*he following is a comprehensive collection of information that you might find helpful, interesting, or even essential in your investigation of low-carbing. Though I have tried to visit virtually every website currently available for low-carb dieting, inevitably by the time this book comes out there will be others. The ones listed here, however, should give you a great place to start. I have also included books that are specifically about low-carbing, as well as what I consider to be essential books about general health and nutrition—the ones I've recommended are very friendly to a low-carb way of life. In this resource section you will also find cookbooks (with the same caveat that applies to websites), links to research, calorie counters, BMI calculators, and vitamins, and even an on-line exercise program. I've also listed a number of newsletters that provide excellent, "non-establishment" medical and health information of interest to low-carbers (and others interested in their health and well-being!) My own website (JonnyBowden.com) will stay up to date with additions in all areas of interest that come out after the book is published. I will also provide links to purchase a number of products—the vitamins recommended here, select foods, and other interesting goodies—so check back often.

www.JonnyBowden.com
Stay in touch with me for the latest updates on the information contained in this book and for information on products, books, tapes, supplements, and new things coming down the pike. Through special arrangements, some of my favorite supplements and foods—many of which are discussed in *Living the Low-Carb Life*—are

available through direct links with the companies that produce them. I've also put together fifteen specially selected vitamin and supplement packages for a variety of health conditions and situations, all containing the finest pharmaceutical-grade supplements from my favorite manufacturers. And you can buy grassfed beef, pemmican (the Paleolithic energy bar made from meat), and completely safe salmon from pristine Alaskan waters plus lots of other goodies. Register for the free newsletter so I can stay in touch with you.

Low-Carbing Websites

www.chtalk.com
★ **Star Feature: Great portal to low-carb forums**
This is a great portal to forums on just about everything of interest to low-carbers. It's a good place to start your exploration into the online world of low-carbing, with discussions on the Atkins diet, the Carbohydrate Addict's Diet, fibromyalgia, thyroid, exercise, and tons of recipes.

www.lowcarbeating.com
★ **Star Features: An amazing databank displays the nutritional content for virtually any food and portion size; also, a busy message board, a plethora of articles on low-carb living and cooking, and pithy editiorials**
LowCarbEating.com is a support and information resource for anyone seriously looking at improving their health through a controlled-carb diet. The100-plus articles (many by published authors), busy message boards, success stories with before and after pix, and hundreds of free recipes are completely searchable, making the site perfect for those who are pressed for time as well as those who like to surf online. The owner of the site, Andrea Mondello, has lost more than 100 pounds on the Atkins diet, has been featured in *USA Today* and *LowCarb Living Magazine*, and has appeared on the *Phil Donahue Show* on low-carb related segments. LowCarbEating.com is all about empowering and educating consumers about the health benefits of and scientific basis behind the controlled-carb lifestlye. Also included: a convenient virtual bookstore featuring the best of low-carb, a product index, and a photo-gallery. Highly recommended.

www.lowcarb.ca (www.lowcarber.org)
★ **Star Features: Terrific carb counter, excellent support forum, "Low-Carb News" current events section**
This is really the mac daddy of all low-carb pages, so if you visit just one, this should probably be it. It's very Atkins-oriented but friendly to all the programs, billing itself (correctly) as an "Atkins diet and low-carb diet resource for low-carb dieters and all healthy weight loss seekers." It has tools, books, a great carb counter, shopping, a review of all the plans, recipes (many by Internet celebrity chef and low-carb cooking

guru Karen Barnaby), research, success stories, and a very busy support forum. The tips section is excellent and includes well-written and quite accurate information by nonprofessionals on a variety of subjects, ranging from constipation to plateaus and more. On this site, you can read the entire text of the very first low-carb diet book ever written, William Banting's *Letter on Corpulence*. One of the highlights is the front-page, frequently updated "Low-Carb News" section with a complete media archive. Highly recommended.

www.dietlowcarb.com
★ **Star Features: Online cookbook and members' pages**
This very friendly site is packed with information. It has a great FAQ section, members' pages complete with pictures, a huge collection of recipes, forums for a large number of topics (including one for those with 100 pounds to lose), and a resources section that contains articles on everything from sugar and stalls to moods and emotions. Nicely done and recommended.

www.lowcarbluxury.com
★ **Star Feature: Free online magazine**
This is the very professionally done personal site of Lora Ruffner, a graphic arts professional who authored two low-carb books and contributes articles to many magazines including *Atlantic Monthly*. The site features a shopping guide, discussion forums, product spotlights, a beginner's guide, tips and ideas, a dining-out section, and a nice, free online magazine called *Low-Carb Luxury*.

www.carbhealth.com
★ **Star Feature: Downloadable tools, such as a grocery list, a meal planner, and more**
Tiffany Anthony, the site's owner and operator, had fibromyalgia, and her doctor suggested lowering her carb intake for the pain. It worked. She has remained pain-free ever since she went low-carb. She started this site in 1998, originally for fibromyalgia sufferers, but soon expanded it into a resource for many different kinds of insulin-related diseases and disorders. The site has morphed into a great general-purpose place to get info, with many news articles, very good recipes (divided by type), and downloadable tools like a grocery list, a daily food diary, and meal planner. Check out the great selection of forums, too.

www.thelowcarblife.com
★ **Star Features: Free weight loss chart, a "clothes swap"**
This is a nice site with most of the usual pages—helpful hints, a quick-start guide, a brief survey of the best-known diets, products, and personal stories. What's unique here are two things: a free weight loss chart that you can use to track your progress, and a "clothes swap" feature that lets dieters who have clothes that no longer fit pass 'em on down the line. Many of the clothes are free for the postage. A really nice feature.

www.geocities.com/alabastercat/lowcarb.html
★ **Star Feature: Plateau-busting section**
This site calls itself the "ultimate low-carb resource page," but it's not. However, it does have a nice beginner's guide, success stories, low-carb in the news, eating-out survival tips, and a very good plateau-busting section. It also has info on specialty concerns like vegetarian low-carb, kosher low-carb, polycystic ovary syndrome, and a research page that links to www.wilstar.net/lowcarb (see below). Very friendly site.

www.wilstar.net/lowcarb
★ **Star Features: Supporting research page, links section**
This is a really good site and a nice example of what you can find on the Internet if you search around and are willing to put up with a little bit of quirkiness. Jerry Wilson is an Internet "character." The basic Wilstar site is a miscellany of everything he's interested in, from history to Christianity to music, but you can bypass all that and go directly to the Low-Carb Pavilion. It has a wonderful page of supportive research, a terrific basics section, a related website links section that is the most extensive I've seen, product links, a concise weight loss plan, nutrition chemistry (fats, proteins, and carbs), and very good FAQs. Definitely worth a visit.

www.bestlowcarbs.com
★ **Star Feature: Articles by Tanya Zilbeter**
This is a pretty cheesy site; although there are a couple of good articles if you search for them, virtually everything brings up a pop-up ad for a product, program, or book, not all of which seem terribly reputable (The "Low-Carb Boot Camp" was "on sale for today only" every day I checked). The site looks like it was put together with papier-mâché and some seed money from a few sponsors. If you've got nothing else to do, you might check it out, but I was singularly underwhelmed.

www.low-carb-diet-safety.com
★ **Star Feature: Scientific answers to criticisms of low-carb diets**
Dr. Jan McBride maintains this very clever little site that answers scientifically many of the criticisms leveled at low-carb diets. She also sells her book, *The Ideal Diet*, which has some very solid and thought-provoking information. The book is downloadable and very inexpensive. Check it out.

www.beyondveg.com
★ **Star Feature: Thought-provoking articles and debate**
This is a rare find—a very thought-provoking and information-dense site dedicated to arguments for and against vegetarian, Paleolithic, and vegan diets, raw foods, and other dietary "orthodoxies." It's an intellectual's dream, with an excellent section on the psychological components of dieting; a wonderful section on Paleo diets, including research; many reasonable and well-argued articles and papers both supporting and questioning the wisdom of vegetarian diets; and a superb section of postings from the files of the great Paleo researcher Dr. Loren Cordain (author of

The Paleo Diet). Two of the many high points on the site are a wonderful article by Cordain called "Comparing High-Protein/Low-Carbohydrate Diets to High-Carbo-hydrate/Low-Fat Diets" and a comprehensive article, superbly referenced and researched, by "ex-vegan" Ward Nicholson called "Paleolithic Diet vs. Vegetarianism: What Was Humanity's Original, Natural Diet?"

www.paleodiet.com
★ Star Features: Comprehensive information on Paleolithic diet, recipe for pemmican
A great resource for information on the Paleolithic diet, which by definition is a low-carb/natural foods approach. Terrific if you like reading the history, science, and anthropology behind low-carbing and the arguments for it as the "natural" human diet. One of the many high points is a recipe section for pemmican, the high-pro-tein, high-fat, low-carb "snack food" that is like a flavorful little cake of pressed meat and can be taken everywhere. This food was a staple of the Eskimo diet discussed in chapter 1 and is highly touted by Ray Audette in *Neanderthin*.

www.carbwire.com
★ Star Feature: Great news section!
This is a cool new site that is like the Google news of the low carb world. Any item of interest that you can imagine is posted here. (On a recent visit I learned that both Olympic gymnast Stephen McCain and rapper Eminem are both low-carb devo-tees!) There's also a section that reviews new low-carb foods and products, a section for recipes, celebrities in the news, the Atkins diet, and much more. Fun to visit.

www.lowcarbfriends.com
★ Star Features: Tops for forums; passions run high and there are some great (and heated) discussions here—an Atkins nutritionist often joins in and answers questions
This site is owned and operated by online retailer Netrition, but even with the com-mercial sheen it's a good place to visit, if for no other reason than the spirited and always interesting forums and bulletin boards, listed by virtually every subject and topic you can imagine. The site also has a BMI calculator, a chat room, an events cal-endar, low-carb news, menus, recipes, and more. And, naturally, a ton of stuff for sale.

www.carbaware.org
★ Star Feature: A nonprofit organization for the support of science and research related to controlled-carb eating
This is a terrific, and very distinct, site. The Carb Awareness Council is the brainchild of Dr. Gil Wilshire and his wife, Regina Schumann. Both are passionate about low-carb eating for both medical and personal reasons (Dr. Wilshire lost 105 pounds by control-ling his carbs, and Ms. Schumann lost 80). Their mission statement says that they are committed to encouraging health and well-being through controlled-carbohydrate nutrition, and that they were founded to support the scientific basis of controlled-carb

diets. They're a nonprofit membership organization which, in 2004, had its first annual conference featuring a roster of superstar speakers from medicine and nutrition. The site has a great news, research, and events section, and publishes a Carb Aware Consumer Bulletin that you can read online. Worth joining.

www.lowcarbtransformation.com
★ **Star Feature: All about the message boards!**
This site is just a really friendly online community with a dozen different message boards ranging from low-carb lifestyle stages to eating plans to health groups. People post their personal journals here, as well as pictures in the "transformation" section. It has a real "town meeting" feel, for those who like that sort of thing.

www.holdthetoast.com
★ **Star Feature: FAQ section**
This is the site of Dana Carpender, author of two well-known books, *How I Gave Up My Low-Fat Diet and Lost 40 Pounds* and *500 Low-Carb Recipes*. The motto of the site is "Fighting the low-fat lie." Carpender also publishes a free newsletter called *Low-carbezine*. Very well-done FAQ section.

www.lowcarb.org
★ **Star Feature: Comprehensive link section**
The Low-Carb Retreat, as this site bills itself, is a low-carb site with a decidedly spiritual spin. For those who might be interested, this is worth a look. If you're not into the religious stuff, don't be put off—there's a lot of good info here. A thought-provoking article on cravings (see "Articles Online by Topic" below) can be found on this site. In addition, it has one of the most comprehensive links sections I've seen.

www.lowcarbiseasy.com
★ **Star Features: Good links to low-carb stores**
Here's another great find, featuring one of the better intros to the low-carb diet, terrific links to articles you won't easily find elsewhere, a support section, and one of the best collections of links to stores selling low-carb products, organized by country (the site originates in England). This also features the opportunity to purchase (for approximately $25) a unique interactive low-carb cookbook that allows you to reset the ingredients or brands, after which the cookbook recalculates the carb and nutrient data for you instantly.

Articles Online by Topic

Body fat: I'm labeling this "only for the adventurous." This article, "Adiposity 101" by Chuck Forsberg, has garnered legendary status on Internet low-carb support sites. It's long, somewhat difficult, and detailed, but it contains just about everything you'd ever want to know about body fat. At least read the executive summary. Forsberg is always updating it, and the latest version can be found at: **www.omen.com/adipos.**

Cholesterol: A long, multipart, and very well-referenced article from the excellent Second Opinions site of Barry Groves (see "Health and General Interest Sites of Value to Low-Carbers," page 296) called "The Cholesterol Myth": **www.second-opinions.co.uk/cholesterol_myth_1.html**

Coconut oil: A great article on the health benefits of *real* coconut oil, titled "What is Virgin Coconut Oil?" by Dr. Mary Enig, author of *Know Your Fats*: **www.coconut-info.com/mary_enig_cholesterol.htm**

Cravings: Learn about cravings, with an emphasis on the emotional and spiritual: **www.angelfire.com/nc/locarb4life/crave.html**

Diet, fat, and cholesterol research: A very good, heavily referenced review, written by a data analyst: **www.ptyza.com/pamstuff/lcjaneen.htm**

Evolutionary diet: A great article outlining the premise that the modern, high-carbohydrate, high-processed food diet is completely out of sync with our ancient genes: **www.thenutritionreporter.com/stone_age_diet.html**

Hidden carbs: This excellent article can be found at: **http://wilstar.com/lowcarb/hiddencarbs.htm**

Ineffectiveness of low-fat/low-cholesterol diet: Reprint of a 1997 article from *The European Heart Journal*: **www.deanesmay.com/corr.html**

Ketogenic diets: Diets that put the body into ketosis have been used successfully for many years in the treatment of epileptic children. If you're interested in reading more about this diet that is supposedly so dangerous, check out the article: **www.jhu.edu/%7Ejhumag/495web/fat.html** Careful with the spelling!

Low-carb dieting: If you've got some time on your hands, this is a really cute "poem" that tells you a lot of what you need to know about low-carb dieting, especially for the newbie: **http://forum.lowcarber.org/showthread.php?t=63363**

Sugar addiction: Thought-provoking article by one of the country's leading experts, Nancy Appleton, Ph.D.: **www.whale.to/w/appleton3.html**

Vegetable oil: "The Oiling of America" is a widely read and circulated paper about the vegetable oil industry. The piece is by Sally Fallon and Dr. Mary Enig, an internationally respected lipid biochemist. You can find it at **www.nexusmagazine.com**, where you will also find many other interesting and thought-provoking second opinion–type papers, including "The Myths of Vegetarianism" by Stephen Byrnes, Ph.D., and "The Health Benefits of Coconut Milk and Oils" by Enig.

Recipes, Food, and Online Cookbooks

Expert Foods: This is the site of Barbara Pollack, an MIT-educated chemical engineer and long-time low-carber. Her company sells products that are low-carbohydrate, high-fiber, and free of sugar, starch, and grain. Especially noteworthy is the Wise Choice line of dessert mixes. Her site has a wonderful collection of recipes, indexed by product, and a menu with a featured recipe section. Her stuff is suitable for dairy-free and low-glycemic diets as well: **www.expertfoods.com**

The Four-Week Carb-Conscious Diet and Cookbook: By Kate Street, M.S., this is a simple, easy-to-follow plan that tells you exactly what to eat and how to make the food without having to follow complicated gourmet recipes. It's not particular to any one dietary plan, like Atkins, but it has great basic stuff in it: **www.lowcarbexercise.com**

I Love Low Carb: Marcie Rathbun started low-carbing in June 2001, dropped four sizes, and became a vocal proponent of the low-carb way of eating. Her website has a nice collection of recipes and a particularly good tip section: **www.ilovelowcarb.com**

Low-Carbohydrate Food Guide: Recipes, foods, diets, stores, and cookbooks. The site motto is "Low-carbohydrate food doesn't have to be boring": **www.low-carbohydrate-food-guide.com**

The Low-Carb Cook: Sharron Long's low-carb recipes are a huge hit on Internet bulletin boards, and she contributes regularly to *CarbHealth* magazine. Lots of tips on candida, fibromyalgia, chronic fatigue, allergies, and food sensitivities: **www.thelowcarbcook.com**

Low-Carbohydrate Cooking—Recipes: An absolutely terrific, comprehensive collection of low-carb recipes of every possible stripe, color, and variety assembled from the hundreds of denizens of the Usenet group alt.support.diet.low-carb: **www.camacdonald.com/lc/LowCarbohydrateCooking-Recipes.htm**

The Low-Carbohydrate Kitchen: A "mom and pop" site featuring some really good recipes and links: **http://members.aol.com/terranova0.diet.index.html**

Pam's Low-Carb Pages: An interesting, do-it-yourself site by a "regular person" that contains some good info and sells the popular cookbook *My Little Black Book of Low-Carb Recipes*, which contains 145 recipes and hints, including lemon meringue pie with real baked meringue, cranberry sauce for holidays, and a bunch of different cheesecakes. An Internet favorite: **www.ptyza.com/pamstuff/lowcarb.htm**

Low-Carb Recipes: Belinda Schwelnhart has two cookbooks available on this site (*Low-Carb Recipes* and *More Low-Carb Recipes*). Her books get rave reviews on Internet low-carb sites and feature recipes that are no-sugar, no-flour, low-carb, and suitable for anyone on Atkins, Protein Power, or any other low-carb diet. She also has a good low-carb cookbook store and a link to the USDA food nutrient database: **www.lowcarbrecipes.com**

Sugar-free Sheila: This site sells cookbooks that are highly recommended by my low-carbing friends who cook. It's particularly interesting because the eponymous

Shelia didn't start out really heavy, so smaller people really relate well to her: www.sugarfreesheila.com

Susan's Low-Carb Resource Page: Recipes galore: **http://members.aol.com/ rowanmoon/cad.html**

Vegetarian Low-Carb: The site for vegetarian low-carbers, with good resources on vegetarian protein sources, tips for following a low-carb diet as a vegetarian, and recipes: **www.immuneweb.org/lowcarb**

Exercise

Let me be very clear: the number one personal trainer in the country is Charles Poliquin, found at **www.charlespoliquin.net**. There's no one else even close. In addition to training countless Olympians, bodybuilders, and sports teams, Poliquin knows so much about nutrition that he frequently lectures at medical and naturopathic schools. If you're really serious about getting in shape, you should visit his website.

For information on exercise specifically designed to work with low-carb diets, **www.lowcarbexercise.com** is actually the best on the Internet. It's run by two exercise physiologists and personal trainers, Graeme and Kate Street, who are also devoted low-carbers. Kate herself was a runner, but found that her body remained flabby on a high-carbohydrate diet despite the amount of exercise she was getting. Her shift to lower carbs, less aerobics, and more weight training transformed her body and gave birth to this site. Their site contains a number of articles on motivation and "low-carb specific" exercise.

The Streets sell an excellent Jumpstart program, which includes their low-carb specific weight training DVD and their *Four-Week "Carb-Conscious Diet" and Cookbook*, which is quite excellent and very user-friendly (the Jumpstart program has its own website as well at **www.lowcarbjumpstart.com**). Kate and Graeme are both extremely knowledgeable, are very passionate about their work, and sell a number of first-rate products related to getting started with exercise. Their basic program requires only an inexpensive stability ball and two sets of dumbbells. This site is an excellent place to get your questions answered regarding carbohydrates in the diet of exercisers. Kate also runs the site **www.healthconsciouswomen.com**, which specializes in addressing the needs of female exercisers.

Low-Carbers: The Dieters Themselves

These sites are low-tech but utterly inspiring personal sites of people who have had spectacular successes with low-carb diets. You can visit them anytime you need a boost.

Angela Stark: This site will show you the transformation of Stark, who went from 196 to 106 pounds with a low-carb lifestyle in just one year. Nice site with interesting links and great before-and-after pics: **www.sugarfreelowcarb.com**

Don Elliott: Elliott lost 165 pounds on a low-carb diet. His story is inspiring, and the pictures are unforgettable. You might show his before-and-after pics to the next person who tells you that all you lose on a low-carb diet is "water weight": **www.dvelliott.com/index1.html**

Jeff's Low-Carb Lifestyle: Jeff went from 317 to 188 pounds, which he has maintained for 3½ years as of this writing. His insights, especially "My Story," "Recollections after a Year of Maintaining," and "Helpful Hints for Anyone Eating Low-Carb," are worth reading: **http://jldavid.paunix.org/lowcarb**

Joyce's Low-Carb Before-and-After Photo Page: This site is exactly what it says it is—an inspiring collection of before-and-after photos from various "regular" people following low-carb diets. A must if you're losing motivation: **http://web-magik.com/beforeafter.html**

Lynne's Low-Carb Page: Short and informative, with some amazing before-and-after pictures. She also has really good links and very thoughtful answers to commonly asked questions: **http://pages.cthome.net/axiak**

"Sugarbane": The alias of a young woman who is a low-carb success story. The motto of the site is "Nothing tastes as good as slim feels." Her site is very personal. The highlight of the site is the single best collection of low-carb links on the Internet, including personal low-carb pages, official sites of all the diets, dozens of recipe sites, newbie guides, and FAQ pages. She also sells her own two-week meal plan with 100 low-carb recipes in Word-document form for a $10 donation to her site. Warning: you have to put up with some very cheesy music: **http://lowcarb4life.sugarbane.com**

Tinakaye's Low-Carb Journey: This is literally an "I can't believe my eyes" experience. Just make sure you scroll down to the last picture at the end of the page. A must-visit: **www.tinakaye.com**

Cooking Truly Low-Carb: Karen went from a size 24 to a size 14 in one year of low-carb eating and was featured on Atkins as a "success story." She also said good-bye to constant fatigue, poor skin tone, heartburn, headaches, a twenty-five-year smoking addiction, and dangerously elevated cholesterol. Her husband also lost a ton of weight. Her site features her personal story, advice, message boards, and more: **www.trulylowcarb.com**

Research Sites

Abstracts of studies on low-carbohydrate diets, posted by Udo Erasmus, author of *Fats that Heal, Fats that Kill*, explore low-carb diets and their relationship to everything from weight loss to epilepsy to exercise. Don't miss this one: **www.udoerasmus.com/abstracts.htm**

Authoritative collection of research papers on everything pertaining to low-carb, assembled by Josh Yelon, who was at University of Illinois when he began compiling this. The purpose of the page is to make published medical research available in one place and to make it understandable to the general public (his commentaries are simple but terrific summaries). He maintains this page for archival purposes. It is an absolutely invaluable resource: **http://finesse.cs.uiuc.edu/users/jyelon/lowcarb.med**

Research related to low-carb eating is organized by subject (kidney health, bone health, caffeine, diabetes, heart disease), and you can read a good general explanation of the research by Laura Richard, a nurse and the author of a low-carb book, or follow a link to the original research and read it for yourself, or print it out and take it to your doctor. This is a great site: **www.lowcarbresearch.org**

Online Stores

Alacarb: Offers a wide range of sugar-free and low-carb products in a nicely laid-out site. Also has featured recipes, but they don't contain nutritional information (calories, carbs, fat, protein): **www.alacarb.com**

CarbSmart: Everything low-carb, arranged by category: foods, protein powders, protein bars, low-glycemic foods, kosher products, books, and shop-by-brand. They have four free newsletters and mailing lists you can subscribe to: *CarbSmart Mailing List*, *CarbSmart Choices*, *CarbSmart Recipe Exchange*, and *CarbSmart Kids*: **http://stores.yahoo.com/carbsmart**

Low-Carb: Started by two sisters who opened a bricks-and-mortar low-carb store (Connoisseur Café) in Anderson, South Carolina, in 1999, and then another in Greenville in 2001. This site is a great place to purchase low-carb products. It also provides a forum for support, information, and education. They are very customer service–oriented and have, among other things, a great recipe section. This site has one of the best collections of low-carb cookbooks that you will find anywhere: **www.low-carb.com**

Ketogenics: This store sells only products that will not interfere with your Atkins or other low-carb diet. Highlight of the site: an interview with Lyle McDonald, author of the definitive book *The Ketogenic Diet*, which tells you everything you could ever possibly want to know about the physiology of ketosis: **www.ketogenics.com**

Low-Carb Grocery: This site sells all kinds of low-carb products. However, there's one caveat: there is no phone number for customer service—just a "Contact Us" link for e-mail. Like most of the stores, there is no label information for the products they sell, so you have only the advertising copy to go on (e.g., "low-carb cereal") and no actual data about what's in the products. Looks good, but I would have liked an easier way of contacting them: **www.lowcarbgrocery.com**

Synergy Diet: A very friendly site specializing in every kind of low-carb food imaginable. It also has an exhaustive listing of articles, most of them taken from popular news media about anything related to low-carb dieting. Like other sites, this does not have label information about exactly what is in the products, but there is an easily accessible customer service department, so I'm sure you could get more information if you were interested in finding out specifics: **www.synergydiet.com**

Vitacost: A recommended high-discount site for low-carb products, foods, and vitamins. It has some good information and articles (including reviews of weight loss products) and a link to HealthNotes, a comprehensive database of nutritional supplements. You can buy almost all the Atkins products here at a discount, and the customer service appears to be exemplary: **www.vitacost.com/lowcarb**

In addition to the sites I've reviewed for this latest edition of *Living the Low Carb Life,* three new ones in particular look like they deserve a visit. All were highly recommended by no less an expert than Andrea Mondello, webmaster for both www.lowcarbeating.com and for the *LowCarb Living* magazine website. Check them out: **www.locarbdiner.com, www.carbtopia.com, www.lowcarbnexus.com**

Helpful Tools

Calculate your BMI (body mass index): BMI is the accepted way of calculating whether or not you are overweight or obese; 25–29.9 is considered overweight and over 30 is obese. **www.halls.md/body-mass-index/bmi.htm**

Glycemic Index and Load: The definitive site for glycemic values is on about.com, but it's buried and you have to look for it. The address is **http://diabetes.about.com /library/mendosagi/hgilists.htm**

The good thing is that if you forget the address, this is the site that usually comes up first on Google when you put in the words "glycemic index" or "glycemic load." Remember, in my opinion, the load is far more important than the index. For a nice, useful list of foods divided into categories of "high," "medium," and "low," go to: **www.mendosa.com/common_foods.htm**

CalorieKing: This superb and very user-friendly site includes a searchable database for any food and nutrition facts, including brand-name foods. It will give you calorie, carb, fat, and protein counts of every food imaginable plus a breakdown of the kinds of fats and minerals found in it. In addition, CalorieKing has a library of useful articles on everything from exercise to emotional eating to motivation, a special section on diabetes, success stories, and a number of forums: **www.calorieking.com**

USDA Nutrient Database: The official site, where you can search for any food and get the most complete nutrient analysis available: carbs, calories, fat, protein, and fiber are just the beginning. It also tells you the amount of every vitamin, mineral, and fatty acid: **www.nal.usda.gov/fnic/cgi-bin/nut_search.pl**

Meal Delivery Service

Home Bistro: This is an interesting company that delivers gourmet low-carb meals straight to your door, nationwide. The meals go from freezer to table in about ten minutes. There are pictures of each meal, along with net carb content and a complete nutritional profile. The company uses a specially developed process for preparing, vacuum-sealing, and then flash-freezing gourmet meals, which you simply warm in the specially designed packaging by placing in simmering water. (Microwaving is not recommended.) There's a special deluxe low-carb sampler, and Home Bistro offers a money-back guarantee: **www.lowcarbmeals.com**

Health and General Interest Sites of Value to Low-Carbers

eDiets: This is the granddaddy of the weight-loss support sites and offers individualized plans of all shapes and sizes (no pun intended). They've recently become very Atkins-friendly, which is definitely a step in the right direction. They have a knowledgeable and committed staff, and have recently added an excellent, free Low-Carb Newsletter to their offerings. And, I'm happy to say, I'm frequently featured on the site doing chats and articles. Definitely worth a visit: **www.ediets.com**

iVillage: This site is the number one destination site for women on the Internet and has been for some years. It has been my home base since 1995; you can find many of my "weight loss coach" articles there, as well as my "Ask Jonny Bowden" message board. At this site, you will find articles, quizzes, and tools about low-carb dieting and supportive message boards where you can share tips and ask questions of fellow low-carb dieters at any hour, day or night. There are boards specifically for Atkins, the Zone, the Carbohydrate Addict's Diet, the Fat Flush Plan, Protein Power, and Somersizing, as well as a more general board for low-carb living and recipes. Very recommended: **www.ivillage.com/diet**

3fatchicks: This is one of the better community sites. It's not technically a low-carb-exclusive site—it's really a very information-dense support site for people who need to lose weight—but it has a lot of low-carb info. The three women who started it don't seem to have any agenda and aren't pushing any program. They have simply tried to beat the bushes for any responsible information they could find on anything, from dietary supplements to dietary programs, that works (or doesn't). Since they get most of their info from mainstream sources (like the *Physicians Desk Reference* and www.WebMD.com), you're not going to find any cutting-edge stuff here, but it's reliable and honest. The site features decent summaries of a bunch of low-carb diets (as well as some low-fat ones), latest health news and updates, a low-fat recipe section *and* a low-carb recipe section, supplement guides, a section on polycystic ovary syndrome, diet tools (including calculators for both BMI and calories burned by walking various distances at various intensities), a plus-size shop, news archives, online journals, and one of the best weblink sections I've seen, especially in the area of obesity. It also has forums where readers can post questions, comments, tips, and more as well as online journals: **www.3fatchicks.com**

The Skinny Daily Post: Julie Ridl, a forty-three-year-old writer, lost more than 100 pounds and maintained her weight loss following a low-carb diet. She began writing to support other obese people who are working hard to lose weight and maintain their losses. The site is composed of daily essays on changing behavior, exercising, rewards, and reviews. Well written and inspiring. Definitely worth a visit. This also has a forum on www.3fatchicks.com (see above): **www.skinnydaily.com** or **http://skinnydaily.blogspot.com**

Mercola: A great site for health information with a tremendous archive. Run by Dr. Joseph Mercola (author of *The No-Grain Diet*), it is a place to hear a thoughtful second opinion on a lot of health information reported by the media. Definitely has an antiestablishment tone, in the best sense of the term. Mercola is not a strict believer in low-carbing, but he is a strict believer in no grains and no sugar, and he is also an advocate of metabolic typing, a system of classifying people as "protein," "veg/carb," or "mixed" types and then designing healing diets for them accordingly. You can order a subscription to his free newsletter. The site *and* the newsletter are highly recommended: **www.mercola.com**

The Nutrition Reporter: This website for the excellent newsletter of the same name (see "Newsletters and Magazines," page 317) offers a large variety of articles on nutritional therapies, sample newsletters, and the complete editorial index of articles that appeared in the magazine since 1996 (you can backorder any copy for $2.50): **www.thenutritionreporter.com**

The Nutrition Physician: Dr. Allen Spreen is one of the most knowledgeable physicians in America when it comes to diet, supplements, and nutritional therapies, and he frequently uses the Atkins diet with patients. This site, sponsored by VitaminUSA, is a free site on which Spreen answers specific nutrition questions. The site also has an extensive archive. Spreen is the author of a number of books, including *Smart Medicine for Healthy Living* and *Nutritionally Incorrect* (see "Recommended Reading," page 318): **www.anutritionphysician.com**

The Omnivore: This little known site is an undiscovered gem. It's got a ton of information, most of it very well referenced, on a number of topics that are of interest to low-carbers. The mission statement of the site says it all: "exposing the myth that saturated fat and cholesterol cause heart disease, cancer, diabetes and obesity." Definitely worth a visit: **www.theomnivore.com**

Price-Pottenger: The Price-Pottenger Nutrition Foundation, a nonprofit educational organization, is a clearinghouse of information on healthful lifestyles, ecology, sound nutrition, alternative medicine, humane farming, and organic gardening: **www.price-pottenger.org**

Ravnskov and THINCS: These are the sites of iconoclast researcher Uffe Ravnskov, M.D., Ph.D., author of *The Cholesterol Myths* (see "Recommended Reading," page 321). His sites are dedicated to disproving the idea that too much animal fat and high cholesterol are dangerous to your heart and vessels. While the establishment dismisses Ravnskov, he is very much worth a listen for low-carb dieters (and other interested people) who want another view of the cholesterol demon. His site is copiously researched and referenced. THINCS is the International Network of Cholesterol Skeptics: **www.ravnskov.nu/cholesterol.htm** and **www.thincs.org**

Second Opinion: Barry Groves, an Englishman with a Ph.D. in nutritional science, runs this site, which was called, by the London *Sunday Times Magazine* (October 2002), one of only five reliable and informative websites for dietary information. Groves devotes his site to "exposing dietary and medical misinformation" about such things as low-calorie diets, fats, cholesterol, heart disease, and other "dietary and medical bits and bobs." The (long) article titled "The Cholesterol Myth," copiously referenced, is a highlight. Highly recommended: **www.second-opinions.co.uk**

Vitamins and Supplements

I once worked in a doctor's office that had the following sign posted:

> The top three things not to bargain shop for:
> Parachutes
> Scuba Equipment
> Vitamins

All vitamin and supplements are not created equal. Two ingredients lists may look similar, but that does not mean they're of the same quality: both Mercedes and Hyundai have engines, but they are hardly the same animal. Fish oils may become rancid or may contain the same pollutants fish do unless they are scrupulously tested—minerals like magnesium and calcium come in a half dozen different chelates (magnesium oxide, magnesium glycinate, etc,), some cheap, some expensive. A supplement may officially contain carnitine, but it may be present in a meaningless amount. The vitamins I recommend are the ones that market to health professionals only, and they are many cuts above what is found in the average store, even a health food store. All the companies linked on my website are of this quality, as are the companies listed below.

Designs for Health: A company founded and run by extremely ethical and science-oriented nutritionists who looked at the products they were using in their own practices and then set out to produce the very best-quality versions that could be found. They are famous for their L-Carnitine, which is among the best in the world. The company website is: **www.designsforhealth.com**

Crayhon Research: Crayhon Research was started by Robert Crayhon, one of the original founders of Designs for Health. The company has dedicated itself to education since 1998, and is famous for putting on amazing seminars and confeences, such as the now legendary annual Boulderfest Nutrition Conference in Colorado, which is attended by doctors, chiropractors, nutritionists, and other health practitioners from all over the country. The company's website is: **www.crayhonresearch.com**

The Life Extension Foundation: One of the oldest and most reliable organizations dedicated to nutritional medicine in the country. The members have been in the forefront of the movement to bring quality supplements and alternative medical protocols to the public for more than twenty-five years. They publish an excellent magazine called *Life Extension*, which is free with membership. They were the first to bring a number of now familiar supplements—such as Policosanol for lowering cholesterol and CLA for its fat- and cancer-fighting properties—to the marketplace. Their supplement line is as good as it gets—superbly made, reliable, well researched, and with the best ingredients: **www.lef.org**

I recommend these products highly and use them in my practice all the time. You can buy these products—along with those from other first-rate manufacturers like Allergy Research, Pure Encapsulations, Phytopharmica, and Douglas Labs—from direct links on my site, www.JonnyBowden.com. These companies do not sell to the general public and you can normally only get their products through health practitioners.

Other excellent companies include **Thorne Research** and **Metagenics**. Thorne is available only through select doctors' offices, but if you see it, it's worth getting. Metagenics is another research- and science-based vitamin company that is widely used by health practitioners. The products are not usually available in stores but once in a while you'll find them in the best high-end pharmacies, usually in big cities.

Newsletters and Magazines

LowCarb Energy is a breezy, fun new glossy mag edited by low-carb veteran Vanesa Sands. Its primary focus is foos, and it's very strong on food and recipes. You can subscribe at: **http: sheknows.com/lowcarb/**

LowCarb Living is a brand new magazine dedicated to all aspects of low-carbing, not just food. It's careful to be evenhanded and fair, and has excellent articles. It's a terrific overall lifestyle magazine with a great look. Since the publication of this book, I've signed on as a member of the editorial advisory board, so look for articles from me on a regular basis! You can subscribe by calling 800-669-1559 or by visiting the website: **www.lclmag.com**

Nutrition and Healing is the newsletter of Dr. Jonathan Wright, one of the great heroes of modern nutritional medicine, who has been at the forefront of the field for more than twenty-five years. He publishes an excellent newsletter, which you can preview and subscribe to at: **www.wrightnewsletter.com**

The Nutrition Reporter bills itself as "the independent newsletter that reports vitamin and mineral therapies," and it is exactly that. It's written by Jack Challen, who has been reporting on nutrition, vitamin, and mineral research since 1974 and has written more than one thousand articles in consumer publications. The publication accepts no advertising, sells no products, and gives excellent summaries of the latest research. Currently a one-year subscription is $26 and is available by writing to *The Nutrition Reporter*, P.O Box 30246, Tucson, AZ 85751 or visiting their excellent website: **www.thenutritionreporter.com**

Real Health, the newsletter, and www.realhealthnews.com are the work of William Campbell Douglass, who has always been an outspoken critic of "business as usual" medicine. This fourth-generation doctor is a medical rebel whose crusading and iconoclastic views on everything from milk to mammograms are always refreshing and interesting. Hint: the antimeat brigade won't get any solace from this site! You can subscribe to the print version of the *Real Health* newsletter through the website.

The Sinatra Health Report: An Insider's Guide to Smart Medicine and Longevity is the monthly newsletter of cardiologist and nutritionist Stephen Sinatra, whose work can be found at **www.drsinatra.com**. A wealth of up-to-date information on a variety of issues of interest to low-carbers and anyone concerned with better health. Telephone: 800-211-7643

Total Health, edited by Lyle Hurd, is a terrific magazine on self-managed natural health, and I am proud to be a contributing editor. You can subscribe by calling 888-316-6051 or visiting **www.totalhealthmagazine.com**, which contains a complete archive of the magazine's articles arranged by condition (from ADD to weight disorders), an online version of the magazine, a "Newsstand" section, and a resource guide.

Recommended Reading
General
Jonny Bowden's Shape Up: The Eight-Week Program to Transform Your Body, Your Health and Your Life: A comprehensive plan, aimed especially at the beginner, to introduce exercise and a lower-carbohydrate eating plan as part of an integrated system of self-care. Lots of emphasis on body image and motivation. Not a prescribed diet—more of a way to gently transition yourself into lower-carb and lower-junk eating. Was wildly successful in its four years on www.ivillage.com, where 75,000 women took part in the Shape Up Challenges. There is also a companion journal, *Jonny Bowden's Shape Up Workbook: Eight Weeks to Diet and Fitness Success with Recipes, Tips and More*, which contains additional writing on hormones, cravings, PMS, and stress.

Heart Sense for Women, Stephen Sinatra, M.D. Sinatra is a cardiologist with multiple board certifications who has written a must-have primer for all women who want to understand the prevention and treatment of heart disease from the point of view of a physician who understands that the conventional wisdom is woefully inadequate. While the diet he recommends is not technically low-carb, he has a lot of great things to say about heart health, mind-body connections, vitamins and supplements, and getting the focus off cholesterol and onto the right kinds of tests.

The Hungry Gene: The Science of Fat and the Future of Thin, Ellen Ruppel Shell. Science journalism at its best. An account of obesity research through the years, it makes a case that obesity is not a matter of weak will or gluttony but of vulnerable genes preyed upon by a hostile environment. It also exposes the unholy alliance between schools and Coke, Pepsi, Pizza Hut, and McDonald's.

Nutritionally Incorrect, Allen Spreen, M.D. A medical gadfly takes on politically correct nutrition, armed with a wealth of knowledge about nutrition, medicine, and health. Definitely worth a read.

Nutrition Made Simple, Robert Crayhon, M.S., C.N. If you buy just one book from which to learn the basics of nutrition, this is the one to get. Crayhon is one of the best and most acclaimed teachers in America, writes in an extremely readable and friendly voice, is deadly accurate, and is quite humorous in the bargain. I cannot recommend this book highly enough.

What Your Doctor May Not Tell You About Hypertension, Mark Houston, M.D., Barry Fox, Ph.D., and Nadine Taylor, M.S., R.D. Mark Houston is to hypertension what Muhammed Ali is to boxing. There is no one I know more knowledgeable about the subject. In addition to being a nationally known and respected cardiologist, he is one of the most expert nutritionists on the planet. Hypertension overlaps with heart disease, diabetes, and obesity in many ways, and this book should be on the shelf of anyone interested in a more modern and enlightened approach to its treatment.

Low-Carb Library Must-Haves

Eat Fat, Grow Slim, Barry Groves, Ph.D. This book is based on the principle that the diet on which it is most difficult to lose weight is a low-fat, high-carbohydrate diet.

Life Without Bread: How a Low-Carbohydrate Diet Can Save Your Life, Christian B. Allan, Ph.D., and Wolfgang Lutz, M.D. A really interesting book that gets slightly technical in spots. It's not exactly a diet (although the authors *do* recommend a daily intake of no more than 72 grams of carbs). Rather, it's a discussion of everything from the basics of low-carb nutrition to heart disease, gastrointestinal disorders, and cancer and their relationship to sugar and a high-carbohydrate diet.

Your Fat Can Make You Thin: The Insulin Control Diet, Calvin Ezrin, M.D. A thinking man's Stillman diet. This is a very low-carb, ketogenic diet that is *also* low-calorie (about 1,000 calories a day) *and* low-fat (and therefore higher in protein). Though that's not my favorite combination, Ezrin really knows what he's talking about and is worth a read. His discussions of ketosis and insulin are particularly good, and a "Doctor to Doctor" chapter is a nice add-on. Good discussion of serotonin and its contribution to weight loss and appetite control.

References on Vitamins and Supplements

The Carnitine Miracle, Robert Crayhon, M.S., C.N. Don't be put off by the unfortunate title, which I believe was the triumph of the marketing director over the author (just a theory). This is an utterly indispensable guide on how to eat, period. Crayhon, in addition to being universally recognized as one of the outstanding nutritionists in the country, was once a stand-up comic; he has the rare ability to write about science and make it seem like beach reading. His wit and user-friendly style shine through this terrific book. Includes top-ten lists such as "the top ten things wrong with the Food Pyramid" and "the top ten things to do to lose weight." Do not miss.

The Encyclopedia of Nutritional Supplements, Michael Murray, N.D. This is exactly what it says it is—a complete encyclopedia of supplements that is thorough, well researched and documented—written by the premiere naturopath in America.

The Real Vitamin and Mineral Book: A Definitive Guide to Designing Your Own Personal Supplement Program, Shari Lieberman, Ph.D., C.N.S. Lieberman literally wrote the book on vitamin and mineral supplementation. This remains the authoritative guide that everyone should have as a reference.

The Vita-Nutrient Solution, Robert Atkins, M.D. A virtual textbook on supplementation for a wide variety of health conditions. The book was actually written, with Atkins' input of course, by Robert Crayhon, who took his name off the cover over a disagreement about the recommended amount of manganese. Other than that, the text is absolutely exemplary.

Sugar and Grains

Dangerous Grains: Why Gluten Cereal Grains May Be Hazardous to Your Health, James Braly, M.D., and Ron Hoggan, M.A. An excellent and thought-provoking book about gluten sensitivity by a renowned food allergy expert and a respected patient advocate. The book goes way beyond the "traditional" model that links gluten sensitivity only to celiac disease; the authors discuss the impact of grains on a range of conditions, including autoimmune disease, chronic pain, osteoporosis, digestive problems, and brain disorders.

Fatland: How Americans Became the Fattest People in the World, Greg Critser. While Critser is not exactly kind to the low-carb gurus like Atkins, the book is nevertheless a fascinating read and a scathing indictment of the sugar industry, the marketing of "supersizing," and the health impact of high-fructose corn syrup.

Get the Sugar Out, Ann Louise Gittleman, M.S., C.N.S. One of America's top nutritionists gives you 501 practical, easy ways to reduce or eliminate sugar from your diet.

Lick the Sugar Habit!, Nancy Appleton, Ph.D. An authority on sugar addiction explains how sugar upsets body chemistry and leads or contributes to a host of diseases and conditions.

The No-Grain Diet, Joseph Mercola, D.O. Mercola runs one of the five most popular sites for health information in the world and the second biggest for "alternative" or "integrative" medicine (see "Mercola," page 314). He is dedicated, passionate, and knowledgeable. If you've ever had a problem with grains or sugar (carbohydrate addiction), you should read this book. While technically not a low-carb advocate, Mercola believes that for the majority of people, sugar and grains are among the worst things you can eat. This book tells you why.

The Sugar Addict's Total Recovery Book and *Your Last Diet: The Sugar Addict's Weight Loss Plan*, Kathleen Des Maisons, Ph.D. Des Maisons, also the author of *Potatoes Not Prozac*, has her Ph.D. in addictive nutrition and takes a unique approach to making brain and body chemistry work for "sugar sensitives." She also maintains **www.radiantrecovery.com,** a website for sugar addicts that contains a ton of terrific information.

Fats
Eat Fat, Lose Weight, Ann Louise Gittleman, M.S., C.N.S. One of America's most popular nutritionists, the creator of the Fat Flush Plan (see page 94), and the former nutrition director of the Pritikin Longevity Center, Gittleman is a reformed low-fat advocate who explains in easy-to-understand terms not only why fat is necessary in the diet but how it can help you lose weight. An excellent introduction to the concept of "good fats" and "bad fats."

Know Your Fats, Mary Enig, Ph.D. This is definitely not an easy book, but if you want the real deal on what's what, this is the source. You can skip a lot of the biochemistry and still find many "news you can use" pearls of wisdom that will definitely cause you to at least question the demonization of all saturated fats. Enig has consistently been an outspoken pioneer in calling for trans-fatty-acid accountability in food labeling and research studies, something that is just now finally beginning to happen.

Food Allergies and Weight Control
The False Fat Diet, Elson Haas, M.D. An excellent book on the connection of food sensitivities and food allergies to weight gain.

Stress and Its Relationship to Fat
Fight Fat After Forty, Pamela Peeke, M.D., M.P.H. Largely responsible for making people aware of the connection of stress to weight gain, this book is based on three years of groundbreaking research on the links between stress and fat that she did as a senior research fellow at the National Institutes of Health. Peeke has made some excellent contributions to the study of obesity. While all of her recommendations are not necessarily in agreement with the low-carb way of life, and some minor points can be argued with (she still recommends limiting egg yolks because they are high

in cholesterol), there is so much good information so brilliantly presented that this book still rates a must-read recommendation.

Tired of Being Tired, Jesse Lynn Hanley, M.D. This book is one of my all-time greatest finds. This primer on stress, adrenal burnout, and healthy eating emphasizes low-carb choices, more protein, and the right kind of fats (which does *not* mean a ban on saturated fats—her section on healthy fats and oils is excellent).

Heart Disease and Cholesterol: Myths and Myth-Conceptions

The Cholesterol Conspiracy, Russell Smith, Ph.D. This may be hard to find, but it's worth the search. You may be able to get it at **www.theomnivore.com** or through Warren Green Medical Publishers at **www.whgreen.com** (go to Current Listings and choose "Medical"). It is a brilliant investigation of how the cholesterol juggernaut has figuratively rolled over the population and forced drastic changes in dietary practices based on, according to the author, "mostly manufactured evidence." Contains more than 2,500 references.

Cholesterolmania: The Greatest Scam in the History of Medicine, Dr. Malcolm Kendrick. This book has not been published as of this writing but will undoubtedly be out soon: be on the lookout for it. Kendrick was kind enough to share the manuscript with me, and it is an utterly spellbinding account, heavily referenced, of the shakiness of the evidence that animal fat and cholesterol are the true causes of heart disease.

The Cholesterol Myths, Uffe Ravnskov, M.D., Ph.D. A detailed, systematic expose in which Ravnskov, a brilliant Swedish scientist and researcher, takes on the cholesterol establishment and literally debunks every major premise of the anti–saturated fat and cholesterol dogma. He also turns his scathing lens on the statin drugs and examines the true reasons why they work (which may very well have little to do with lowering cholesterol). A highly condensed version of this brilliant book is available on Ravnskov's website: **www.ravnskov.nu/cholesterol.htm**.

Diabetes and Syndrome X

Atkins Diabetes Revolution, Mary C. Vernon, M.D., C.M.D., and Jacqueline A. Eberstein, R.N. This book was essentially written by two highly respected medical associates of Dr Robert Atkins, and if there is any justice in the world, it will become the bible for diabetes treatment. Dr. Mary Vernon and Jacquline Eberstein, a nurse, built on Dr Atkins' copious notes and treatment protocols, added their own spin, and came up with nothing less than a blueprint for the way diabetes should be treated. An absolute must-read.

Diabetes: Prevention and Cure, C. Leigh Broadhurst, Ph.D. Much more than a primer on diabetes (though it should be read by everyone who is at risk), this is a terrific handbook for healthy lower-carb eating based on the principles of the evolutionary diet. Broadhurst is a brilliant researcher with a flair for writing accessible stuff. Includes a lot of information on vitamins and supplements.

Dr. Bernstein's Diabetes Solution, Richard Bernstein, M.D. Bernstein, himself a diabetic, developed a method of normalizing his blood sugars and regaining his health, then entered medical school at forty-five so that he could publish his findings and treat other diabetics. His book, which advocates a very low-carb diet, is indispensable for diabetics and the physicians who treat them.

Syndrome X, Jack Challem, Burton Berkson, M.D., and Melissa Diane Smith. Though there have been a number of books written about metabolic syndrome, or Syndrome X (a precursor to diabetes that centers around insulin resistance), this is one of the best. In addition to discussing all of the ways in which too much insulin contributes to the diseases of aging, it also contains two different dietary approaches: a moderate-carb, moderate-protein approach for prevention and a higher-protein, low-carb diet for treatment of both Syndrome X and type 2 diabetes. Also contains an excellent discussion on supplements and herbs and how they fit into a treatment plan.

Everything You Ever Wanted to Know About Ketosis But Were Afraid to Ask

The Ketogenic Diet, Lyle McDonald. This is probably the most complete and detailed book on ketosis ever written and is only for those who really care about the details. McDonald has a huge following among athletes and bodybuilders, and focuses more on how to use the diet in those populations than he does on how to use it for weight loss. He has, however, the single biggest collection of scientific references on ketosis from serious, peer-reviewed journals assembled in one place that I've ever seen. The book, now out of print and selling for well over $150 used online, is available in a downloadable version ($29.95) from: **www.theketogenicdiet.com**

Cookbooks

15 Minute Low-Carb Recipes: Instant Recipes for Dinners, Desserts, and More, Dana Carpender. The latest by the popular author of *How I Gave Up My Low-Fat Diet and Lost 40 Pounds* and *500 Low-Carb Recipes*. Carpender also runs the popular low-carb site: **www.holdthetoast.com**

101 Low-Carb and Sugarfree Dessert Recipes, April S. Fields. Comfort food without sugar. One highlight: butter pecan brittle.

500 Low-Carb Recipes: 500 Recipes from Snacks to Dessert That the Whole Family Will Love, Dana Carpender. From the proprietor of the popular site **www.holdthetoast.com** and the author of *How I Gave Up My Low-Fat Diet and Lost 40 Pounds*. Some sample fare: Heroin Wings (so named because they are supposedly addictive!), Mockahlua Cheesecake, Meatza (pizza without the crust), and the secret to low-carb stuffing.

501 Recipes for a Low-Carb Life, Gregg Gillespie. An outstanding collection of recipes for every possible occasion, including a superb section on one-dish meals. Most recipes have 20 grams or less of carbs per serving. Personal faves: napa slaw and Caribbean steamed vegetables.

Baking Low Carb, Diana Lee. Dana Carpender of **www.holdthetoast.com** says that this book "is utterly indispensable for the low-carber who is tired of eggs for breakfast, for the vegetarian low-carber who doesn't want to live on tofu, and for anyone who just wants to eat muffins and brownies and zucchini bread again." 'Nuff said.

Back to Protein: The Low-Carb, No-Carb Meat Cookbook, Barbara Doyen. More than 450 protein recipes, including things like lasagna without pasta, beef stroganoff without noodles, crusted beef Wellington without pastry, BLT chicken without the bread, and chimichangas without tortillas. No sugar, no refined flour, and no artificial sweeteners (except for two recipes). Also includes twenty-two "exotic" recipes using alligator, bison, etc.

Eat Yourself Thin Like I Did Low-Carb Cookbook, Nancy Moshier, R.N. Developed by a registered nurse, also a successful low-carber, who lost 130 pounds and has kept it off for three years as of this writing.

A Complete Low-Carb Lifestyle: An Executive Chef's Low-Carb Lifestyle Culinary Guide, Gregory Pryor. Gregory Pryor is a certified executive chef who worked directly with the Atkins group for many years. This is a great, no-nonsense approach to cooking, offering the insights of a professional chef who has been eating and cooking this way for a decade. His website is: **lowcarbchef.net**

Eat Yourself Thin With Fabulous Desserts, Nancy Moshier, R.N. Every recipe is under 10 grams of carbs, and more than half are below 5.

Everyday Low-Carb Cooking, Alex Haas. This has 240 recipes from two dozen cuisines transformed into low-carb fare. Includes hamburgers, chicken wings, pizza, clam chowder, and chocolate pudding (all recommended by **www.low-carbohydrate-food-guide.com)**

The Everything Low-Carb Cookbook, Patricia M. Butkus. Rates recipes as low-to-no carb and low-to-moderate carb. Offers alternatives to pasta, bread, and cake recipes and features such fare as chicken cacciatore, beef teriyaki with mixed vegetable stir-fry, arugula salad with grilled beef medallion, and Pacific coast seafood stew; **www.low-carbohydrate-food-guide.com** calls it "one of our favorites."

Fabulous Lo-Carb Cuisine, Ruth Glick. Glick is an award-winning author of thirteen cookbooks and an expert at designing recipes for special diets. She's been a low-carber herself for more than a year at the time of this writing. Some samples: shrimp bisque, toffee-flavored pecans, and an especially outstanding dessert section with recipes that all use Splenda (sucralose) as a sweetener.

The Gourmet Prescription for Low-Carb Cooking, Deborah Friedson Chud. By a physician who writes about food and scored big with her first book, *The Gourmet Prescription*, this book has recipes that emphasize high-fiber vegetables and fruits.

Lauri's Low-Carb Cookbook: Rapid Weight Loss with Satisfying Meals! 2nd edition, Lauri Ann Randolph. The more than 230 recipes all have less than 10 grams of carbs per serving. Recipes for both the beginner and the gourmet.

Lose Weight the Smart Low-Carb Way: 200 High-Flavor Recipes and a 7-Step Plan to Stay Slim Forever, Bettina Newman, R.D.. Features "Smart Low-Carb food substitutions."

Lose Weight the Smart Low-Carb Way, Bettina Newman, R.D., David Joachim and Leslie Revsin. This book is a more moderate approach to low-carb. It explains why low-carb does not mean no-carb, promotes low-glycemic foods, and emphasizes unsaturated fat. It's especially useful for those homemakers who want to incorporate low-carb dishes into family meals and make low-carb substitutions for conventional recipes. Nice charts, including one of flours listed in descending order of effective carb counts (ECC). At least 200 good recipes.

The Low-Carb Cookbook: The Complete Guide to the Healthy Low-Carbohydrate Lifestyle with Over 250 Delicious Recipes, Fran McCullough. Written by a well-known cookbook editor and writer who lost more than 60 pounds herself the low-carb way, this book has been a favorite for a long time and has an introduction by Drs. Michael and Mary Dan Eades.

Low-Carb Meals in Minutes, Linda Gassenheimer. This book is not really low-carb compared to most on the market, but it's definitely lower-carb compared to traditional cookbooks. Considered a good choice for ongoing weight loss and maintenance phases. Particularly good for busy people.

Low-Carb Recipes Fast and Easy and *More Low-Carb Recipes Fast and Easy*, Belinda Schweinhart. Known to be especially easy to follow, these recipe books have a nice following on the Internet and are also featured on Belinda's site, **www.lowcarbrecipes.com**. The first volume has FAQs like "How do you make almond flour?" and a chart for using sugar substitutes of your choice in the recipes.

Nourishing Traditions: The Cookbook That Challenges Politically Correct Nutrition and the Diet Dictocrats, Sally Fallon and Mary Enig, Ph.D. While this is technically a cookbook, it is also a lot more. Wonderful recipes using whole natural foods (no fat-free varieties here) and a running commentary that challenges conventional dietary wisdom. Be forewarned that this is not specifically a low-carb book, but it belongs on your bookshelf anyway.

Sugarfree New Orleans: A Cookbook Based on the Glycemic Index, Deanie Comeaux Bahan. A compilation of favorite New Orleans recipes including shrimp remoulade, crabmeat au gratin, seafood in wine sauce, and voodoo chocolate sauce.

The Smart Guide to Low-Carb Cooking, Mia Simms. 150 recipes with an emphasis on the "antiaging" effects of low-carb eating. Nice touch: how to make your own protein bars.

The Ultimate Low-Carb Diet Cookbook: Over 200 Fabulous Recipes to Add Variety and Great Taste to Your Low-Carbohydrate Lifestyle, Donna Pliner Rodnitzky. A nice section on definitions and basics makes this a good gift for cooks who just want some very brief and basic low-carb background to go with their recipes.

End Notes

Chapter 1: The History and Origins of Low-Carb Diets

1. William Banting, *Letter on Corpulence*, 1864; full text available at www.lowcarb.ca/corpulence/corpulence_1.html.
2. Phil McGraw, *The Ultimate Weight Solution* (New York: The Free Press, 2003).
3. Vance Thompson, *Eat and Grow Thin* (New York: E.P. Dutton, 1914).
4. Alfred Pennington, *New England Journal of Medicine* 248 (1953): 959.
5. Alfred Pennington, *American Journal of Digestive Diseases* 21 (1954): 69.
6. Alfred Pennington, *Holiday Magazine*. Quoted in Richard MacKarness, *Eat Fat and Grow Slim* (London: Harvill Press, 1958).
7. Vilhjalmur Stefansson, "Adventures in Diet," *Harpers Monthly Magazine* (November 1935, December 1935, January 1936).
8. Ibid.
9. Ibid.
10. Evelyn Stefansson, preface to *Eat Fat and Grow Slim*, by Richard MacKarness (London: Harvill Press, 1958).
11. Ibid.
12. Blake Donaldson, *Strong Medicine* (New York: Doubleday, 1960).
13. Alan Kekwick and Gaston L.S. Pawan, "Calorie Intake in Relation to Body Weight Changes in the Obese," *Lancet* 2 (156): 155.
14. Alan Kekwick and Gaston L.S. Pawan, "Metabolic Study in Human Obesity with Isocaloric Diets High in Fat, Protein or Carbohydrate," *Metabolism* 6 (1957): 447–60.
15. Alan Kekwick and Gaston L.S. Pawan, "The Effect of High Fat and High Carbohydrate Diets on Rates of Weight Loss in Mice," *Metabolism* 13, no 1 (1964): 87–97.
16. B. Brehm, et al., "A Randomized Trial Comparing a Very Low Carbohydrate Diet and a Calorie-Restricted Low Fat Diet on Body Weight and Cardiovascular Risk Factors in Healthy Women," *Journal of Clinical Endocrinology and Metabolism* 88 (2003): 1617–23.
17. Richard MacKarness, *Eat Fat and Grow Slim* (London: HarvillPress, 1958).
18. C.B. Allan and W. Lutz, *Life Without Bread.* (Los Angeles: Keats Publishing, 2000).
19. Richard MacKarness, *Eat Fat and Grow Slim* (London: HarvillPress, 1958).
20. Anonymous, *Beyond Our Wildest Dreams: A History of Overeaters Anonymous as Seen by a Cofounder* (Rio Rancho, New Mexico: Overeaters Anonymous, Inc, 1996).
21. Herman Taller, *Calories Don't Count* (New York: Simon & Schuster, Inc., 1961).
22. Ibid.

23. Ancel Keys, "Coronary Heart Disease in Seven Countries," *Circulation* 41, suppl. 1 (1970): 1–211.

24. Uffe Ravnskov, *The Cholesterol Myths* (Washington, D.C.: New Trends Publishing, 2000).

25. Malcolm Kendrick, "Why the Cholesterol-Heart Disease Theory Is Wrong," www.redflagsweekly.com/kendrick/2002_nov28.html (28 November 2002).

26. Uffe Ravnskov, "Is Atherosclerosis Caused by High Cholesterol?" *QJM* 95, no. 6 (June 2002): 397–403.

27. Mary Enig, "The Oiling of America," www.westonaprice.org/know_your_fats/oiling.html.

28. C.V. Felton et al., "Dietary Polyunsaturated Fatty Acids and Composition of Human Aortic Plaques," *Lancet* 344 (1994): 1195.

29. P.A. Godley et al., "Biomarkers of Essential Fatty Acid Consumption and Risk of Prostatic Carcinoma," *Cancer Epidemiology Biomarkers & Prevention* 5, no. 11 (November 1996): 889–895.

30. M.S. Micozzi and T.E. Moon, *Investigating the Role of Macronutrients*, vol. 2, Nutrition and Cancer Prevention Series (New York: Marcel Dekker, 1992).

31. Laura Fraser, *Losing It: False Hopes and Fat Profits in the Diet Industry* (New York: Plume, 1998).

32. Irwin Stillman, *The Doctor's Quick Weight Loss Diet* (New York: Dell, 1967).

33. "Popular Diets: A Scientific Review," *Obesity Research* 9 (2001): 5S–17S.

34. Ancel Keys, "Atherosclerosis: A Problem in Newer Public Health," *Journal of Mount Sinai Hospital NY* 20 (1953): 118–39.

35. Ancel Keys, "Coronary Heart Disease in Seven Countries," *Circulation* 41, suppl. 1 (1970): 1–211.

36. G. Mann, *Coronary Heart Disease: The Dietary Sense and Nonsense* (London: Janus Publishing, 1993)

37. Ibid.

38. Uffe Ravnskov, *The Cholesterol Myths* (Washington D.C.: New Trends Publishing, 2000).

39. G. Mann, et al, "Atherosclerosis in the Masai," *American Journal of Epidemiology* 95 (1972): 26–37.

40. John Yudkin, *Sweet and Dangerous* (New York: Wyden, 1972).

41. Ancel Keys, "Letter: Normal Plasma Cholesterol in a Man Who Eats 25 Eggs a Day," The New England Journal of Medicine, 325 (1991): 584.

42. National Heart, Lung, and Blood Institute, National Cholesterol Education Program, www.nhlbi.nih.gov/about/ncep.

43. Apex Fitness Group, *Apex Fitness Systems Certification Manual*, 3rd ed. (Thousand Oaks, Calif.: Apex Fitness Group, 2001).

44. Dean Ornish, "Intensive Lifestyle Changes for Reversal of Coronary Heart Disease," *Journal of the American Medical Association* 280, no. 23 (16 December 1998): 2001–7.

45. "Popular Diets: A Scientific Review," *Obesity Research* 9 (2001): 5S–17S, tables 6 and 7, www.obesityresearch.org/cgi/content/full/9/suppl_1/5S.

46. Walter Willett, "R&D: Discover Dialogue," *Discover* 24, no. 3 online edition, www.discover.com (March 2003).

47. "Too Many Carbs in Your Diet?" www.ABCnews.com (9 January 2002).

48. Walter Willett, *Eat, Drink, and Be Healthy* (New York: Fireside, 2002).

49. USDA Millennium Lecture Series Symposium on the Great Nutrition Debate, www.usda.gov/cnpp/Seminars/GND/Proceedings.txt (24 February 2000).

Chapter 2: Why Low-Carb Diets Work

1. Woodson Merrell, "How I Became a Low-Carb Believer," *Time* (1 November 1999).
2. Gary Taubes, "What If It's All Been a Big Fat Lie?" *New York Times* Magazine, (7 July 2002).
3. Sharon H. Saydah et al., "Abnormal Glucose Tolerance and the Risk of Cancer Death in the United States," *American Journal of Epidemiology* 157 (15 June 2003): 1092–1100.
4. B.A. Stoll, "Upper Abdominal Obesity, Insulin Resistance and Breast Cancer Risk," *International Journal of Obesity & Related Metabolic Disorders* 26, no. 6 (June 2002): 747–53.
5. Nancy Appleton, *Lick the Sugar Habit* (New York: Avery, 1996).
6. C. Leigh Broadhurst, *Diabetes: Prevention and Cure* (New York: Kensington Books, 1999).
7. Christian Allan and Wolfgang Lutz, *Life Without Bread* (New York: McGraw-Hill, 2000).
8. Walter Willett, *Eat, Drink, and Be Healthy* (New York: Fireside, 2001).
9. C. Leigh Broadhurst, *Diabetes: Prevention and Cure* (New York: Kensington Books, 1999).
10. W. Ringsdorf et al., *Dental Survey* 52, no. 12 (1976): 46–48.
11. E. Kijak et al., *Southern California State Dental Association Journal* 32, no. 8 (September 1964).
12. Ron Rosedale, "Insulin and Its Metabolic Effects," lecture given at Boulderfest Nutrition Conference, Boulder, Colo., 1999.
13. J. Lemann, "Evidence That Glucose Ingestion Inhibits Net Renal Tubular Reabsorption of Calcium and Magnesium," *American Journal of Clinical Nutrition* 70 (1967): 236–45.
14. John Yudkin et al., "Effects of High Dietary Sugar," *British Journal of Medicine* 281 (22 November 1980): 1396.
15. Ron Rosedale, "Insulin and Its Metabolic Effects," lecture given at Boulderfest Nutrition Conference, Boulder, Colo., 1999.
16. J. Michael Gaziano, "Fasting Triglycerides, High-Density Lipoprotein and Risk of Myocardial Infarction," *Circulation* 96 (1997): 2520–25.
17. Gerald Reaven, "An Interview with Gerald Reaven," interview by Louise Morrin, *The Canadian Association of Cardiac Rehabilitation Newsletter*, September 2000.
18. Calvin Ezrin, with Kristin Caron, *Your Fat Can Make You Thin* (Lincolnwood, Ill.: Contemporary Books, 2001).
19. Adam Marcus, "Low-Fat Mice Hold Clue to Obesity Treatment," Reuters (7 December 2000).
20. Mitchell Lazar et al, *Nature* (18 January 2001).
21. N. Seppa, "Protein May Tie Obesity to Diabetes," *Science News* 159 (20 January 2001): 36.
22. Calvin Ezrin, with Kristin Caro, *Your Fat Can Make You Thin* (Lincolnwood, Ill.: Contemporary Books, 2001).
23. D.K. Layman et al., "A Reduced Ratio of Dietary Carbohydrate to Protein Improves Body Composition and Blood Lipid Profiles During Weight Loss in Adult Women," *Journal of Nutrition* 133, no. 2 (February 2003): 411–17.
24. D.K. Layman et al., "Increased Dietary Protein Modifies Glucose and Insulin Homeostasis in Adult Women During Weight Loss," *Journal of Nutrition* 133, no. 2 (February 2003): 405–10.
25. D.K. Layman et al., "The Role of Leucine in Weight Loss Diets and Glucose Homeostasis *Journal of Nutrition* 133, no. 1 (January 2003): 261S–267S.

26. Y.O. Chang and C.C. Soong, "Effect of Feeding Diets Lacking Various Essential Amino Acids on Body Composition of Rats," *International Journal for Vitamin and Nutrition Research* 45, no. 2 (1975): 230–36.

27. D.K. Layman et al., "A Reduced Ratio of Dietary Carbohydrate to Protein Improves Body Composition and Blood Lipid Profiles During Weight Loss in Adult Women," *Journal of Nutrition* 133, no. 2 (February 2003): 411–17.

28. C.S. Johnson et al., "Postprandial Thermogenesis Is Increased 100% on a High-Protein Low-Fat Diet Vs. a High-Carbohydrate, Low-Fat Diet In Healthy, Young Women," *Journal of the American College of Nutrition* 21, no. 1 (February 2002): 55–61.

29. American Association of Clinical Endocrinologists, "Findings and Recommendations on the Insulin Resistance Syndrome" (American Association of Clinical Endocrinologists, Washington, D.C., 25–26 August 2002).

30. Ibid.

31. Ibid.

32. Ibid.

33. National Diabetes Fact Sheet, Centers for Disease Control, 20 August 2003.

34. American Association of Clinical Endocrinologists, "Findings and Recommendations on the Insulin Resistance Syndrome" (American Association of Clinical Endocrinologists, Washington, D.C., 25–26 August 2002).

35. John E. Gerich, "Contributions of Insulin-Resistance and Insulin-Secretory Defects to the Pathogenesis of Type 2 Diabetes Mellitus," *Mayo Clinic Proceedings* 78 (April 2003): 447–56.

36. E.S. Ford et al., "Prevalence of the Metabolic Syndrome Among US Adults" JAMA 287 (2002): 356–359.

37. Dara Myers, "Diabetes Diet War," *U.S. News & World Report* (14 July 2003): 48–49.

38. Richard Bernstein, *The Diabetes Solution* (New York: Little, Brown, 1997).

39. C. Leigh Broadhurst, *Diabetes: Prevention and Cure* (New York: Kensington Books, 1999).

40. American Association of Clinical Endocrinologists, "Findings and Recommendations on the Insulin Resistance Syndrome" (American Association of Clinical Endocrinologists, Washington, D.C., 25–26 August 2002).

41. Laure Morin-Papunen, "Insulin Resistance in Polycystic Ovary Syndrome," (Ph.D. diss., University of Oulu, Finland, 2000).

42. Mark Perloe, M.D. "Polycystic Ovary Syndrome" available at: http://www.ivf.com/pcostreat.html

43. Ron Rosedale, "Insulin and Its Metabolic Effects," lecture given at Boulderfest Nutrition Conference, Boulder, Colo., 1999.

44. V. Marigliano et al., "Normal Values in Extreme Old Age," *Annals of the New York Academy of Sciences* 673 (22 December 1992): 23–28.

45. J. Salmeron et al., "Dietary Fat Intake and Risk of Type 2 Diabetes in Women," *American Journal of Clinical Nutrition* 73, no. 6 (June 2001): 1019–26.

46. B.V. Mann, "Metabolic Consequences of Dietary Trans Fatty Acids," *Lancet* 343 (1994): 1268–71.

47. Elson Haas, *The False Fat Diet* (New York: Ballantine Books, 2000).

48. Joseph Mercola, "Celiac Disease (Wheat Intolerance) More Common," www.mercola.com (2 July 2003).

49. James Braly with Ron Hoggan, *Dangerous Grains* (New York: Avery, 2002).

50. Joseph Mercola with Alison Levy, *The No-Grain Diet* (New York: Dutton, 2003).

51. S. Liu et al., "A Prospective Study of Dietary Glycemic Load, Carbohydrate Intake, and Risk of Coronary Heart Disease in U.S. Women," *American Journal of Clinical Nutrition* 71, no. 6 (June 2000): 1455–61.
52. Walter Willett et al., "Glycemic Index, Glycemic Load, and Risk of Type 2 Diabetes," *American Journal of Clinical Nutrition* 76, no. 1 (July 2002): 274S–280S.

Chapter 3: Fourteen Low-Carb Diets and What They Can Do For You

1. "Popular Diets: A Scientific Review," *Obesity Research* 9 (2001): 5S–17S.
2. Kathleen Des Maisons, personal communication with author, August 2003.
3. B. Golomb et al., "Insulin Sensitivity Markers: Predictors of Accidents and Suicides in Helsinki Heart Study Screenees," *Journal of Clinical Epidemiology* 55, no. 8 (August 2002): 767–73.
4. Calvin Ezrin, with Kristen Caron, *Your Fat Can Make You Thin* (Lincolnwood, Ill.: Contemporary Books, 2001).
5. David Leonardi, personal communication with author, August 2003.
6. Richard Bernstein, *The Diabetes Solution* (New York: Little, Brown, 1997), 43.
7. Loren Cordain, "Cereal Grains: Humanity's Double-Edged Sword," *World Review of Nutrition and Dietetics* 84 (1999): 19–73.
8. Michael Eades and Mary Dan Eades, *The 30-Day Low-Carb Diet Solution* (New York: John Wiley and Sons, 2002): 11.
9. P. Webb, "The Measurement of Energy Exchange in Man, an Analysis," *American Journal of Clinical Nutrition* 33, no. 6 (1980): 1299–1310.

Chapter 4: Supplements and Diet Drugs

1. C. Wilhelm, "Growing the Market for Anti-Obesity Drugs," *Chemical Market Reporter* (15 May 2000).
2. Steven Peikin, Complete Book of Diet Drugs, Kennsington Books 2000 NYC p.62.
3. *Physicians' Desk Reference*, 55th ed. (Montvale, N.J.: Medical Economics, 2001).
4. F. Kelly et al., "Sibutramine: Weight Loss in Depressed Patients," *International Journal of Obesity & Related Metabolic Disorders* 19, suppl. 2 (1995): 145.
5. Donna Ryan, "Review Article: Use of Sibutramine to Treat Obesity," www.MDConsult.com.
6. W.P. James et al., "Effect of Sibutramine on Weight Maintenance After Weight Loss: A Randomised Trial," *Lancet* 356 (December 2000): 2119–25.
7. Frederick Samaha et al., "A Low-Carbohydrate as Compared with a Low-Fat Diet in Severe Obesity," *New England Journal of Medicine* 348, no. 21 (22 May 2003): 2074–81.
8. G. Foster et al., "A Randomized Trial of a Low-Carbohydrate Diet for Obesity," *New England Journal of Medicine* 348, no. 21 (22 May 2003): 2082–90.
9. Poston and Foreyt, "Review Article: Successful Management of the Obese Patient," www.MDConsult.com.
10. D.H. Ryan et al., "Sibutramine: A Novel New Agent for Obesity Treatment," *Obesity Research* 3, suppl. 4 (1995): 553S–559S.
11. George Bray et al., "A Double Blind Randomized Placebo Controlled Trial of Sibutramine," *Obesity Research* 4 (1996): 263–70.
12. Gary Glazer, "Long-Term Pharmacotherapy of Obesity 2000: A Review of Efficacy and Safety," Archives of Internal Medicine 161, no. 15 (13 August 2001): 1814–24.

13. E. Wooltorton, "Obesity Drug Sibutramine (Meridia): Hypertension and Cardiac Arrhythmias," *Canadian Medical Association Journal* 166 (14 May 2002): 10.

14. S. Rossner et al., "Weight Loss, Weight Maintenance and Improved Cardiovascular Risk Factors After 2 Years Treatment with Orlistat for Obesity," *Obesity Research* 8 (2000): 49–61.

15. L. Sjostrom et al., "Randomized Placebo-Controlled Trial of Orlistat for Weight Loss and Prevention of Weight Regain in Obese Patients," *Lancet* 352 (1998): 167–72.

16. M. Davidson et al., "Weight Control and Risk Factor Reduction in Obese Subjects Treated for 2 Years with Orlistat: A Randomized Controlled Trial," *Journal of the American Medical Association* 281, no. 3 (1999): 235–42.

17. Poston and Foreyt, "Review Article: Successful Management of the Obese Patient," www.MDConsult.com.

18. C.N. Boozer et al., "Herbal Ephedra/Caffeine for Weight Loss: A 6-Month Randomized Safety and Efficacy Trial," *International Journal of Obesity & Related Metabolic Disorders* 26, no. 5 (May 2002): 593–604.

19. D. Kalman et al., "An Acute Clinical Trial Evaluating the Cardiovascular Effects of an Herbal Ephedra-Caffeine Weight Loss Product in Healthy Overweight Adults," *International Journal of Obesity & Related Metabolic Disorders* 26, no. 10 (October 2002): 1363–66.

20. John Hernandez, "Weight Loss Protocols," lecture at Boulderfest Nutrition Conference, Boulder, Colo., 2002.

21. The complete list of studies can be found in Dr. Michael Murray's *Encyclopedia of Nutritional Supplements* (Rocklin, Calif.: Prima Publishing, 1996, p. 318) or in Dr. Murray's *Encyclopedia of Natural Medicine*, 2nd ed. (Rocklin, Calif.: Prima Publishing, 1998, p. 690).

22. Andrea Sparti et al., "Effects of Diets High or Low in Unavailable and Slowly Digestible Carbohydrates on the Pattern of 24-h Substrate Oxidation and Feelings of Hunger in Humans," *American Journal of Clinical Nutrition* 72, no. 6 (2000): 1461–68.

23. G.A. Spiller, *Dietary Fiber in Health and Nutrition* (Boca Raton, Fla.: CRC Press, 1994).

24. Manisha Chandalia, et al., "Beneficial Effects of High Dietary Fiber Intake in Patients with Type 2 Diabetes Mellitus," *New England Journal of Medicine* 342 no. 19 (11 May 2000): 1392–98.

25. D.S. Ludwig et al., "Dietary Fiber, Weight Gain, and Cardiovascular Disease Risk Factors in Young Adults," *Journal of the American Medical Association* 282 (1999): 1539–46.

26. G.S. Kelly, "Nutritional and Botanical Interventions to Assist with the Adaptation to Stress" *Alt Medicine Review* 4:4 (1999): 249–65.

27. Robert Atkins, *The VitaNutrient Solution* (New York: Simon & Schuster, Inc., 1998).

28. D.P. Rose et al., "Effect of Oral Contraceptives and Vitamin B$_6$ Deficiency on Carbohydrate Metabolism" *American Journal of Clinical Nutrition* 28 (1975): 872–78.

29. Maurice Shils et al., *Modern Nutrition in Health and Disease*, 9th ed. (Baltimore: Lippincott, Williams & Wilkins, 1999).

30. Ron Rosedale, personal communication with author, August 2003.

31. Maurice Shils et al., *Modern Nutrition in Health and Disease*, 9th ed. (Baltimore: Lippincott, Williams & Wilkins, 1999).

32. Ibid.

33. D.W. Laight et al., *Cardiovascular Research* 47, no. 3 (2000): 457–64.

34. A. Ceriello, *Metabolism* 49, 2 suppl. 1 (February 2000): 27–29.

35. P. Faure et al., *Journal of Nutrition* 127, no. 1 (1997): 103–7.

36. A.A. Rivellese et al., "Long-Term Effects of Fish Oil on Insulin Resistance and Plasma Lipoproteins in NIDDM Patients with Hypertriglyceridemia" *Diabetes Care* 19, no. 11 (November 1996): 1207–13.

37. C. Popp-Snijders et al., "Dietary Supplementation of Omega-3 PUFAs Improves Insulin Sensitivity in Non-Insulin Dependent Diabetes," *Diabetes Research* 4, no. 3 (March 1987): 141–47.

38. M.T. Behme, "Dietary Fish Oil Enhances Insulin Sensitivity in Miniature Pigs," *Journal of Nutrition* 126, no. 6 (1996): 1549–53.

39. E. De Stefani, "Alpha-Linolenic Acid and Risk of Prostate Cancer: A Case-Control Study in Uruguay" *Cancer Epidemiology Biomarkers & Prevention* 9, no. 3 (March 2000): 335–38.

40. J.M. Ramon et al., "Dietary Fat Intake and Prostate Cancer Risk: A Case-Control Study in Spain" *Cancer Causes and Control* 11, no. 8 (September 2000): 679–85.

41. L.M. Newcomer et al., "The Association of Fatty Acids with Prostate Cancer Risk" *Prostate* 47, no. 4 (June 2001): 262–68.

42. Y. Takahashi et al., "Dietary Gamma-Linolenic Acid in the Form of Borage Oil Causes Less Body Fat Accumulation Accompanying an Increase in Uncoupling Protein 1 mRNA Level in Brown Adipose Tissue," *Comp Biochem Physiol B Biochem Mol Biol* 127, no. 2 (October 2000): 213–22.

43. K. Vaddadi et al., *Journal of Medical Science* 7 (1979): 52.

44. Ron Rosedale, "Insulin and Its Metabolic Effects," lecture at Boulderfest Nutrition Conference, Boulder, Colo., 1999.

45. S. Humphries et al., "Low Dietary Magnesium Is Associated with Insulin Resistance in a Sample of Young, Nondiabetic Black Americans," *American Journal of Hypertension* 12, no. 8 (August 1999): 747–56.

46. F. Corica et al., "Effects of Oral Magnesium Supplementation on Plasma Lipid Concentrations in Patients with Non-Insulin-Dependent Diabetes Mellitus," *Magnesium Research* 7, no. 1 (March 1984): 43–47.

47. J. Lal et al., "Effect of Oral Magnesium Supplementation on the Lipid Profile and Blood Glucose of Patients with Type 2 Diabetes Mellitus," *Journal of the Association of Physicians of India* 51 (January 2003): 37–42.

48. S. Jacob et al., "Oral Administration of RAC-alpha-lipoic Acid Modulates Insulin Sensitivity in Patients with Type 2 Diabetes Mellitus: A Placebo-Controlled Pilot Trial," *Free Radical Biology & Medicine* 27 (1999): 309–14.

49. J.L. Evans et al., "Alpha-Lipoic Acid: A Multifunctional Antioxidant That Improves Insulin Sensitivity in Patients with Type 2 Diabetes," *Diabetes Technology & Therapeutics* 2, no. 3 (autumn 2000): 401–13.

50. Burt M. Berkson, "A Conservative Triple Antioxidant Approach to the Treatment of Hepatitis C," *Medizinische Klinik* 94, suppl. 3 (15 October 1999): 84–89.

51. V. Crawford et al., "Effects of Niacin-Bound Chromium Supplementation on Body Composition in Overweight African-American Women," *Diabetes, Obesity & Metabolism* 1, no. 6 (November 1999): 331–37.

52. R.A. Anderson et al., "Elevated Intakes of Supplemental Chromium Improve Glucose and Insulin Variables in Individuals with Type 2 Diabetes," *Diabetes* 46, no. 11 (November 1997): 1786–91.

53. B.E. Wilson and A. Gondy, "Effects of Chromium Supplementation on Fasting Insulin Levels and Lipid Parameters in Healthy, Non-Obese Young Subjects," *Diabetes Research and Clinical Practice* 28, no. 3 (June 1995): 179–83.

54. D.D. Hepburn et al., "Nutritional Supplement Chromium Picolinate Causes Sterility and Lethal Mutations in *Drosophila melanogaster*," *Proceedings of the National Academy of Sciences of the United States of America* 100, no. 7 (April 2003): 3766–71.

55. D.M. Stearns et al., "Chromium Picolinate Produces Chromosome Damage in Chinese Hamster Ovary Cells," *FASEB Journal* 9, no. 15 (December 1995): 1643–48.

56. K.R. Manygoats, et al., "Ultrastructural Damage in Chromium Picolinate-Treated Cells: A TEM Study," *Journal of Biological Inorganic Chemistry* 7 (September 2002): 791–98.

57. R.A. Anderson et al., "Lack of Toxicity of Chromium Chloride and Chromium Picolinate in Rats," *Journal of the American College of Nutrition* 16, no. 3 (June 1997): 273–79.

58. H.G. Preuss and R.A. Anderson, "Chromium Update: Examining Recent Literature 1997–1998," *Current Opinion in Clinical Nutrition and Metabolic Care* 1, no. 6 (November 1998): 487–89.

59. W. Mertz, "Chromium in Human Nutrition: A Review," *Journal of Nutrition* 123 (1993): 626–33.

60. A. Reddi et al., "Biotin Supplementation Improves Glucose and Insulin Tolerances in Genetically Diabetic KK Mice," *Life Sciences* 42 (1998): 1323–30.

61. M. Maebashi et al., "Therapeutic Evaluation of the Effect of Biotin on Hyperglycemia in Patients with Non-Insulin Dependent Diabetes Mellitus," *J Clin Biochem Nutr* 14 (1993): 211–18.

62. J.C. Coggeshall et al., "Biotin Status and Plasma Glucose in Diabetics," *Annals of the New York Academy of Sciences* 447 (1985) 389–92.

63. M.F. McCarty, "High-Dose Biotin, an Inducer of Glucokinase Expression, May Synergize with Chromium Picolinate to Enable a Definitive Nutritional Therapy for Type II Diabetes." *Medical Hypotheses* 52, no. 5 (May 1999): 401–6.

64. Stephen Sinatra, *L-Carnitine and the Heart* (New Canaan, Conn.: Keats Publishing, 1999).

65. G. Kelly, "L-Carnitine: Therapeutic Applications of a Conditionally Essential Amino Acid," *Alternative Medicine Review* 3 (1998): 345–60.

66. G. Derosa et al., "The Effect of L-Carnitine on Plasma Lipoprotein(a) Levels in Hypercholesterolemic Patients with Type 2 Diabetes Mellitus," *Clinical Therapeutics* 25, no. 5 (2003): 1429–39.

67. M.T. Abdel-Aziz et al., "Effect of Carnitine on Blood Lipid Pattern in Diabetic Patients," *Nutrition Reports International* 29 (1984): 1071–79.

68. G. Mingrone et al., "L-Carnitine Improves Glucose Disposal in Type 2 Diabetic Patients," *Journal of the American College of Nutrition* 18, no. 1 (1999): 77–82.

69. He Zhi-Qian et al., "Body Weight Reduction in Adolescents by a Combination of Measures Including Using L-Carnitine," *Acta Nutrimenta Sinica* 19, no. 2 (1997): 146–51.

70. Patrick Quillin, *Healing Nutrients* (New York: Vintage Books, 1987).

71. D.M. Muller et al., "Effects of Oral L-Carnitine Supplementation on In Vivo Long-Chain Fatty Acid Oxidation in Healthy Adults," *Metabolism* 51, no. 11 (November 2002): 1389–91.

72. S.A. Center et al., "The Clinical and Metabolic Effects of Rapid Weight Loss in Obese Pet Cats and the Influence of Supplemental Oral L-Carnitine," *Journal of Veterinary Internal Medicine* 14, no. 6 (November–December 2000): 598–608.

73. K. Owen et al., "Effect of L-Carnitine and Soybean Oil on Growth Performance and Body Composition of Early-Weaned Pigs," *Journal of Animal Science* 74, no. 7 (1996): 1612–19.

74. Diana Schwarzbein, personal communication with author, August 2003.

75. C.J. Rebouche, "Carnitine," in *Modern Nutrition in Health and Disease*, 9th ed., by Maurice Shils et al. (Baltimore: Lippincott, Williams & Wilkins, 1999), 505.

76. L. Van Gall et al., "Exploratory Study of Coenzyme Q10 in Obesity," in *Biomedical and Clinical Aspects of Coenzyme Q10*, 4th ed., edited by Fokers and Yamamura (Amsterdam: Elsevier Science Publishers, 1984), 369–74.

77. S. Greenberg and W.H. Frishman, "Coenzyme Q10: A New Drug for Cardiovascular Disease," *Journal of Clinical Pharmacology* 30 (1990): 596–608.

78. Shari Lieberman with Nancy Bruning, *The Real Vitamin and Mineral Book* (New York: Avery, 1997).

79. J.R. Cronin, "Green Tea Extract Stokes Thermogenesis: Will It Replace Ephedra?" *Altern Comp Ther* 6 (2000): 296–300.

80. S.J. Bell, "A Functional Food Product for the Management of Weight," *Critical Reviews in Food Science and Nutrition* 42, no. 2 (March 2002): 163–78.

81. A.G. Dulloo et al., "Efficacy of a Green Tea Extract Rich in Catechin Polyphenols and Caffeine in Increasing 24-h Energy Expenditure and Fat Oxidation in Humans," *American Journal of Clinical Nutrition* 70, no. 6 (December 1999):1040–45.

82. M. Yoshikawa et al., "*Salacia reticulata* and Its Polyphenolic Constituents with Lipase Inhibitory and Lipolytic Activities Have Mild Antiobesity Effects in Rats," *Journal of Nutrition* 132 (2002): 1819–24.

83. R.A. Anderson and M.M. Polansky, "Tea Enhances Insulin Activity," *Journal of Agricultural and Food Chemistry* 50, no. 24 (20 November 2002): 7182–86.

84. E.A. Sotaniemi et al., "Ginseng Therapy in Non-Insulin-Dependent Diabetic Patients," *Diabetes Care* 18, no. 10 (October 1995): 1373–75.

85. J.T. Xie et al., "Ginseng Berry Reduces Blood Glucose and Body Weight in db/db Mice," *Phytomedicine* 9, no. 3 (April 2002): 254–58.

86. S.A. Attele et al., "Antidiabetic Effects of Panax Ginseng Berry Extract and the Identification of an Effective Component," *Diabetes* 51, no 6 (June 2002): 1851–58.

87. T. Zhang et al., "Ginseng Root: Evidence for Numerous Regulatory Peptides and Insulinotropic Activity," *Biomedical Research* 11 (1990): 49–54.

88. V. Vuksan et al., "American ginseng improves glycemia in individuals with normal glucose tolerance," *Journal of the American College of Nutrition* 19, no. 6 (November–December 2000): 738–44.

89. C. Cangiano et al., "Eating Behavior and Adherence to Dietary Prescriptions in Obese Adult Subjects Treated with 5-Hydroxytryptophan," *American Journal of Clinical Nutrition* 56, no. 5 (November 1992): 863–67.

90. C. Cangiano et al., "Effects of Oral 5-HTP on Energy Intake and Macronutrient Selection in Non-Insulin Dependent Diabetic Patients," *International Journal of Obesity & Related Metabolic Disorders* 22, no. 7 (July 1998): 648–54.

91. F. Ceci et al., "The Effects of Oral 5-HTP on Feeding Behavior in Obese Female Subjects," *Journal of Neural Transmission* 76, no. 2 (1989): 109–17.

92. Natural Medicines Comprehensive Database, *Monograph: Bitter Orange* (Stockton, Calif.: Therapeutic Research, 2003).

93. M. Blumenthal et al., *Herbal Medicine Expanded Commission E Monographs* (Atlanta: Integrative Medicine Communications, 2000).

94. G. Calapai et al., "Antiobesity and Cardiovasculartoxic Effects of Citrus Aurantium Extracts in the Rat: A Preliminary Report," *Fitoterapia* 70 (1999): 586–92.

95. Natural Medicines Comprehensive Database, *Patient Handout: Bitter Orange* (Stockton, Calif.: Therapeutic Research, 2003).

96. L. Rogers and R. Pelton, *Quarterly Journal of Studies of Alcohol* 18, no. 4 (1957): 581–87.

97. F Goodwin, *APA Psychiatric News* (5 December 1986).

98. Robert Atkins, *The VitaNutrient Solution* (New York: Simon & Schuster, Inc., 1998).

99. Ron Rosedale, "Insulin and Its Metabolic Effects," lecture given at Boulderfest Nutrition Conference, Boulder, Colo., 1999.

100. F. Sampalis et al., "Evaluation of the Effects of Neptune Krill Oil on the Management of Premenstrual Syndrome and dysmenorrhea," *Alternative Medicine Review* 8, no. 2 (May 2003): 171–79.

101. C. Ip et al., "Mammary Cancer Prevention by Conjugated Dienoic Derivative of Linoleic Acid" *Cancer Research* 51, no. 22 (15 November 1991): 6118–24.

102. M. Belury, "Dietary CLA in Health," *Annual Review of Nutrition* 22 (2002): 505–31.

103. U. Riserus et al., "Treatment with Dietary Trans10cis12 Conjugated Linoleic Acid Causes Isomer-Specific Insulin Resistance in Obese Men with the Metabolic Syndrome," *Diabetes Care* 25, no. 9 (September 2002): 1516–21.

104. U. Riserus et al., "Supplementation with Conjugated Linoleic Acid Causes Isomer-Dependent Oxidative Stress and Elevated C-Reactive Protein: A Potential Link to Fatty Acid-Induced Insulin Resistance," *Circulation* 106, no. 15 (October 2002): 1925–29.

105. D.S. Kelley and K.L. Erickson, "Modulation of Body Composition and Immune Cell Functions by Conjugated Linoleic Acid in Humans and Animal Models: Benefits vs. Risks," *Lipids* 38, no. 4 (April 2003): 377–86.

106. T.M. Larsen et al., "Efficacy and Safety of Dietary Supplements Containing CLA for the Treatment of Obesity," *Journal of Lipid Research* (16 August 2003).

107. U. Riserus, personal communication with author, August 2003.

108. E. De Stefani, "Alpha-Linolenic Acid and Risk of Prostate Cancer: A Case-Control Study in Uruguay," *Cancer Epidemiology Biomarkers & Prevention* 9, no. 3 (March 2000): 335–38.

109. J.M. Ramon et al., "Dietary Fat Intake and Prostate Cancer Risk: A Case-Control Study in Spain" *Cancer Causes and Control* 11, no. 8 (September 2000): 679–85.

110. L.M. Newcomer et al., "The Association of Fatty Acids with Prostate Cancer Risk," *Prostate* 47, no. 4 (June 2001): 262–68.

111. K. Cusi et al., "Vanadyl Sulfate Improves Hepatic and Muscle Insulin Sensitivity in Type 2 Diabetes," *Journal of Clinical Endocrinology and Metabolism* 86, no. 3 (2001): 1410–17.

Chapter 5: The Five Biggest Myths About Low-Carb Diets

1. Donald Voet and Judith Voet, *Biochemistry* (New York: John Wiley and Sons, 1998).

2. R.L. Veech et al., "Ketone Bodies: Potential Therapeutic Uses," *IUBMB Life* 51 (2001): 241–47.

3. M.J. Sharman et al., "A Ketogenic Diet Favorably Affects Serum Biomarkers for Cardiovascular Disease in Normal-Weight Men," *Journal of Nutrition* 132, no. 7 (July 2002): 1879–85.

4. E.C. Westman et al., "Effect of 6-Month Adherence to a Very Low Carbohydrate Diet Program," *American Journal of Medicine* 133, no. 1 (2002): 30–36.

5. B. Brehm et al., "A Randomized Trial Comparing a Very Low Carbohydrate Diet and a Calorie-Restricted Low Fat Diet on Body Weight and Cardiovascular Risk Factors in Healthy Women," *Journal of Clinical Endocrinology and Metabolism* 88 (2003): 1617–23.

6. M.T. Hannan et al., "Effect of Dietary Protein on Bone Loss in Elderly Men and Women: The Framingham Osteoporosis Study," *Journal of Bone and Mineral Research* 15, no. 12 (December 2000): 2504–12.

7. J.E. Kerstetter et al., "Dietary Protein, Calcium Metabolism, and Skeletal Homeostasis Revisited," *American Journal of Clinical Nutrition* 78, no. 3 (September 2003): 584S–592S.

8. J.E. Kerstetter et al., "Dietary Protein Affects Intestinal Calcium Absorption," *American Journal of Clinical Nutrition* 68 (1998): 859–65.

9. Ibid.

10. A. Rosenvinge Skov et al., "Effect of Protein Intake on Bone Mineralization During Weight Loss: A 6-Month Trial," *Obesity Research* 10 (2002): 432–38.

11. R.P. Heaney, "Editorial: Protein and Calcium—Antagonists or Synergists?" *American Journal of Clinical Nutrition* 75, no. 4 (2002): 609–10.

12. E.L. Knight et al., "The Impact of Protein Intake on Renal Function Decline in Women with Normal Renal Function or Mild Renal Insufficiency," *Annals of Internal Medicine* 138 (2003): 460–67.

13. T.B. Wiegmann et al., "Controlled Changes in Chronic Dietary Protein Intake Do Not Change Glomerular Filtration Rate," *American Journal of Kidney Diseases* 15, no. 2 (February 1990): 147–54.

14. A. Rosenvinge Skov et al., "Changes in Renal Function During Weight Loss Induced by High vs. Low-Protein Low-Fat Diets in Overweight Subjects," *International Journal of Obesity* 23, no. 11 (November 1999): 1170–77.

15. "Popular Diets: A Scientific Review," *Obesity Research* 9 (2001): 5S–17S.

16. S.B. Sondike et al., "Effects of a Low-Carbohydrate Diet on Weight Loss and Cardiovascular Risk Factor in Overweight Adolescents," *Journal of Pediatrics* 142, no. 3 (March 2003): 253–58.

17. G. Foster et al., "A Randomized Trial of a Low-Carbohydrate Diet for Obesity," *New England Journal of Medicine* 348, no. 21 (22 May 2003): 2082–90.

18. Frederick Samaha et al., "A Low-Carbohydrate as Compared with a Low-Fat Diet in Severe Obesity," *New England Journal of Medicine* 348, no. 21 (22 May 2003): 2074–81.

19. Alain Golay et al., "Weight-Loss with Low or High Carbohydrate Diet?" *International Journal of Obesity & Related Metabolic Disorders* 20, no. 12 (December 1996): 1067–72.

20. Alain Golay et al., "Similar Weight Loss with Low- or High-Carbohydrate Diets," *American Journal of Clinical Nutrition* 63, no. 2 (February 1996): 174–78.

21. Walter Willett, "Dietary Fat Plays a Major Role in Obesity: No," *Obesity Reviews* 3, no. 2 (May 2002): 57–58.

22. Walter Willett and R.L. Leibel, "Dietary Fat Is Not a Major Determinant of Body Fat," *American Journal of Medicine* 113, suppl. 9B (30 December 2002): 47S–59S.

23. J.L. Boucher et al., "Weight Loss, Diets, and Supplements: Does Anything Work?" *Diabetes Spectrum* 14 (2001): 169–75.

24. Ibid.

25. John Yudkin, "Diet and Coronary Thrombosis: Hypothesis and Fact," *Lancet* 2 (1957): 155–62.

26. Uffe Ravnskov, *The Cholesterol Myths* (Washington, D.C.: New Trends Publishing, 2000).

27. Malcolm Kendrick, "Why the Cholesterol-Heart Disease Theory Is Wrong," www.redflagsweekly.com/kendrick/2002_nov28.html (28 November 2002).

28. Ancel Keys, "Letter-Normal Plasma Cholesterol in a Man Who Eats 25 Eggs a Day," *New England Journal of Medicine* 325 (1991): 584.

29. E. Braunwald, "Shattuck Lecture—Cardiovascular Medicine at the Turn of the Millennium: Triumphs, Concerns, and Opportunities," *New England Journal of Medicine* 337, no. 19 (1997): 1360–69.

30. I.A. Prior et al., "Cholesterol, Coconuts, and Diet on Polynesian Atolls: A Natural Experiment," *American Journal of Clinical Nutrition* 34, no. 8 (August 1981): 1552–61.
31. A. Ascherio and Walter Willett, "Health Effects of Trans Fatty Acids," *American Journal of Clinical Nutrition* 66, suppl. 4 (October 1997): 1006S–1010S.
32. Mary Enig, *Know Your Fats* (Brookhaven, Penn.: Bethesda Press, 2000).
33. Ibid.
34. Gary Taubes, "The Soft Science of Dietary Fat," *Science* 291 (March 2001).
35. D.M. Dreon et al., "A Very Low Fat Diet Is Not Associated with Improved Lipoprotein Profiles in Men with a Predominance of Large, Low-Density Lipoproteins," *American Journal of Clinical Nutrition* 68, no. 3 (1999): 411–18.
36. J. Michael Gaziano, "Fasting Triglycerides, High-Density Lipoprotein and Risk of Myocardial Infarction," *Circulation* 96 (1997): 2520–25.
37. Dean Ornish, "Intensive Lifestyle Changes for Reversal of Coronary Heart Disease," *Journal of the American Medical Association* 280, no. 23 (16 December 1998): 2001–7.
38. A. Ascherio and Walter Willett, "Health Effects of Trans Fatty Acids," *American Journal of Clinical Nutrition* 66, suppl. 4 (October 1997): 1006S–1010S.
39. A. Ascherio et al., "Dietary Fat and Risk of Coronary Heart Disease in Men: Cohort Follow Up Study in The United States," *British Medical Journal* 313 (13 July 1996): 84–90.
40. Alain Golay et al., "Weight-Loss with Low or High Carbohydrate Diet?" *International Journal of Obesity & Related.*

Chapter 6: Frequently Asked Questions

1. "Health and Medicine," *U.S. News & World Report* (14 July 2003).
2. Ibid.
3. Ibid.
4. Calvin Ezrin, with Kristen Caron, *Your Fat Can Make You Thin* (Lincolnwood, Ill.: Contemporary Books, 2001).
5. E.R. Shell, *The Hungry Gene: The Science of Fat and the Future of Thin* (New York: Atlantic Monthly Press, 2002).
6. Natural Medicines Comprehensive Database, *Monograph: Bitter Orange* (Stockton, Calif.: Therapeutic Research, 2003).
7. M. Blumenthal et al., *Herbal Medicine Expanded Commission E Monographs* (Atlanta: Integrative Medicine Communications, 2000).
8. G. Calapai et al., "Antiobesity and Cardiovasculartoxic Effects of Citrus Aurantium Extracts in the Rat: A Preliminary Report," *Fitoterapia* 70 (1999): 586–92.
9. Natural Medicines Comprehensive Database, *Patient Handout: Bitter Orange* (Stockton, Calif.: Therapeutic Research, 2003).
10. J. Carroll and D. Koenigsberger, "The Ketogenic Diet: A Practical Guide for Caregivers," *Journal of the American Dietetic Association* 98, no. 3 (1998): 316–21.
11. Lyle McDonald, *The Ketogenic Diet* (www.theketogenicdiet.com, 1998).
12. Donald S. Robertson, *The Snowbird Diet* (New York: Warner Books, 1986).
13. Mary Enig, "Letter to Dr. Mercola," www.mercola.com (Jan. 16, 2000).
14. S. Sadeghi et al., "Dietary Lipids Modify the Cytokine Response to Bacterial Lipopolysaccharide in Mice," *Immunology* 96, no. 3 (March 1999): 404–10.
15. Mary Enig, *Indian Coconut Journal* (September 1995).
16. I.A. Prior et al., "Cholesterol, Coconuts, and Diet on Polynesian Atolls: A Natural Experiment," *American Journal of Clinical Nutrition* 34, no. 8 (August 1981): 1552–61.

17. Jordan Rubin, "Extra Virgin Coconut Oil—the Good Saturated Fat," *Total Health* 25, no. 3 (June/July 2003): 30.
18. Mary Enig, "Coconut: In Support of Good Health in the 21st Century," www.apcc.org.sg/special.htm.
19. Mary Enig, *Know Your Fats* (Silver Spring, Maryland: Bethesda Press, 2000).
20. Kathleen Des Maisons, *The Sugar Addict's Total Recovery Program* (New York: Ballantine, 2000).
21. Kathleen Des Maisons, *Your Last Diet* (New York: Ballantine, 2001).
22. Jennie Brand-Miller et al., *The New Glucose Revolution* (New York: Marlowe & Co., 2002).
23. Joseph Mercola, *The No-Grain Diet* (New York: Dutton, 2003).
24. John Hernandez, "Weight Loss Protocols," lecture given at Boulderfest Nutrition Conference, Boulder, Colo., 2000.
25. G.B. Keijzers et al., "Caffeine Can Decrease Insulin Sensitivity in Humans," *Diabetes Care* 25, no. 2 (February 2002): 399–400.
26. M. Sachs et al., "Effect of Caffeine on Various Metabolic Parameters In Vivo," *Zeitschrift fur Ernahrungswissenschaft* 23, no. 3 (September 1984): 181–205.
27. Grahm et al., "Caffeine Ingestion Elevates Plasma Insulin Response in Humans During an Oral Glucose Tolerance Test," *Canadian Journal of Physiology and Pharmacology* 79, no. 7 (July 2001): 559–65.
28. S.P. Tofovic et al., "Renal and Metabolic Effects of Caffeine in Obese Diabetic, Hypertensive Rats," *Renal Failure* 23, no. 2 (March 2001): 159–73.
29. K. Muroyama et al., "Anti-Obesity Effects of a Mixture of Thiamin, Arginine, Caffeine and Citric Acid in Non-Insulin Dependent Diabetic KK Mice," *Journal of Nutritional Science and Vitaminology* 49, no. 1 (February 2003): 56–63.
30. A. Pizziol et al., "Effects of Caffeine on Glucose Tolerance: A Placebo-Controlled Study," *European Journal of Clinical Nutrition* 52, no. 11 (November 1998): 846–49.
31. R.M. van Dam et al., "Coffee Consumption and Risk of Type 2 Diabetes Mellitus," *Lancet* 360 (9 November 2002): 1477–78.
32. L. Tllefson et al., "An Analysis of FDA Passive Seizures Associated with Consumption of Aspartame," *Journal of the American Dietetic Association* 92, no. 5 (May 1992): 598–601.
33. R. Blaylock, *Excitotoxins: The Taste That Kills* (Albuquerque, N.M.: Health Press, 1996).
34. David Voreacos, "Experts Tell Panel of Continued Concern Over Use of Aspartame," *Los Angeles Times*, 4 November 1987, p. 19.
35. Kathleen Des Maisons, *The Sugar Addict's Total Recovery Program* (New York: Ballantine, 2000).
36. S. Elliott et al., "Fructose, Weight Gain, and the Insulin Resistance Syndrome," *American Journal of Clinical Nutrition* 76, no. 5 (November 2002): 911–22.
37. M. Dirlewanger et al., "Effects of fructose on hepatic glucose metabolism in humans," *American Journal of Physiology, Endocrinology and Metabolism* 279, no. 4 (October 2000): E907–E911.
38. Elson Haas, *The False Fat Diet* (New York: Ballantine Books, 2000).
39. L.H. Leung, "Pantothenic Acid as a Weight-Reducing Agent: Fasting Without Hunger, Weakness and Ketosis," *Medical Hypotheses* 44, no. 5 (May 1995): 403–5.
40. Alan Kekwick and Gaston L.S. Pawan, "Metabolic Study in Human Obesity with Isocaloric Diets High in Fat, Protein or Carbohydrate," *Metabolism* 6 (1957): 447–60.

Chapter 7: Tricks of the Trade:
The Top 50+ Tips for Making Low-Carb Work for You

1. C.D. Summerbell et al., "Relationship Between Feeding Pattern and Body Mass Index in 220 Free-Living People in Four Age Groups," *European Journal of Clinical Nutrition* 50 (1996): 513–19.
2. R.M. Ortega et al., "Differences in the Breakfast Habits of Overweight/Obese and Normal Weight Schoolchildren," *International Journal for Vitamin and Nutrition Research* 68 (1998): 125–32.
3. R.M. Ortega et al., "Associations Between Obesity, Breakfast-Time Food Habits, and Intake of Energy and Nutrients in a Group of Elderly Madrid Residents," *Journal of the American College of Nutrition* 15 (1996): 65–72.
4. F. Halberg, "Chronobiology and Nutrition," *Contemporary Nutrition* 8, no. 9 (1983): 2 pages (unpaginated).
5. D.K. Layman et al., "A Reduced Ratio of Dietary Carbohydrate to Protein Improves Body Composition and Blood Lipid Profiles During Weight Loss in Adult Women," *Journal of Nutrition* 133, no. 2 (February 2003): 411–17.
6. D.K. Layman et al., "Increased Dietary Protein Modifies Glucose and Insulin Homeostasis in Adult Women During Weight Loss," *Journal of Nutrition* 133, no. 2 (February 2003): 405–10.
7. D.K. Layman et al., "The Role of Leucine in Weight Loss Diets and Glucose Homeostasis," *Journal of Nutrition* 133, no. 1 (January 2003): 261S–267S.
8. Joseph Mercola, *The No-Grain Diet* (New York: Dutton, 2003).
9. B.K. Hope et al., "An Overview of the *Salmonella enteritidis* Risk Assessment for Shell Eggs and Egg Products," *Risk Analysis* 22, no. 2 (April 2002): 203–18.
10. Joseph Mercola, "Raw Eggs for Your Health—Major Update," www.mercola.com/2002/nov/13/eggs.htm
11. B.K. Hope et al., "An Overview of the *Salmonella enteritidis* Risk Assessment for Shell Eggs and Egg Products," *Risk Analysis* 22, no. 2 (April 2002): 203–18.
12. L.A. Tucker and M. Bagwell, "Television Viewing and Obesity in Adult Females," *American Journal of Public Health* 81 (1991): 908–11.
13. W.H. Dietz and S.L. Gortmaker, "Do We Fatten Our Children at the Television Set?" *Pediatrics* 75 (1985): 807–12.
14. Michael Murray et al., *Encyclopedia of Natural Medicine*, 2nd ed. (Rocklin, Calif.: Prima Health, 1998): 681.

Bibliography of Diets

The Atkins Diet

Atkins, Robert C., M.D. *Dr. Atkins' New Diet Revolution*. Pbk. ed. New York: Quill, 2002.

———. *Atkins for Life: The Complete Controlled Carb Program for Permanent Weight Loss and Good Health*. New York: St. Martin's Press, 2003.

———. *Dr. Atkins' Health Revolution: How Complementary Medicine Can Extend Your Life*. Pbk ed., New York: Bantam, 1990.

———. *Dr. Atkins' New Carb Gram Counter*. Rev. ed. New York: M Evans & Co., 2002.

———. *The Vita-Nutrient Solution: Nature's Answer to Drugs*. New York: Simon & Schuster, 1999.

Atkins, Robert C., M.D., and Sheila Buff. *Dr. Atkins' Age-Defying Diet Revolution: A Powerful New Dietary Defense Against Aging*. New York: St. Martin's Press, 2001.

Atkins, Robert C., M.D., and Fran Gare. *Dr. Atkins' New Diet Cookbook*. New York: M Evans & Co., 1995.

The Carbohydrate Addict's Diet

Heller, Richard F., M.D., and Rachael F. Heller, M.D. *The Carbohydrate Addict's Carbohydrate Counter*. New York: Signet, 2000.

———. *The Carbohydrate Addict's Cookbook: 250 All-New Low-Carb Recipes That Will Cut Your Cravings and Keep You Slim for Life*. New York: John Wiley & Sons, 2000.

———. *The Carbohydrate Addict's Diet: The Lifelong Solution to Yo-Yo Dieting*. New York: E P Dutton, 1991; Reprint, New York: New American Library, 1999.

———. *The Carbohydrate Addict's Fat Counter*. New York: Signet, 2000.

———. *The Carbohydrate Addict's Gram Counter*. New York: Signet, 1993.

———. *The Carbohydrate Addict's Lifespan Program: A Personalized Plan for Becoming Slim, Fit and Healthy in Your 40s, 50s, 60s and Beyond*. New York: E P Dutton, 1997; Reprint, New York: Plume, 1998.

———. *The Carbohydrate Addict's Program for Success: Taking Control of Your Life and Your Weight*. New York: Plume, 1993.

———. *Carbohydrate-Addicted Kids: Help Your Child or Teen Break Free of Junk Food and Sugar Cravings—for Life!* New York: HarperCollins, 1998.

————. *Healthy for Life: The Scientific Breakthrough Program for Looking, Feeling, and Staying Healthy Without Deprivation*. New York: E P Dutton, 1995; Reprint, New York: Plume, 1996.

Heller, Richard F., M.D., Rachael F. Heller, M.D., and Ellen Edwards. *The Carbohydrate Addict's Calorie Counter*. New York: Signet, 2000.

Heller, Richard F., M.D., Rachael F. Heller, M.D., and Frederic J. Vagnini, M.D. *The Carbohydrate Addict's Healthy Heart Program: Break Your Carbo-Insulin Connection to Heart Disease*. New York: Ballantine Publishing Group, 1999.

The 7 Day Low Carb Rescue and Recovery Plan

Heller, Richard F., M.D., and Rachael F. Heller, M.D. *The 7-Day Low Carb Rescue and Recovery Plan*. New York: Dutton, 2004.

Curves

Heavin, Gary, with Carol Colman. *Curves: Permanent Results Without Permanent Dieting*. New York: Putnam, 2003.

————. *Curves on the Go: The Planner Companion to Curves*. New York: Putnam, 2003.

The Fat Flush Plan

Gittleman, Ann Louise, M.S., C.N.S. *The Complete Fat Flush Program*. Package ed. New York: McGraw-Hill/Contemporary Books, 2002.

————. *The Fat Flush Cookbook*. New York: McGraw-Hill/Contemporary Books, 2002.

————. *The Fat Flush Journal and Shopping Guide*. New York: McGraw-Hill/Contemporary Books, 2002.

————. *The Fat Flush Plan*. New York: McGraw-Hill/Contemporary Books, 2001.

Gittleman, Ann Louise, M.S., C.N.S., and Joanie Greggains. *The Fat Flush Fitness Plan*. New York: McGraw-Hill/Contemporary Books, 2003.

The GO-Diet: The Goldberg-O'Mara Diet Plan

Goldberg, Jack, Ph.D., and Karen O'Mara, D.O. *The GO-Diet: The Goldberg-O'Mara Diet Plan*. N.p. : Go Corp, 1999.

The Hamptons Diet

Pescatore, Fred, M.C., *The Hampton's Diet: Lose Weight Quickly and Safely with the Doctor's Delicious Meal Plans*. New York: John Wiley & Sons, 2004.

The Lindora Program: Lean for Life

Graff, Cynthia Stamper, and Jerry Holderman. *Lean for Life Phase One: Weight Loss*. 2d ed. Irvine, Calif.: Griffin Publishing Group, 2002.

Graff, Cynthia Stamper, and Jerry Holderman. *Lean for Life Phase Two: Lifetime Solutions*. 2d ed. Irvine, Calif.: Griffin Publishing Group, 2001.

Graff, Cynthia Stamper, and Jerry Holderman. *Lean for Life Recipe Book*. Irvine, Calif.: Griffin Publishing Group.

Neanderthin
Audette, Ray. *Neanderthin: Eat Like a Caveman to Achieve a Lean, Strong, Healthy Body*. New York: St. Martin's Press, 1999.

The Paleo Diet
Cordain, Loren. *The Paleo Diet: Lose Weight and Get Healthy By Eating the Food You Are Designed to Eat*. New York: John Wiley & Sons, 2002.

Protein Power
Eades, Michael R., M.D., and Mary Dan Eades, M.D. *The 30-Day Low-Carb Diet Solution*. New York: John Wiley & Sons, 2002.
———. *Protein Power: The High-Protein, Low-Carbohydrate Way to Lose Weight, Lower Cholesterol and Blood Pressure, and Restore Your Health—in Just Weeks!* New York: Bantam Books, 1996; Reprint, New York: Bantam Books, 1999.
———. *The Protein Power Lifeplan*. New York: Warner Books, 2001.
Eades, Michael R., M.D., Mary Dan Eades, M.D., and Ursula Solom. *The Low-Carb Comfort Food Cookbook*. New York: John Wiley & Sons, 2002.

The Scarsdale Diet
Tarnower, Herman, M.D., and Samm Sinclair Baker. *The Complete Scarsdale Medical Diet: Plus Dr. Tarnower's Lifetime Keep-Slim Program*. New York: Bantam Books, 1995.

The Schwarzbein Principle
Schwarzbein, Diana, M.D., and Nancy Deville. *The Schwarzbein Principle: The Truth About Losing Weight, Being Healthy, and Feeling Younger*. Deerfield Beach, Fla.: Health Communications, 1999.
Schwarzbein, Diana, M.D., and Marilyn Brown. *The Schwarzbein Principle II—The Transition: A Regeneration Program to Prevent and Reverse Accelerated Aging*. Deerfield, Fla.: Health Communications, 2002.
Schwarzbein, Diana, M.D., Nancy Deville, and Evelyn Jacob Jaffe. *The Schwarzbein Principle Cookbook*. Deerfield, Fla.: Health Communications, 1999.
———. *The Schwarzbein Principle Vegetarian Cookbook*. Deerfield, Fla.: Health Communications, 1999.

Somersizing
Somers, Suzanne. *Eat Great, Lose Weight*. New York: Crown Publishers, 1997; Reprint, Running Press, 2001.
———. *Somersize Desserts* New York: Crown Publishing, 2001.

————.*Somersize by Suzanne Somers*. Starring Suzanne Somers. Twentieth Century Fox, 1996. Videocassettes.

————. *Suzanne Somers' Eat, Cheat, and Melt the Fat Away*. New York: Crown Publishers, 2001.

————. *Suzanne Somers' Fast and Easy: Lose Weight the Somersize Way with Quick, Delicious Meals for the Entire Family!* New York: Crown Publishers, 2002.

————. *Suzanne Somers' Get Skinny on Fabulous Food*. New York: Crown Publishing, 1999.

The South Beach Diet

Agatston, Arthur, M.D. *The South Beach Diet: The Delicious, Doctor-Designed, Foolproof Plan for Fast and Healthy Weight Loss*. Emmaus, Pa.: Rodale Press, 2003; Large print ed., New York: Bantam Books, 2003.

————. *The South Beach Diet Cookbook*. Emmaus, Pa.: Rodale Press, 2004.

————. *The South Beach Diet Good Fats/Good Carbs Guide*. Emmaus, Pa.: Rodale Press, 2003.

Sugar Busters!

Andrews, Samuel S., M.D., Morrison C. Bethea, M.D., Luis A. Balart, M.D., and H. Leighton Steward. *Sugar Busters! for Kids*. New York: Ballantine Books, 2001.

Steward, H. Leighton, Morrison C. Bethea, M.D., Sam S. Andrews, M.D., and Luis A. Balart, M.D. *The New Sugar Busters! Cut Sugar to Trim Fat*. Rev. ed. New York: Ballantine Books, 2002. Large print ed., New York: Random House, 2002.

————. *Sugar Busters! Quick & Easy Cookbook*. New York: Ballantine Books, 1999.

————. *Sugar Busters! Shopper's Guide*. New York: Random House, 1999.

The Zone

Sears, Barry, Ph.D. *The Anti-Aging Zone*.

————. *The Zone: a Dietary Road Map*. New York: Regan Books, 1995.

————. *Mastering the Zone: The Next Step in Achieving SuperHealth and Permanent Fat Loss*. New York: Regan Books, 1996.

————. *The Soy Zone: 101 Delicious and Easy-to-Prepare Recipes*. New York: Regan Books, 2001.

————. *The Omega Rx Zone: The Miracle of the New High-Dose Fish Oil*. New York: Regan Books, 2002.

————. *A Week in the Zone: A Quick Course in the Healthiest Diet for You*. New York: Regan Books, 2000.

————. *Zone Food Blocks: The Quick and Easy, Mix-and-Match Counter for Staying in the Zone*. New York: Regan Books, 1998.

Index